THE
UNSPEAKABLE
MIND

THE UNSPEAKABLE MIND

*Stories of Trauma and Healing from
the Frontlines of PTSD Science*

Shaili Jain, M.D.

HARPER

An Imprint of HarperCollinsPublishers

The views expressed here are the author's and do not necessarily reflect the official policy or position of the US Department of Veterans Affairs or the US government. This discussion of post-traumatic stress disorder (PTSD) in soldiers, veterans, and civilian survivors of war in no way implies a political opinion about a particular war or foreign policy decision. To protect patients' privacy, the patients' stories depicted are composites of various real encounters brought together to illustrate a situation. If these composites bear resemblance to any person, living or dead, this is entirely coincidental and unintentional. Reading this book does not substitute for seeking medical attention and treatment for PTSD and related conditions, and these chapters do not constitute medical advice for any one individual. Please see the Resources section for recommended readings, online resources, and organizations that may be able to help PTSD sufferers and their families connect with health care professionals who can provide an in-person evaluation and specific advice regarding treatment.

FIRST EDITION

Designed by Bonni Leon-Berman

Library of Congress Cataloging-in-Publication Data has been applied for.

ISBN 978-0-06-246906-9

19 20 21 22 23   LSC   10 9 8 7 6 5 4 3 2 1

THIS BOOK IS DEDICATED TO

My mother, that rarest of souls who gives of
herself to others with pure joy.
&
My father, who insisted on preserving a precious inheritance.
In a larger sense, you are the author of this book.

The ordinary response to atrocities is to banish them from consciousness. Certain violations of the social compact are too terrible to utter aloud: this is the meaning of the word *unspeakable*.

—JUDITH HERMAN, *TRAUMA AND RECOVERY: THE AFTERMATH OF VIOLENCE—FROM DOMESTIC ABUSE TO POLITICAL TERROR*

CONTENTS

PROLOGUE

No story lives unless someone wants to listen.

—J. K. Rowling

The interview room at Milwaukee's veterans medical center[*] is small, so before our patient Josh enters, we rearrange the seating so as not to overwhelm him and settle on a circle formation. Our team consists of a serious, bespectacled medical student; the psychiatry intern dressed in her standard VA-issued royal blue scrubs; me, the chief resident, on the cusp of graduating from residency; and our attending physician, a seasoned senior psychiatrist. Josh has our undivided attention; none of us is preoccupied with our to-do lists or glances at the clock to check if it is time to move on to the next patient. We are, in a way, entranced, unified in knowing that we are witnessing something significant.

Josh's appearance sets him apart. Self-assured with a muscular build, Josh has a slight tan, his brown hair is cut short, and he has piercing blue eyes. All of twenty-one, he tells us how, along with so many of his friends, he was moved to action by the events of 9/11. He joined the marines not long after graduating from high school, because that was what was expected in his family. Both

---

[*] Veterans Affairs (VA) medical centers or hospitals are run by the Veterans Health Administration, a branch of the Department of Veterans Affairs (a cabinet-level government agency) and offer care to anyone who has served in the armed forces.

his grandfathers, a couple of uncles, and a handful of cousins had joined the service, and so had he. Josh was born and raised in a rural town a couple hundred miles north of Milwaukee. He was sent to the "hospital in the city" because his local VA did not have an inpatient psychiatric hospital.

He tells us how happy he was to come home after his military discharge and how good it felt to see family and friends. But those feelings were brief and quickly gave way to strange thoughts and emotions. Josh articulates his story with disarming poise. As he talks, I begin a mental diagnostic checklist.

"Not long after coming home I started having nightmares. I would say they are worse than nightmares because they are a replay of stuff that *really* happened in Afghanistan, stuff I want to forget. I feel everything I felt when I was in Afghanistan: fear, panic, my heart thumping in my throat. I wake up screaming, and my sheets are drenched. This happens almost every night, and I dread going to sleep."

Nightmares. Check.

"Weird stuff is happening when I'm awake, too. I can't trust my eyes and ears anymore. I look at everything again and again to be sure that I'm safe. I always feel something bad is going to happen. I can't just relax."

Hypervigilance.

"I went to the store with my kid brother once, and we were loading up the truck with groceries when a car backfired. I just hit the ground. My body just reacted. I wasn't in control. When I realized it was a car, I calmed myself down . . . there were a bunch of people staring at me, and some were laughing. I don't care about them; it was the look on my kid brother's face that just killed me. He was scared and looked shocked, like he didn't recognize me. I just felt so ashamed."

Exaggerated startle response.

"After that I just started to hang out more at home; I didn't want to do any of the things I used to love doing. Before Afghanistan, my mom always complained how I could never sit still and that I was always out with my buddies, at the movies, bowling, fishing, playing ball, and now I didn't want to do any of that. I just sat at home for weeks at a time, drinking beer and staring at the TV watching dumb reality shows, sort of zoned out and feeling numb."

Markedly diminished interest or participation in significant activities.

"Then I started getting a lot of thoughts about Afghanistan during the day. The slightest thing took me right back. If I happen to flick to news covering the war, then *bam!* I'm suddenly lost in this other world. Sometimes, family or friends would come over to visit, and some even asked, "Did you kill anyone?" or "Did you see anyone get killed?" Their questions made me want to puke. I felt so sick I would just get up and leave. I started to feel pissed all the time, like I was looking for an excuse to knock someone out! Whisky calms me down, and it helps me sleep, too. I don't have the nightmares when I drink, or if I do I don't remember them as much, so I started drinking more."

Avoidance of external reminders that arouse distressing memories, thoughts, or feelings about the traumatic event.

Persistent negative emotional state such as anger, guilt, shame. Check.

"I was doing that for months, and then my mom was having a birthday party for my grandpa. The whole family was coming over. I love my grandpa, but the thought of all those people, the noise, it was too much. I started drinking the morning of the party. By the afternoon I was drunk. It was a barbecue, and this is where it gets vague, because I'm telling you I can't remember. I remember the decorations, the cake, and then the smoke from the meat on the grill, it just hit me, and I was back in Afghanistan again, like really there, fighting for my life. I swear I could not help it. If I could have, I would have. I have no idea what is happening to me."

The team knows what happened at the birthday party; we read the eyewitness accounts, police report, and emergency room evaluation before we met Josh. He had a flashback, a quintessential symptom of post-traumatic stress disorder (PTSD), where he felt a combat experience was happening again in real time. Once the flashback was under way, he lacked the ability to stop it, and he relived all the original emotions of rage and terror. During the flashback, he assaulted family members. He kicked and punched and grabbed one by the neck so hard that it took three grown men to pull him off. The police were called, ambulances arrived, and that was what led to his hospital admission.

If this had been the 1970s, after the Vietnam War and before such flashbacks came to be viewed as a hallmark feature of PTSD, Josh probably would have been misdiagnosed with schizophrenia. But this was 2004, and our understanding was much deeper.

The VA patients I had met before Josh were typically middle-aged Vietnam War–era veterans whose PTSD looked different. For some, it had been treated and tamed over the decades and was not a major issue. For others, it was entrenched and layered with decades of severe alcohol and drug addiction, homelessness, and suicide attempts. For those patients, their PTSD was buried under all the other problems and was not the main focus. Josh's PTSD was fresh, florid, and untreated.

Josh stares at his hands with disbelief after revealing this altered version of himself. His earlier poise caves in to reality, and his face falls to anguish. To my left, the medical student has teared up, and even our attending physician, with all her years of experience, seems struck by his story.

I abandon my mental checklist.

INTRODUCTION

We are on the verge of becoming a trauma-conscious society.
—Bessel van der Kolk, *The Body Keeps the Score: Brain, Mind, and Body in the Healing of Trauma*

Imagine, if you will, a circle. Entering this circle is every American who has survived a trauma. By trauma* I don't mean a messy breakup, losing a job, or having a home repossessed, even though these are all thoroughly stressful. Traumatic events go beyond that to a moment when your life is threatened, you are rendered helpless, and your sense of normalcy is shattered. Perhaps the most obvious image that comes to mind is the soldier back from war, but that is only part of the story. Being raped, being robbed at gunpoint, surviving a fatal car accident, escaping a deadly fire, or witnessing a spouse, child, or parent be brutally assaulted can also be a trauma.

More than half of Americans will say that at some point in their life they have lived through such an event, and large numbers of them will report experiencing many such traumas. Indeed, exposure to danger appears essential to being human. Tragic stories of deadly floods, fires, hurricanes, and earthquakes fill the pages of history books with alarming regularity, and the horrors that result from human-made disasters such as war, terror, and torture provide

* The terms *trauma*, *traumatic event*, and *trauma exposure* are used interchangeably in this book.

bountiful evidence of humans' seemingly endless capacity to be inhumane toward one another.

For the people in this circle, once the danger has ebbed, distress is natural. They may feel on edge, have nightmares, and be overwhelmed by traumatic memories. They may feel like this for hours, days, or weeks, but humans, by design, are psychologically resilient. The clear majority will heal with the tincture of time.

Now imagine within this circle a second, smaller circle of those who *don't* heal. At any given moment, a snapshot of this second circle would capture more than 6 million people. Despite no longer being in danger, they are unable to transcend their traumatic pasts. Instead, they suffer every day with invisible wounds; some fall into oblivion, and others seek revenge. This book is about the inhabitants of this second, smaller circle. These people have PTSD.

It's important to also note the thick fringe around that second circle—a no-man's-land between the larger circle of trauma-exposed Americans, who have healed naturally, and those with full-blown PTSD. This fringe represents the millions of trauma-exposed Americans who might not quite meet the textbook definition of PTSD but nonetheless suffer and also need help.

Post-traumatic stress** is a constellation of symptoms that have been described since ancient times, yet the condition remains elusive. Humans are hardwired to deny the unpalatable, and this denial has taken a toll on understanding the impact of trauma on the human psyche. PTSD was not formally recognized by the psychiatric establishment until 1980, and no doubt this delay came at a large price.

Traumatic stress cuts to the heart of life, interfering with one's capacity to love, create, and work—incapacity brought on not by poor

** The terms *post-traumatic stress*, *PTSD*, and *traumatic stress* are used interchangeably in this book.

lifestyle choices, moral weakness, or character flaws but by a complex interplay among biology, genes, and environment. PTSD is a disorder of memory famous for causing nightmares, flashbacks, and an exaggerated startle reaction. Lesser known, but equally devastating, is how it renders a person's emotional life barren. It mutes happiness and yields, instead, to an irritability that keeps sufferers on the perpetual verge of withdrawal from the world and alienation from those who love them.

Eighty percent of PTSD sufferers have at least one other psychiatric condition, typically depression, alcoholism, drug abuse, or anxiety, and all have a higher risk of death by suicide. PTSD seeps beyond the confines of the mind or brain; it impacts cells, organs, and bodily systems and has emerged as a risk factor for various diseases from cancer to heart disease to obesity.

PTSD is so widespread that it can impact any of us, but the socially disadvantaged are most vulnerable. Unfortunately, only a third of PTSD sufferers receive treatment because it is tough to diagnose and a challenge to treat, a situation further complicated by the fact that sufferers are often hard to reach.

Traumatic stress can spread to anyone with whom the sufferers share their lives. Trauma begets trauma. Most commonly affected are the sufferer's family members, who are at higher risk of developing depression, anxiety, and PTSD themselves. In cases of mass traumatization, such as torture, slavery, and genocide, we now know that PTSD's deep footprint can last for generations.

The statistics speak for themselves: most of us will, sooner or later, experience a potentially traumatic event. If you are fortunate enough not to have such an experience, the odds are that a loved one or others with whom your life is inextricably intertwined—in the community where you live, at the place where you work, where your children go to school or play—will be affected.

None of us can afford to ignore PTSD.

Today is a unique moment in the story of PTSD. Its formal recognition was followed by mountains of research, driven in part by a scientific community that remained skeptical. By the late 1990s, an astounding 16,000 PTSD research publications were indexed in the medical literature. The first two decades of the twenty-first century then saw the horror of the September 11, 2001, terrorist attacks; wars in Afghanistan and Iraq; terrorist attacks in Boston, London, Madrid, Moscow, Mumbai, and Paris; the December 26, 2004, Asian tsunami; Hurricane Katrina; civil war in Syria; and many other human-made and natural disasters. These events further consolidated scientific discoveries about PTSD into a body of evidence that continues to grow exponentially. Add to this parallel advances in neuroscience, which enable us to probe the brain's neurocircuitry, and the scientific world has made dramatic advances in understanding the biological basis of PTSD. Encouragingly, what was once considered an incurable and disabling condition is today very treatable.

Our society has also evolved and appears more willing to listen to the traumatized. Today people are held in rapt attention when the unthinkable strikes. We want to hear from survivors, make sense of the senseless, and learn about tragedies. In the public dialogue that ensues, words such as *traumatized, psychological wounds,* and *traumatic stress* are often used. There appears to be an acceptance of the link between exposure to trauma and psychological symptoms. Still, although the term *PTSD* may have become part and parcel of our modern vernacular, it is often sloppily invoked and steeped in confusion and hearsay.

For these reasons, there has never been a better time for an interpretative work on PTSD that is grounded in science and ultimately aims to serve all humanity—a book that will spark a healthy societal discourse and also serve to clarify and integrate the various perspectives of PTSD that are already out there.

The Unspeakable Mind offers the reader a textured portrait of PTSD from my perspective as a trauma scientist and, most important, from my real-world experience as a psychiatrist and PTSD specialist who has spent almost two decades caring for thousands of patients who have survived child abuse, rape, intimate partner violence, life-threatening accidents, or war.

Through the millennia, artists, writers, musicians, religious scholars, and philosophers have been driven to make sense of such traumas and help the traumatized heal. I write about traumatic stress as a medical professional who seeks to understand the deep imprint trauma leaves on the brain and body and who is trained to intervene so that such lives, marred by tragedy, might eventually be recovered. Being a physician offers intimate glimpses into human life. In the sacred space between doctor and patient, fundamental truths are revealed by people from all walks of life. During this process, it is hoped, patients experience some catharsis and the physician is left with the privilege of bearing witness. It is from this multitude of intimate experiences that I paint a portrait of PTSD that is accessible for all who seek to know more about this condition.

The Unspeakable Mind is divided into seven parts. Part 1, "Discovering Traumatic Stress," opens with my personal connection to the field and introduces the reader to the scope of the PTSD problem and why it is such a pressing public health concern. I also highlight the many dichotomies and complexities that surround the diagnosis and invariably influence the way it is detected and treated. Part 2, "The Brain," consists of vividly recounted patient stories that deconstruct PTSD symptom by symptom. The last few decades have seen stunning advances in the neuroscience of PTSD, and although this world is rapidly evolving and newer technologies continue to shift the landscape, there is much that we already know about the neurobiology of traumatic stress. Part 3, "The Body," illuminates the long-term implications of psychological adversity and exposure to trauma on physical health and how this exposure has consequences across the life span from childhood through old age. Part 4, "Quality of Life," presents a wider view of how traumatic stress is closely intertwined with race, gender, and poverty. It also deconstructs the dangerous repercussions of PTSD and how it destroys the quality of life and human relationships. Part 5, "Treating Traumatic Stress," presents the many avenues via which PTSD sufferers can heal. It goes beyond effective traditional PTSD treatments to include cutting-edge innovation and experimental and alternative approaches. Part 6, "Our World on Trauma," describes more than two decades of research done by trauma scientists, working globally, to understand how PTSD manifests in civilian survivors of war, disaster, and terrorism. There is now a clear sense of how PTSD intersects with culture, societal expectations, and human rights issues. Finally, in part 7, "A New Era: An Ounce of Prevention," I draw on a decade of my own research and clinical innovation and propose a promising paradigm shift. A paradigm that allows us to approach the problem of PTSD in the new millennium with hope.

The Unspeakable Mind tells the complete story of PTSD, deconstructing its impact on many levels: cellular, emotional, psychological, behavioral, societal, cultural, and global. This book is for anyone who wishes to understand PTSD and especially for people who are living with it and their loved ones. For readers who have experienced traumatic events and are still trying to fathom the impact on their lives, this book provides answers. Moreover, I hope such readers will also find reassurance: they are not alone, and there is much that can be done to alleviate their distress. Not only does PTSD affect us on an individual level, it also infiltrates our society and culture. This infiltration allows for a penetrating and honest inspection of its global impact. It is my hope that the reader will emerge with a precise sense of traumatic stress and why it is an inescapable part of all our lives and the world we live in.

PART 1

Discovering
Traumatic Stress

THE ROAD TRIP
WITH MY FATHER

Life can only be understood backwards; but it must be lived
forwards.
—Søren Kierkegaard

For as long as I remember, I have been drawn to those who have
suffered the unspeakable. This is not because it is, in any way,
easy to be around such souls, and there is certainly little comfort
to be derived from such exposure. What fuels my compulsion is
a reassuring sense that this position of bearing witness is where I
was always meant to be. The seeds of this compulsion were sown
decades before I was born, during the 1947 Partition of India. In
the terrifying violence that occurred during this bloody chapter
of history, my paternal grandfather was murdered. That act of
violence meant his young children would, for years to come, endure a harrowing social descent.

I felt the aftershocks of 1947 decades before I knew much about
this calamitous event in the history of South Asia. My father was
born in the northern region of India, known as the Punjab, at a time
when Indians were fighting for freedom from British colonial
supremacy. The last thing the British did before they quit India in
1947 was an act known as the Partition, which resulted in the birth
of the Republic of India, with a Hindu majority, and East and West
Pakistan,[*] both with a Muslim majority. The Partition was a negligently

---

[*] In 1971, East Pakistan became the independent country of Bangladesh.

orchestrated British plan that required millions of people to move at a moment's notice. The new nations were grossly unprepared for what would become the largest refugee crisis of the twentieth century. Nearly 2 million people perished, and seventy-five thousand women were raped and mutilated in the accompanying chaos and violence. Up to 14 million people were forced to flee their ancestral homelands.

My father was ten years old when he was orphaned and forced to live as a refugee in the newly independent India. Two decades later, he would emigrate to England, where I was born and raised. I spent chunks of my youth living in the shadow Partition had cast on his life and with a feeling that no matter how much I loved him and he loved me, a part of him, forever changed in 1947, remained inaccessible.

Growing up as the daughter of Indian immigrants, I was mostly unaware of the details of this traumatic legacy and more preoccupied with the racial tensions that were part and parcel of my everyday life in England, a life lived in two worlds. In the first, England was my meritocratic savior, rewarding hard work and dedication with a life of opportunity and promise. In the second, my brown skin and foreign name rendered my citizenry second rate.

To my teenage mind, becoming a physician offered a way out of that unpleasantness. The solidarity of a profession that stood for a higher calling that transcended race, social status, and religion was alluring. I did not know it at the time, but the seeds of a traumatic past and my childhood experiences were converging and guiding my life's choices. Becoming a physician submerged me into a world of suffering, and choosing to specialize in psychiatry, a field dedicated to alleviating psychological distress, meant I would learn how to make sense of such suffering and acquire the skills to relieve it.

As a child, I had been aware of my family's traumatic history only in a vague sense. Dad had delivered it as snippets dropped into conversation at inopportune moments and, more rarely, as startling declarations. Often accompanied by his anger or fear, those comments sat awkwardly until they came to represent little more than an intrusion into my life. Now, as a PTSD specialist, I understand the way this family story of trauma had manifested. Those snippets were a by-product of the way Dad had processed the events. After surviving the unspeakable— a violent act, devastating loss, or shocking atrocity—the mind is confronted with a dilemma. There is a natural inclination to bury such an event. Yet there is an opposing desire to narrate, out loud, what has befallen us, so that the world may know of it, too. This dilemma creates an oscillation between the two, which explains the fragmented way his story had permeated my childhood.

Over the years, the path toward becoming a physician took me farther from home and eventually to the United States for psychiatric residency training, and my already tenuous connection to my family history weakened. By 2007, I had graduated from residency and was comfortably ensconced in private practice in Milwaukee. In my day-to-day work, I took care of patients with many types of mental illnesses, from eating disorders to psychosis. I was neither a researcher nor a specialist in the treatment of any particular illness. In the spring of that year, my parents visited from England, and we took a two-week road trip through Orlando, Washington, D.C., and New York City, a gift to celebrate Dad's seventieth birthday. It was during that road trip that I first heard the full story of my father's life before the Partition and the tragic events of 1947.

I remember listening to his story unfold, his careful words hinting to me that he had been contemplating the details for quite some time. His story was stripped of the bitterness that I had experienced as a child. His tone was reflective, and the story was infused with details he had collected from his return visits to India, which were more frequent in his postretirement life. I was drawn to his narration because I could sense it was beyond the casual. By then Dad was the sole surviving member of his family of origin, and what he was offering me was testimony.

He spoke of his father, mother, brothers, and sisters, who were virtually unknown to me as my childhood home in England had been bereft of family heirlooms and photographs and I had visited India only twice in my life. The relatives Dad now spoke of had all lived in India, and many of them had died decades before my birth. Dad's act of disclosure opened a gate to a world that was, in many ways, utterly foreign. His road trip revelations changed everything. The events of 1947 meant that members of my family had had their hopes aborted and dreams destroyed and were in psychological despair when they died.

After the road trip, I returned to laying down roots and forging new connections in my American life, but I could not shake the feeling that I was leaving something precious behind. I could not name what it was, but I knew that if I did not go back to collect it, my journey forward would be fruitless. It dawned on me that many factors had sealed my ancestors' fate during that period of history. There was the reality of the times they lived in, a fragile world in which it was to be expected that loved ones could be snatched away in an instant by infection, accident, a merciless act of God, or a human-made atrocity. There was the sheer bad luck that my family had lived under colonial rule, where their destiny had never been their own to begin with. Their lives may have ended in 1947, but now, separated by six decades and more than seven thousand miles, I felt overwhelmed by the legacy of vulnerability that was my inheritance.

As a physician, I often met people living with similar vulnerabilities: the single mom living in the inner city, consumed with anxiety that her young son will become collateral damage in the gang warfare that has devastated their neighborhood; the young woman who survived a childhood of abuse and neglect only to languish in an abusive marriage; and the recent immigrant who witnessed a massacre in his hometown and now struggles to build an American life. A new reality started to sink in: I would devote my career to helping those who lived every day with such vulnerability and to healing those who were required to live in the aftermath of trauma. After all, I myself, all along, had been one of those people.

In the months that followed, I felt a need to know more about traumatic stress. Becoming a researcher held allure, as it offered an objectivity that was missing from my day-to-day work. I craved objective proof that what I was doing for my patients was *really* working, and I was no longer satisfied with the feel-good factor associated with my patients' feedback or my self-appraisal. I was familiar with PTSD in my everyday clinical practice, but there was one health care organization where I trained as a resident that cared about PTSD more than any other hospital I had ever worked in. It was the VA system.

When I had first arrived in the United States, my first job had been as an intern at the Clement J. Zablocki Veterans Affairs Medical Center in Milwaukee. Until that point, I had never worked in a hospital that existed for the sole purpose of caring for retired military, and, as a new immigrant, I was humbled by how seriously Americans took their debt to the men and women who had made that ultimate patriotic commitment.

I spent a good part of that internship navigating the corridors of the Milwaukee VA hospital and caring for hospitalized veterans. That was also my first year living in the United States, so, in parallel, I was undergoing the metamorphosis that adapting to a new country demands. I was learning about the United States less from neighbors or the news media and more from my veteran patients and my colleagues who cared for them. It was not long before I found myself in awe at the unique promise and huge heart of my adopted country. Once during morning ward rounds, a senior VA physician told me how he felt a sense of purpose when he stepped into a VA hospital; by the end of my internship year I felt that sense of purpose, too.

The VA is charged with taking care of the health of all veterans, so whatever the main health issues are for this population becomes the areas in which the VA will place priority, money, and resources. With one in three veterans carrying a diagnosis of at least one psychiatric condition, the treatment of mental illness has long been a VA priority—a priority that has only intensified in the years that followed the tragic September 11, 2001, terrorist attacks and the subsequent wars in Afghanistan and Iraq.

For these reasons, when I left private practice to get advanced training in PTSD, it made no sense to go anywhere other than a VA hospital. Within two years of the road trip, I moved across the country to the California site of the National Center for PTSD, a VA-funded consortium widely regarded as a world leader in PTSD research. There I would spend the better part of three years as a fellow and postdoctoral scholar at the Stanford University School of Medicine. There was, however, a price to pay for working in such a brilliant brain trust. Within weeks, I went from being a respected doctor with a very comfortable life to living off savings in an academic environment that was stiff with competition and full of unpredictability.

Years after his road trip revelations, Dad told me that he had deliberately revealed the details of our family story to me that day because he was perturbed by a sense that I was getting complacent. He said, "I wanted to jolt you out of your slumber" and added, "You had all this expertise and training, and I needed to know you were going to use it for something essential." Indeed, before the road trip, the many obstacles were enough to deter me from embarking upon an academic career. But now a deeper connection to my work helped spur me forward on that new career path, engaged in advancing the science of PTSD and unlocking the secrets of what fosters resilience in the aftermath of unspeakable traumas.

A PRESSING PUBLIC
HEALTH CONCERN

Trauma remains a much larger public health issue, arguably the greatest threat to our national well-being.

—Bessel van der Kolk, *The Body Keeps the Score: Brain, Mind, and Body in the Healing of Trauma*

To understand traumatic stress, we must first examine the nature of the events that lead to it. Unlike regular stressful events, such as moving to a new house, living with a chronic illness, suffering financial loss, or dealing with marital discord, traumatic events are so tremendous that individuals are rendered helpless by the force of the situation. The trauma shatters their sense of normalcy, control, and meaning and typically involves being threatened directly with death, being sexually assaulted, or witnessing such traumas as they occur to other people.

The human response to such trauma is universal and visceral. In her landmark 1992 text *Trauma and Recovery*, Dr. Judith Herman, a psychiatrist and PTSD expert at Harvard University, described this response:

> The ordinary human response to danger is a complex, integrated system of reactions, encompassing both body and mind. Threat initially arouses the sympathetic nervous system, causing the person in danger to feel an adrenaline rush and go into a state of alert. . . . People in danger are often

able to disregard hunger, fatigue, or pain. Finally, threat evokes intense feelings of fear and anger. These changes in arousal, attention, perception, and emotion are normal, adaptive reactions. They mobilize the threatened person for strenuous action, either in battle or in flight.

Numerous studies document rates of exposure to such traumas in the general population. In the US civilian adult population, six out of every ten men and five out of every ten women report having experienced at least one significant traumatic event during their lives. The most frequently reported are physical and sexual assaults, accidents, and fires. By age forty-five, most Americans have experienced one such trauma, and a subset will experience multiple such events. Worldwide, more than 70 percent of adults experience a trauma at some point in their lives, and over 30 percent experience four or more such events.

When I was a research fellow at the National Center for PTSD, one of the first tools I was trained to use was the Clinician-Administered PTSD Scale, a thirty-item interview deemed the gold standard in making this diagnosis. The protocol required me to start the interview by screening for *any* traumatic events the patient might have experienced over a lifetime. This screening was done with a checklist that asked specifically about exposure to a whole slew of traumatic events from witnessing a violent, sudden death to being raped to being involved in a life-threatening accident.

The first patient I screened was Rita, a middle-aged woman veteran, originally from Puerto Rico, who calmly cooperated with my lengthy evaluation. Rita spoke with a timid voice. Her English was good but heavily accented. She listened carefully to my questions, leaning in and cocking her ear toward me to ensure she fully understood what I was trying to say. Then she would sit in silence, her brow furrowed, as her brain sifted through five decades of life events and memories.

As we proceeded, I grew astounded by what was unfolding. I had fully expected that she would answer no to most of the screening questions, but the reality was quite different. Starting from age eight, when she had witnessed the death of her cousin in an accident on her uncle's farm, she went on to the time when as a senior in high school she had been date-raped, to a period of three years when her then partner had beaten her so badly that she had been hospitalized twice for internal bleeding, to the most recent trauma of being a passenger in a car wreck that had cost the driver his life. When the interview was over, Rita seemed exhausted and even surprised by some of her answers. "I've been through a lot!" As she forced a half smile, tears started to fall, and she said, "No one has ever asked me about all those things before today."

Over several weeks I continued to interview dozens of patients. Though each story was unique, the overarching theme was similar: exposure to many traumas, across a lifetime, was the norm. Alarmed and concerned that I was somehow administering the checklist incorrectly, I consulted with a senior researcher, who dismissed my caution by vigorously shaking her head no. "You have to realize," she explained, "these traumatic experiences are not actually unusual events, they are an expected part of life for millions of people. If you haven't experienced a traumatic event in your life, you are part of a very, *very* lucky minority."

Of the large percentage of Americans exposed to trauma, only 20 percent of the women and 8 percent of the men will go on to develop PTSD. So although it is true that the overall *risk* of developing PTSD remains low, the number of PTSD cases in the general population is high because the rate of exposure to trauma is so high. At any given moment, in the United States alone, there are over 6 million *active* cases of PTSD that require treatment. PTSD is a pressing public health concern.

A couple irrefutable facts about trauma exposure and the development of PTSD are worth highlighting. First, the higher the "dose" of trauma one experiences, the higher the odds of developing PTSD. So the lifetime prevalence of PTSD in the general population is about 7 percent, but higher rates of PTSD are found in some high-risk populations. For every one hundred service members who served in the current wars in Afghanistan and Iraq, almost twenty will develop PTSD, and the lengthier their deployments and the more intense their combat exposure, the higher this rate climbs. Higher rates of PTSD are also found in police officers, firefighters, and other first responders. Similar statistics are seen among low-income women and teenagers living in high-crime inner-city areas.

Second, the type of trauma matters. The capacity of humans to assign meaning to traumatic life events differentiates us from other living creatures. This is why traumatic injuries of human design such as rape, war, and child abuse leave such deep wounds. In contrast, after enduring an act of God such as a random accident or natural disaster, the odds of developing PTSD drop to half of what is seen after traumas perpetrated by other humans. Rape is the trauma most likely to lead to PTSD, closely followed by combat exposure, child abuse, sexual molestation, and physical assault.

PTSD rarely lives alone. It is often found among the depressed, alcohol and drug addicted, and anxiety ridden. PTSD symptoms can improve spontaneously, particularly in the first year after exposure to trauma, but for about one-third of sufferers, symptoms remain high for many years. There also can be a delayed expression where, for weeks, months, and even years after the trauma, the person reports no complaints and then one day develops full-blown symptoms. Regardless of the pattern of onset, the implication of not getting timely treatment is clear: if one is untreated and still has PTSD after one to two years, the chance of remission is reduced. These statistics take on chilling significance when one considers that only a third of people with PTSD receive mental health treatment, and among those who do, it takes an average of twelve years after the first onset of symptoms for them to get help.

The psychiatrist and trauma expert Dr. Jonathan Shay wrote about the plight of Vietnam veterans in his 1994 book *Achilles in Vietnam: Combat Trauma and the Undoing of Character*, "Such unhealed PTSD can devastate life and incapacitate its victims from participation in the domestic, economic, and political life of the nation. The painful paradox is that fighting for one's country can render one unfit to be its citizen." Shay's anecdotal observations seem prophetic when considered in the light of 2015 research findings from a study of Vietnam veterans led by Dr. Charles Marmar, a psychiatrist and PTSD expert at New York University. The results, published in *The Journal of the American Medical Association*, found a *current* prevalence of PTSD in 4.5 percent of male and 6.1 percent of female combat Vietnam War–era veterans. Extrapolating these figures suggests that *more than a quarter-million Vietnam veterans still struggle every day with the consequences of PTSD forty years after that war ended.*

Marmar shared his thoughts about the quality of life for Vietnam War veterans:

> The effect on quality of life is profound. The nightmares and flashbacks, the startle reactions—these positive symptoms are very disturbing. But the negative symptoms, which include numbing, detachment, inability to express and receive affection, erosion of the ability to enjoy things, often lead to withdrawal, fractured family, and alienation, and they

are often associated with heavy alcohol and drug misuse. For every war fighter who is traumatized, there are 10 to 20 people in their lives that are part of their social fabric that are also affected to varying degrees: parents, siblings, spouses, children, grandchildren. That is a huge network.

A BRIEF HISTORY OF
TRAUMA

The conflict between the will to deny horrible events and the will to proclaim them aloud is the central dialectic of psychological trauma.
—Judith Herman, *Trauma and Recovery: The Aftermath of Violence—From Domestic Abuse to Political Terror*

"Stat consult for patient in room 12, agitated patient throwing food trays at nursing staff," reads the text message on my pager.

It's six o'clock on a Saturday evening. I have just left the hospital and am driving home. The urgency forces me to turn my car around and abandon my dinner plans. In the doctors' lounge, I review the patient's electronic record. My disappointment turns to irritation as I scan records faxed from another hospital where she was a recent patient: "Multiple admissions," "Unexplained abdominal pain, likely irritable bowel syndrome," "Negative workups," "Pending litigation outcome." Between the lines of these reports is a sinister suggestion: this patient is making up or exaggerating her symptoms for some external gain, possibly a payout from a legal case. This suggestion fuels my irritation; if this is true, this consult is futile.

When I arrive on the ward and head toward room 12, I overhear a nurse talking to a student in the hallway. "Can you believe her? She's acting as though irritable bowel syndrome is gonna kill her!" she exclaims. Her trainee rolls her eyes in agreement. Her comment stops me in my tracks. The urgency of the consult, the hopeless chart entries, the exasperated nurse, my disappointment and irritation—

all are indicators of how the patient is feeling. My irritation at my disrupted evening made me miss that sign. As a psychiatric consultant, I should have known better.

For the second time that day, I change direction and speak to the nurse and her student about their challenging day caring for this patient. Her relentless requests and never-ending questions about her diagnosis and treatment. Her dramatic posturing when in pain, so flagrant that she accidently knocked a dinner tray off a table, its hot contents splattering all over a nurse's aide—the last straw. The reason for the stat psych consult.

"Tough patient," I offer.

The nurse nods and adds with an embarrassed tone, "I didn't mean to talk so loudly in the hallway. I was frustrated."

Back on course, I head toward the patient's room. I pause at the open doorway before knocking. Inside the darkened, quiet room a middle-aged woman lies on her back, both hands resting on her belly, eyes closed, moaning quietly. I scan the room for flowers, cards, or slippers from home, the items people bring when a loved one is hospitalized. Nothing. When I announce myself as a psychiatrist, her face drops and she turns her head. Talking to the wall, she scoffs, "Oh, I suppose they think this is all in my head!"

Still I push through, inviting her to tell me why she is here. In detail she describes her frustration with a different hospital where, for a year, she was treated for abdominal pain. She saw gastro-enterologists, gynecologists, and urologists and had blood tests, ultrasounds, CTs, and MRIs but to no avail. "They could not help me there. That's why I came here." She pauses as her face screws up in pain and she clutches her belly harder. "I met with my new gastro-enterologist yesterday. I like him. I know he can help me." I am leaning back against the wall, arms crossed, as I listen to her story. My arms and neck tense as I think to myself, *Why is she doing this?*

Prematurely, I jump in: "Are you involved in some type of legal dispute?"

Her face falls as she tells me about a car accident eighteen months ago. She admitted she had been at fault and was being sued. She was very stressed by the subsequent legal wrangling. A few months later, the stomach pains started. Things only went downhill after that. Her poor health meant she gave up a job she loved, and her husband was working two jobs to make ends meet. As a result, she hardly ever saw him. I am filled with shame at my inquisitorial judgment of her.

Determined to turn things around, I take a chair and sit at her eye level. In a more relaxed tone, I ask her about her life. She tells me about her twenty-year career as a creative director at a local company, her lifelong passion for art, and how she regularly hosted parties for local artists. As she talks, I imagine her stylishly dressed, surrounded by the chinking of wineglasses and the chatter of guests. As she reminisces, her hands leave her tummy and augment her conversation in gestures. She sits up. The pain disappears from her face and is quickly replaced with smiles. We have connected!

It seems she has read my mind. The talking stops, her hands move up to around her head, this time clenching the bed rails, and her body starts to writhe in pain.

"Doctor, why is this happening to me?"

I have a theory; the anguish in her eyes says it all. At some unknown time, she was traumatized. The stress of the car accident triggered memories of the trauma, but the hurt from that unspeakable injury was so intense that the only way it could manifest was with this complaint of stomach pains. Can my theory heal her? No, but it cements my empathy for her, and empathy is something that can heal. I rack my brain for a way to keep her connected, maintain her trust, and try to make her curious about her psyche. My thoughts are interrupted by the arrival of her gastroenterologist. Her eyes light up. "Oh, Doctor, I am so glad you have come. I wanted to know more about those tests you were thinking of ordering."

I watch as her hope for a cure becomes fixated upon him. The gastroenterologist and I exchange an awkward glance; our combined presence in this room is contradictory. I take my cue from the patient and say good-bye. As I exit room 12, I realize I disappeared for her the moment he came in.

***

As far back as the late 1800s, physicians started to offer explanations of what happens in the human mind after exposure to psychologically traumatic events. During that era figures such as Pierre Janet and Sigmund Freud discovered *traumatic hysteria* and provided dramatic demonstrations of the powerful ways that "forgotten memories" could manifest as physical symptoms in patients. Those early pioneers garnered formal recognition from the wider medical community as they proposed a radical shift: *to study and treat trauma victims from a psychological perspective.*

Prior to their audacious proposal there was no formal acknowledgment of psychological stress, so such symptoms were misattributed to discrete lesions in the brain or body. For instance, survivors of railway accidents were thought to have suffered microscopic lesions of the spine or brain, and veterans of the Civil War had lesions in their heart that explained the constellation of symptoms reported after their combat experiences. Now those pioneering physicians were asserting that an emotional "shock" caused symptoms that manifested as physical complaints but were actually "hysterical" in nature.

The idea of traumatic hysteria showcases a fascinating narrative of how the prevailing culture is intertwined with the way traumatic stress manifests in an individual. For instance, symptoms of traumatic stress tend to become somatized (i.e., present as genuine physical complaints as opposed to complaints of emotional distress) when the psychological nature of the symptoms is not understood by the physician, is too scary or daunting for the patient to accept, or is considered taboo by society. A classic example of this is how centuries of societal denial of childhood sexual abuse meant that symptoms of post-traumatic stress related to such horror were neatly contained as a physical symptom instead: paralysis of a limb, unexplained pain, or bizarre attacks of dizziness.

Freud and Janet might well have used the term *hysteria* to describe the patient I had seen that Saturday. They, too, might have hypothesized that some type of early psychological trauma had been buried deep for decades only to be triggered by the stress of her recent car accident. Unable to accept the earlier trauma, she could only express her distress as abdominal pain. As a psychiatrist, I would have offered her a talking cure: a way for her to understand the origin of her pain, give words to her symptoms, and make the process of accessing her emotions less frightening. But in today's medical environment such an offer often disappoints. Instead, in an era of hyperspecialization that offers limitless procedures and tests and the allure of experimental technologies, such patients often embark on a quest to pinpoint the source of their pain, their journey driven by a conviction that the source is embodied somewhere in the physical structures of their body.

OLD WINE IN A NEW BOTTLE?

From Shell Shock to Battered Women to PTSD

In World War One, they called it shell shock. Second time around, they called it battle fatigue. After 'Nam, it was post-traumatic stress disorder.

—Jan Karon, *Home to Holly Springs*

Traumatic stress has accrued various names over the centuries. Some of these labels capture the physical impact of PTSD on the body: soldier's heart, effort syndrome, shell shock, neurocirculatory asthenia, irritable heart. Others emphasize the psychological impact: nostalgia, combat fatigue, war neurosis, combat hysteria, combat neurasthenia, war psychoneurosis, traumatic neurosis. This push and pull between the two theories of physical and psychological origins of traumatic stress continued until World War I, when the horrors of warfare coincided with a modern psychiatry better prepared to understand the phenomenon.

Shell shock, a term that began to be used around 1915, described the effects of exploding artillery shells on soldiers. British soldiers were complaining of tinnitus, amnesia, headaches, dizziness, tremor, and hypersensitivity to noise, and it was assumed that those symptoms were caused by brain damage produced by shock waves from explosions. This theory was questioned when it became apparent that many of these soldiers had not, in fact, been exposed to artillery fire or exploding shells, nor did they have physical signs of a head injury; the majority of such cases were, upon closer inspection, found to have emotional origins. Shell shock would go on to become the signature psychological injury of World War I.

The psychiatrist Dr. Abram Kardiner was the first to integrate explanations for traumatic reactions. Based on his work with World War I veterans, Kardiner insisted that there were *both* psychological and physiological parts to a traumatic reaction. Despite his contributions, the study of post-traumatic stress languished for decades following the World Wars. Dr. Bessel van der Kolk, a psychiatrist and PTSD expert, attributes this in part to the fact that "Psychiatry as a profession has a very troubled relationship with the idea that reality can profoundly and permanently alter people's psychology and biology."

The 1970s saw a renewed interest in trauma and spurred scientific studies that followed traumatized individuals over time with researchers methodically documenting what they were observing. Furthermore, beyond war, many traumas were being studied— natural disasters, rape, domestic violence, and child abuse—and critical similarities were highlighted among all of them. The human response to trauma was appearing to be universal. More labels followed such as rape trauma syndrome, battered women's syndrome, and child abuse syndrome.

PTSD was formally recognized by the psychiatric establishment in 1980, when it was first acknowledged in the latest revision of the field's *Diagnostic and Statistical Manual of Mental Disorders*, or *DSM*. PTSD was classified as an anxiety disorder with four key criteria (exposure to a traumatic event and three resultant symptom clusters) that were necessary for the diagnosis to be made. These criteria were applicable to all cases of PTSD, not just combat-related PTSD.

Unlike other psychiatric disorders, the decision to include PTSD in the *DSM* was highly attributable to many forces external to the medical field such as Vietnam War veterans' organizations, advocacy groups for women's rights, and advances in legislation that acknowledged the rights of victims of trauma and the need to protect them. Suspicion about these external influences meant it took time for PTSD to be accepted by the wider scientific community, and what followed was mountains of compensatory research to test its legitimacy. Still, two decades after its official acceptance as a medical condition, PTSD was still being denied within the field of psychiatry, with arguments that social forces and politics had colluded to "invent" the condition.

Controversy aside, defining PTSD in the pages of the *DSM* offered a standard from which research and treatment advances could be made. In the scientific community, giving PTSD a name solidified the connection between exposure to traumatic events and subsequent changes in human thought, emotion, and behavior. The illumination of that pathway would, in the ensuing decades, advance our understanding about the fundamental impact of psychological stress on many levels: cellular, hormonal, genetic, behavioral, psychological, and social. Perhaps of most value, inclusion in the *DSM* meant that mental health professionals could grant their patient's experience an "official" name, an act that helped provide legitimacy, validation, and even a sense of commonality with fellow sufferers. For the PTSD sufferer, who may be having an unfathomable experience of "losing my mind," this label, in and of itself, is a reassuring thing to be able to offer.

Since its formal recognition, PTSD's legitimacy has been established and reestablished in a mammoth body of cross-sectional and longitudinal research. Today, clinicians have at their disposal various validated structured interviews to improve diagnostic accuracy.

Epidemiological, clinical, and biological markers support the PTSD diagnosis, markers as strong as those used to support the existence of other mental health conditions.

In the latest *DSM*, the definition of PTSD remains at its core true to the original description except that it is no longer classified as an anxiety disorder and has earned a place in a category called "trauma- and stress-related disorders."* At the heart of making a correct diagnosis of PTSD is the discovery that the patient has survived a traumatic, often life-threatening event, either personally or by witnessing it happen to another. In the aftermath, the patient suffers from four clusters of symptoms: intrusive (unwanted and upsetting) memories of the event, avoidance of people or places associated with it, negative mood changes, and an agitated state of constantly feeling in danger. Timing matters, because for PTSD to be diagnosed, symptoms must have lasted more than one month and caused so much distress that they have disrupted how the individual lives, works, and interacts with the world. Moreover, a PTSD diagnosis can be made only when the clinician is certain that all these symptoms cannot be explained by other medical or psychiatric conditions.

---

* Stress-related disorders result from exposure to a specific event, whereas anxiety disorders relate to fear, worry, and anxiety that are disproportionate to actual occurrences in a person's life.

ROCKY ROADS

Overdiagnosis and Underrecognition

PTSD can unfortunately mimic virtually any condition in Psychiatry.

—Jonathan Shay, *Achilles in Vietnam: Combat Trauma and the Undoing of Character*

Almost forty years after its 1980 recognition, PTSD remains steeped in controversy, and there are complaints that it is being overemphasized by society and overdiagnosed in hospitals. These grumblings can be explained, in part, by a widespread misunderstanding about the natural human response to trauma.

It is common, immediately after enduring trauma, for survivors to experience symptoms that are frequently associated with PTSD. It is crucial to understand that in this context, such symptoms often represent the brain's natural healing process. Take, for instance, the common experience of unwanted, intrusive trauma memories. The brain, by playing the trauma over and over, allows the original emotions associated with the trauma (e.g., fear, anger, or horror) to become blunted. With time, the survivor builds a tolerance to the emotional angst associated with the memories. Moreover, this replay reminds us to learn from the experience, perhaps to adapt our lifestyle accordingly or spark a change in attitude. For the majority of people, once the immediate posttrauma period has passed, memories of the trauma are not much more intrusive or memorable than any other memories. Time really can heal.

The same can be said of trauma-related nightmares, the scary dreams that make you cry out in your sleep or wake up in a blind panic, soaked in sweat and with your heart pounding in your throat. Many trauma survivors report having these even if they do not have PTSD. Such dreams can also contribute to the brain's natural healing process and with time will eventually disappear.

The experience of having nightmares, feeling jumpy or on edge, or being troubled by reminders of the trauma will often resolve spontaneously within days and weeks.[*] We must take solace in the fact that the human brain has a remarkable capacity to heal itself. Indeed, beyond the normal healing process, survivors may even find that they have grown emotionally or spiritually, a phenomenon referred to as *post-traumatic growth*. They report new life priorities, a deepened sense of meaning, and an enhanced connection with others or with a higher power. It is not only premature but inaccurate to pathologize this period and label it as PTSD. Only if symptoms persist with intensity and disruption for longer than a month after the trauma is a diagnosis of PTSD considered.

Somewhat related is another incorrect belief that serving in a war zone or being raped or surviving a natural disaster *must* mean that a combat soldier or sexual assault survivor or flood victim has PTSD. This misleading belief prevails even though study after study has shown otherwise. As Dr. Charles Marmar, a psychiatrist and PTSD expert at New York University, told me about the results of his 2015 National Vietnam Veterans Longitudinal Study, "Approximately 3/4 of Vietnam veterans who served in the warzone *never* developed significant levels of stress, anxiety, or depression related

---

[*] Acute stress disorder is a syndrome of PTSD-type symptoms that lasts from three days to one month following trauma exposure. It is typically a transient stress response that remits itself within one month. That said, about half of the trauma survivors who develop PTSD present first with acute stress disorder.

to their military service." In other words, the majority of Vietnam War combat veterans never suffered from PTSD linked to war.

Genetic factors probably account for one-third of the overall risk of developing PTSD following exposure to traumatic events. Research studies suggest the following additional markers of vulnerability: the severity of the trauma, being female, being younger, having a history of childhood abuse, having other psychiatric problems, belonging to a minority group, having lower socioeconomic status, and having a lower education level. Though these markers hint at a profile of survivors who might develop PTSD after trauma exposure, it is a profile that is far from being fully fleshed out.

Another erroneous notion is that the only mental health problem that one can develop after surviving trauma is PTSD. Just as cigarette smoking can not only cause lung cancer but also contribute to heart disease and a host of other diseases, traumatic events can serve as triggers for a variety of psychological conditions such as depression, panic disorder, substance abuse, and, in some vulnerable individuals, a psychotic break or episode of mania. The problem is that many of these conditions share common features with PTSD, and so professional skill is required to distinguish one from another. It is crucial to make this distinction, though, because to offer a patient the right treatment you must first make the correct diagnosis.

Current screening questionnaires and checklists undoubtedly increase the scientific precision with which PTSD is detected and diagnosed. These screens are often used to try to quantify the severity of symptoms and also to track response to treatment. Still, Dr. Matthew Friedman, a psychiatrist and PTSD expert at the Geisel School of Medicine at Dartmouth University, told me about the dangers of overrelying on such screening tools: "What many people do not understand is that screens are designed to be biased toward false positives. The expectation with the screen is that many of the people who screened positive are not going to have the diagnosis, but you do not want to leave out anybody who might."

The fact remains that we still need well-trained clinicians, tuned in to the subtle manifestations of human behaviors, to interpret the data such tests generate.

***

An opposing dilemma faced by clinicians is what to do when we meet someone who, after experiencing traumatic events, may not complain of textbook PTSD symptoms but nonetheless is suffering significantly more than someone who has not been traumatized. These people are stuck in a sort of no-man's-land with a hazy condition that has been referred to as partial PTSD.

My patient Alfonzo, an immigrant from Mexico, had spent the better part of thirty years driving long-distance trucks for a transport company based in Wisconsin. He had been referred by his primary care doctor, who had told me how, a couple of years prior, Alfonzo had sustained a back injury during a minor road traffic accident. Two spinal surgeries and several courses of physiotherapy later, Alfonzo had reported little improvement and had been forced into early retirement. His back pain was hard to control despite receiving vast quantities of oxycodone, tramadol, and gabapentin. When asked to rate his pain on a scale of numbered cartoon faces moving from 0 (smiling and pain free) to 10 (weeping in agony), Alfonzo always checked the 10. Stuck at an impasse, his doctor wondered if depression was in some way exacerbating his pain.

Alfonzo certainly looked depressed. A short man with a slight build, casually dressed in a leather jacket and jeans, he offered a weak grip when we shook hands and made little eye contact. He relayed his story in a timid, deeply accented voice. His expression was blank, and he seemed to stare right past me, his eyes moist and red. He smelled of cigarettes and musky aftershave and presented with a gloomy aura, as though nothing I could do would ever help him.

He told me how he had worked hard all his life and had always been on the road, often volunteering for overtime and going for days with barely enough sleep. He was the sole provider not only for his wife and five children but also for his extended family back home in Mexico, who relied on him to subsidize the costs of school supplies, weddings, medical bills, and funerals.

When we first met, I asked my standard questions that screened for trauma exposure, and his response came in the form of a shrug. "No, nothing, Doctor. I have had a pretty normal life."

Since retirement, he told me, he felt sad most of the time, he found little enjoyment in life, he had lost his interest in sex and food, and he slept poorly. What followed was months of trials of antidepressant medications, ramped up to maximum doses, and talk therapy for his depression. All this had made little dent in his misery. One morning, I found myself taking a deep sigh when I read his name on the clinic schedule. I felt gloomy about his upcoming appointment, during which, I was sure, he would have nothing positive to report. However, that day he appeared different; his usual apathy was replaced by anger.

A hidden story emerged that started to cast light on why his treatment, thus far, might have been so ineffective. Alfonzo told me of his revelation: he had worked so hard his entire life because he was more comfortable being on the road, alone for weeks at a time, than he was in family life. Now that he was retired, he found it hard to be around his children and wife all the time.

"Doctor, I have always had a tough time showing my emotions . . . I don't think I have ever felt that emotion of love."

Work had served as a distraction from having to acknowledge that startling fact, but now, in his retirement, he was left with little choice but to face it. I was aware that Alfonzo had lost his father when he was young, but what he now revealed was that when he was five, his father had been killed in a hit-and-run accident. The whole extended family, children included, had rushed to the local community hospital, where Alfonzo, peering between the gaps of his frantic clan, had caught a glimpse of his father's mangled corpse. At the funeral, his uncle had taken him to one side and, amid the sobs and wails of the funeral party, had whispered in his ear, "Alfonzo, you are the head of your family now . . . you are the man of your house. Don't forget that." Not long after, Alfonzo had started to work to contribute to the household, and it was the role of provider that would come to define him.

He told me that after his own road traffic accident, he had lost confidence in his ability to drive, a fact he had never revealed to anyone until now. He found himself thinking more and more about his father's accident and would be lost for stretches of time, staring into space, imagining what his father might have experienced in the moments before and after the hit and run. He admitted that he thought a lot about his own death and that every time he stepped into his vehicle, he would fantasize about hastening his death by using his car as a weapon.

What can one do for patients like Alfonzo who fall short of meeting the textbook definition of PTSD? His memories of his father's death were faded, and he had contorted much of his life to avoid the emotional pain of that early trauma. Still, a clinician has a responsibility to assist and heal even when textbooks don't offer definitive guidance. Treating Alfonzo required that I become at ease with the ambiguity of the situation and take an eclectic approach to his treatment.

Psychiatrists are different from physicians in other medical specialties. We rarely wear white coats, and we tend to avoid physically touching our patients. Instead of listening for breath and heart sounds, we've mastered the skill of listening (really listening) to what patients say, a procedure that, if done expertly, can yield volumes of critical information. Being a psychiatrist has taught me that *how* patients share their story is almost as important as *what* they share. The way the dialogue unfolds, where they pause, what causes a tear to fall or a brow to furrow, a misplaced laugh, a moment of hesitation or irritation, how a voice softens, and the ease with which the narrative flows are all vital clues that provide me with hints on where to go to unearth the hallmark features of PTSD.

Using these skills, I can delve into the details of my patients' answers to questions and sift through and discard what will add little to our quest for the truth. While listening, my brain automatically organizes and catalogues a patient's narrative, weaving it together into a coherent outline. Additional touches are always needed: dabs of inference, keeping his or her story in social perspective, and paying as much attention to what is said as to what is *not* said, all the while searching for patterns and clues in the raw data that are being offered to me. I rarely get complete answers to my questions, but becoming a psychiatrist has primed my brain to tolerate ambiguity when searching for the essential truths in a story.

One of the frustrations of diagnosing PTSD is that there is no blood or urine test, ultrasound, or sophisticated imaging technique that we can rely on to confirm our suspicions. Still, although psychiatry's diagnostic system may seem lacking when compared to other fields of medicine, this does not mean it is invalid when used properly. I understand that psychiatry is in the midst of a revolution, heading toward a time when it will diagnose with blood tests and brain scans and offer tailored treatments, but I also accept my duty to heal the pain of those suffering *today* from a condition that has been documented since ancient times. I often hold two opposing facts in my brain: that PTSD is overdiagnosed in some people *and* underdiagnosed in others. If warranted, I offer a diagnosis of PTSD knowing that some may find it meaningful and be filled with relief whereas others might be skeptical and reject me for it.

Making the diagnosis of PTSD is the first step. There is no pill or elixir that can be dispensed after the diagnosis is made, no magic bullet that can eradicate all the symptoms in a matter of days. Treatment is delivered within the confines of a professional relationship, and, for treatment to work, I have to earn the trust of my patients and keep their faith. As one of my bosses told me when I was in training and still mastering the skill of psychiatric diagnosis, "The ultimate goal is that your diagnostic interview should not just be diagnostic, it should be therapeutic, too." So by the time a skilled clinician is done diagnosing a patient, the patient should have gotten something out of the experience, too. It may just be catharsis, the relief of feeling understood, or perhaps an inkling of hope that relief from their tortured circumstances may be in sight. Whatever it is, the patient should emerge with some sense that the interview itself was, even if just to a small degree, healing.

Over the years, I have come to value the importance of getting off to a good start because it invariably helps smooth the way for the journey ahead. Starting well involves exercising compassion in caring for a clientele whose pathologies often render them mistrustful, avoidant, and even hostile; tolerance in handling ambivalence or outright rejection of treatment; the tenacity to hang in there even when one's limits are tested by irritable rants; obsessive attention to maintaining a healthy distance between oneself and one's patients yet retaining a flexibility in accommodating patients' personal preferences; and finally, an empathic commitment to being a faithful companion on a road made bumpy by a condition that can rarely be cured but can certainly be ameliorated and managed well.

PART 2

The Brain

A DISORDER OF MEMORY

The Past is never dead. It's not even past.

—William Faulkner, *Requiem for a Nun*

When the receptionist buzzes to inform me that my new patient is already here, I note that she is almost an hour early. Time serves as an invisible boundary encircling the whole visit, and any breach demands my attention. The breach provides me with invaluable data about my patient's psyche. Is it her personal habit to be early? Does it have something to do with a bus schedule? Why no access to a car? An accident or a drunken driving charge? Dire financial straits? Or does she have difficulty remembering the contents of the appointment letter the clinic sent her? If so, why? A neurological problem or a learning disability? Experience has taught me the most likely explanation: her timing is simply a reflection of the way she is feeling, desperate and anxious for help.

I go out to the busy waiting room, calling only her first name to preserve confidentiality. Maria is middle-aged, short, plumpish, and neatly dressed in a skirt and blouse. Her clothes are immaculately ironed, and as she walks toward me, I take in the coral hues of her nail polish, her jewelry, and the leather of her designer handbag. Maria has large brown eyes that have been artfully accentuated with mascara and eyeliner. Her olive skin is unblemished, and her hair is dark, lush, and long, lending her a youthful appearance. As she takes a seat in my office, I notice her face. It is tight, almost devoid of expression, and her eyes look terrified, a look I've seen hundreds of times before. It is the look of a person who is overwhelmed by a tsunami of emotions and unfathomable thoughts. I make a mental note to listen carefully for any hints of trauma in her story and to use such openings in her narrative to dig for a deeper truth.

I scan my desk in search of a box of tissues and then start with the usual introduction: who I am, what I do, and what she can expect by coming to see me.

"Maria, in your own words, please tell me how you think I may be able to help you today."

"Umm, well . . . I need something to help me sleep."

Tears start to well up in her eyes. I offer her a tissue, which she silently accepts and uses to dab gently at the corners of her eyes.

"Please, in your own time, go on . . ."

We sit in silence for a minute as she tries to control her tears.

"I've got a lot going on, you know, family stuff. I have been stressed and am not sleeping well. The problem is that it is impacting my work; I am tired and can't focus during the day. My boss is the head of our department, so I can't afford to mess up. I love my job and don't want to lose it. One of the other secretaries suggested I come see you for a sleeping pill."

"I'm sorry to hear you have been having a tough time, Maria. Can you tell me more about what happens when you sleep?"

The tears start rolling fast, and it becomes harder for her to talk. "I've been having these bad dreams for the past few weeks; they happen two, maybe three times a week. In the dream I am in a pitch-black room, lying on a bed, and I just feel trapped and suffocated. Then I wake up because I can't breathe . . . I sit up and am gasping for air. I can't remember any other details, but I'm starting to feel scared to go to sleep."

"Can you tell me if you have ever had these dreams before?"

"Yes . . . years ago, in my twenties. I think I was pretty depressed at that time, and I saw a counselor at our church. It helped, and I got better. Then I started a new job, got married, and had my kids, and it all seemed to go away."

"So tell me, what else has been going on in your life lately?"

Maria tells me how her marriage of more than twenty-five years just ended in divorce. Being born and raised in a conservative, Catholic family, she experienced the divorce as a major blow. She and her husband had been happy for many years, raising their two children, a boy and a girl, in the neighborhood where she had grown up. Maria prided herself on being an excellent homemaker. Even though she always worked full-time outside the home, she never let her kids or husband lift a finger. Meals were made from scratch every evening, and for holidays she would spend hours cooking, cleaning, and organizing elaborate events for the extended family.

Over the last decade her husband had been cheating on her. Maria had been devastated and there had been arguments, but nothing had been resolved. She had decided to "look the other way," and the infidelity had continued. Finally, one day, her husband asked her for a divorce because his girlfriend was pregnant and he wanted to marry her. Maria had granted him his wish, but the whole ordeal had been agonizing.

"You see, Doctor, in my life, family is my number one, number two, and number three priorities. It's all that really matters."

The interview went on, and I asked the myriad questions that are the basic part of a psychiatric evaluation: How is your mood? Appetite? Motivation? Concentration? Sex drive? Are you menopausal? Do you have any illnesses such as diabetes, a seizure disorder, any heart problems? Have you ever been hospitalized in a psychiatric hospital? Have you ever tried to kill yourself? How much alcohol do you drink? Do you use street drugs? Were you abused in any way as a child? Physically? Emotionally? Sexually?

I pause at the last question, look up from my checklist, and face Maria directly.

"Yes, I was sexually abused by my uncle, my aunt's husband, for the two years before I went to middle school."

Her face is blank, and she reports the fact without emotion.

"Actually, that uncle, he died a few weeks ago. I went to his funeral."

"Oh, was that difficult?"

"Well, no, not really, I did not feel much about the fact that he was dead. I was there more to support my aunt and cousins, you know? But now that you mention it, after the funeral was over, I sat in my car and had this weird experience. I could not stop shaking, and my heart was racing. I felt like I was suffocating. I sat there for fifteen minutes before I could drive the car home."

Words from thick medical texts drift into my mind: *physiological reactions to cues that symbolize the trauma.*

"Maria, did anyone know about the abuse? Did you ever tell anyone?"

"When I was a kid? No. But later, in my twenties, during that time that I told you about when I was depressed, the abuse came up during the sessions with the therapist and so I told my mom . . ."

"What did she say?"

"Not much . . . 'Are you sure it happened, Maria? Has it stopped?' When I answered yes, it stopped the year I went to middle school, she just left it at that: 'Leave it in the past, Maria, no point in bringing this kind of thing up now.'"

"How did her response make you feel?"

Maria shrugged her shoulders. "Not great, of course, but like I told you, Dr. Jain, for the women in my family, you don't ever do anything to split the family apart. My mom and her sister are very close; it would have caused too many problems to bring it up after all this time. I did distance myself from that uncle, only saw him when I had to, at Thanksgiving, Christmas, and that sort of thing. When my daughter was young, I always made sure she was never alone with him."

The tears dry up, and Maria resumes her composure and then looks at me with a curious expression. "Do you think my sleep problems have to do with this abuse?"

"It's quite possible; you have been under a lot of stress lately, and perhaps between your divorce and this uncle's funeral some unresolved issues have been stirred up."

"Hmm, but the thing is, even though I *know* he abused me, I don't remember much about that time in my childhood."

Random words from a PTSD textbook filter to the forefront of my mind: *amnesia is common for traumatic events.*

I end the session by prescribing Maria a short course of sleep medication and schedule her next appointment for the following week at eleven o'clock.

A week later, the wall clock shows ten minutes after eleven, yet Maria has not arrived. Our first session generated more questions than I could answer, and this, paired with Maria's absence, bothers me. During that first visit I was unsure what was happening, so all I could suggest was we take a "wait and see" approach. I wonder if my lack of a definitive response to her predicament was unsatisfying. Perhaps she will not come back to see me, or she has sought help elsewhere. My ruminations are interrupted by the receptionist, who tells me Maria has just checked in. I glance at the clock; it is twenty minutes after eleven.

I go out to the waiting room to greet her and am taken aback by her appearance. She is wearing jeans with a stained T-shirt and dark sunglasses, presumably to cover up the fact that she has been crying. Her unbrushed hair is tied up in a careless bun. We have barely entered the office when she pours out all her worries: how she has reported in sick for work, how the nightmares are worse, the suffocating feeling more real, and she is frightened to take the medication because she fears she will stop breathing in her sleep. She tells me that memories of the sexual abuse are coming back to her during the day. She can be doing the simplest of things like washing the dishes, buying groceries, or answering calls at her desk when she has a memory of the abuse.

"I have no control. They come to me! I feel like I am going crazy! Why is this happening to me? What did I do to deserve this?"

She tells me that she has been remembering childhood trips to the park, family birthday celebrations, Thanksgiving dinners, and sleepovers that were marred by her uncle's violations. Her speech is stilted, her narrative disjointed. Even as she tells her story, she does not seem to be telling it to me; she just stares into space. I try to intervene with reassuring explanations, but Maria's eyes betray the truth that her mind is pulling her elsewhere. Her brain's networks are misfiring, awry, and depleted.

A week later, Maria misses her appointment. When the receptionist calls her, Maria reports she completely spaced on the time and day of her appointment. Concerned about her rapid decline, I schedule her as an add-on to my clinic. The boundary of time has been completely breached, and I take this rupture to be a reflection of Maria's inner chaos and unraveling. During the visit she cries uncontrollably and tells me how she is on sick leave from work, her house is neglected, and her mother has become so concerned that she has moved in with her. This is all I am able to glean, as Maria struggles to answer direct questions. She is distracted, and when she does talk, she finds it hard to keep herself from discussing details of her sexual abuse. She touches parts of her body as though to protect herself from an imaginary attacker and murmurs to herself, "Please don't touch me" in a timid voice. Other times, she seems angry and yells out through sobs, "No, no, don't do that!"

It is horrifying to watch. I am losing Maria as she drowns in a flood of traumatic memories. Her past appears to have become so overpowering that I, along with everything else in the present, have simply ceased to exist.

A line from Jonathan Shay's *Achilles in Vietnam* enters my head: "So long as the traumatic moment persists as a relivable nightmare, consciousness remains fixed upon it. The experiential quality of reality drains from the here and now; the dead are more real than the living."

***

Psychological distress triggered by reminders of trauma, marked physiological reactions (such as sweating, breathing difficulties, or heart palpitations), intrusive memories, nightmares, and flashbacks are the five quintessential intrusive features of PTSD. These intrusions are known for imposing themselves at any moment when the individual is awake or, in the case of nightmares, during sleep. Some sufferers experience just one symptom, others all five. Trauma-related intrusive symptoms typically begin in the first month after the trauma but, as was the case for Maria, in 15 percent of cases there can be a lag period of days, weeks, months, and even years before they announce themselves. This lag further confuses an already jarring experience and can complicate efforts to make a correct diagnosis.

Each of these intrusive symptoms manifests differently. The most startling are the intrusive memories, nightmares, and flashbacks. This trio is akin to the torrential rain, thunder, and lightning of a storm: shocking and thoroughly disruptive. The remaining intrusion symptoms are like a heavy, steady rain that pours day after day and inhibits life in less obvious ways. Regardless of how they present, they all arrest the course of an individual's life in the present.

Crucial to understanding what occurs in the brain when it experiences intrusive symptoms is an awareness of what happens when humans remember and forget traumatic events. In other words, we need to understand memory. Indeed, PTSD is often described as a disorder of memory.

Fundamentally different in their quality and form, there are two types of memory in PTSD. First are the involuntary intrusions that are unwanted, vivid, and emotional and involve a sense of reliving the trauma. An essential function for the human brain is to consolidate our memories. This process involves stabilizing memories and allowing them to ripen and mature. After a traumatic event, the consolidation process goes into overdrive. It is this over-consolidation that lends traumatic memories their intrusive and unforgettable quality and explains how they can invade a survivor's life, weeks, months, and years later in a highly visual manner. An example would be Maria's memories of child sex abuse intruding into her workday. These involuntary intrusions can be so intense that they have been described as indelible images.

The second type of PTSD memory is voluntarily recalled trauma narratives. These memories are not as emotionally intense as involuntary intrusions and their content is notable for being disorganized. This disorganization is attributable not to poor recall but to the very nature of the traumatic memories. In essence, there is an inability to put into words the most emotional part of a traumatic event, a period of time that could have lasted anywhere from several seconds to several hours. This explains how Maria *knows* she was sexually abused as a child but can voluntarily recall very few memories from that period in her life.

These two types of PTSD memories present an instant paradox:

involuntary and vivid intrusive memories are a quintessential feature of PTSD, but PTSD sufferers can also report vague memories when they voluntarily recall their trauma narrative and, in some cases, total amnesia. This paradox has been at the heart of the controversies that have surrounded PTSD. How reliable can a survivor's story be if the memory of the event is hazy? How does one go about measuring the capacity to forget? The facts of a trauma can dominate a life, yet the specific trauma memories can be excluded from consciousness. How can this be? Recent advances in our understanding of the neuropsychology of normal memories shed some light on this paradox.

Neuropsychology categorizes normal memories as either explicit or implicit. Explicit memories consist of autobiographical facts. In Maria's case, these facts would include the birth date of her firstborn or her telephone number at work. Such memories are deliberately retrieved. In contrast, implicit memories are activated through environmental or internal cues, not by deliberate retrieval. An example is driving a car, an act that does not require deliberate recall and is often done in autopilot fashion. Traumatic memories are similar to these implicit memories in that they do not require deliberate retrieval and can be triggered by environmental cues.

Traumatic memories are also stored in the brain alongside the sensory information that was experienced during the trauma. When Maria experienced an episode of sexual abuse by her uncle during a sleepover at her cousin's home, it was encoded not only with what she saw but also with what she smelled (his aftershave), touched (she clenched her fists until her nails left indentations on the palms of her hands), tasted (her undigested dinner of macaroni and cheese regurgitating into her mouth), and heard (the Supremes playing on the neighbor's radio).

All this information is encoded together in interconnected neural networks. In his pioneering work investigating what happens in the brains of people with anxiety disorders, the psychologist Dr. Peter J. Lang coined a term for these neural networks: *fear structures*. Dr. Edna Foa, a psychologist at the University of Pennsylvania, further developed this concept, applying it to the neuropsychology of PTSD. She noted that the fear structures encoded in PTSD are particularly large and the interconnection between these neural networks is strong. If one element is triggered, all related trauma memories could come flooding back. Indeed, a full-blown flashback means the entire network has been activated, which explains why people with PTSD feel as though they are reliving the trauma. It is precisely the strength and size of these fear structures that cause so many of the problems faced by people living with PTSD.

Because many of the sensory elements of these fear structures are commonly encountered in everyday life, they unwittingly act as triggers. For Maria, buying groceries from a clerk who resembles her uncle, sitting next to a colleague who wears the same aftershave, seeing macaroni and cheese, and hearing the Supremes on the radio during her daily commute are all sensory cues that may trigger the thoughts, emotions, and bodily experiences that surrounded the original sexual abuse. The truly harrowing aspect is that rarely can trauma survivors spontaneously connect the dots between such triggers and the intrusive memories that result. Maria may not even register the resemblance between the grocery store clerk and her uncle. Instead, she simply feels overcome by fear and nausea as she leaves the store. This random triggering lends these symptoms their out-of-the-blue quality. PTSD treatment involves helping survivors become more aware of their triggers so that the resulting intrusive symptoms feel less jarring.

Where in the brain are these memories made? The hippocampus, located in the temporal lobe, processes the storage and retrieval of our long-term memories. We know that the hippocampus is smaller in people who have PTSD, but why this is so remains a mystery. Some theories suggest that traumatic stress leads to overproduction of the body's stress hormones, which causes the death of the nerve cells in the hippocampus, and hence it shrinks in size. Other findings hint to a reverse relationship in that having a smaller hippocampus renders a person more vulnerable to developing PTSD after trauma exposure. In other words, it is a risk factor that has simply lain dormant until the brain becomes traumatized.

From what molecular building blocks are memories made? Unlike taking a blood test, a saliva swab, or a sample of bone marrow, there is no simple way to take brain tissue from a live human. For this reason, neuroscientists have relied on animal models, and the work of Dr. Eric R. Kandel forms the basis of much of what we understand about how memories are formed. Kandel was awarded the 2000 Nobel Prize in Physiology or Medicine for his pioneering research investigating the synaptic connections between nerve cells in the sea slug *Aplysia*. Synapses are found where nerve cells connect to other nerve cells and are key to brain function and especially to memory. *Aplysia* is a species of sea slug that has a simple neuroanatomy and large nerve cells that render it ideal for scientific study. *Aplysia* also shows a withdrawal reflex in response to an aversive or "traumatic" stimuli, and this attribute proved fundamental to understanding how memory and learning are intertwined. Kandel and his colleagues were able to show that memories were formed when *Aplysia* was exposed to an aversive stimulus and that those memories left a physical trace in the form of proteins in the synapses.

More recently, Kandel and his colleagues at Columbia University identified a prion protein called cytoplasmic polyadenylation element-binding protein (CPEB) that plays a key role in the maintenance of long-term memories in mice. In a 2015 study, the team trained mice to memorize a way to navigate through a maze. They then rendered the mice CPEB gene nonfunctional. Without the gene, the mice forgot how to navigate the maze. Regarding the role of such prion proteins specifically in PTSD, Kandel told me, "PTSD very likely has prion mechanisms. We have so far identified a second prion that seems to play a role as a protective factor in PTSD." Though Kandel and his team are only in the preliminary stages of learning about the precise role of this prion in PTSD, such discoveries offer fascinating insights into its molecular basis.

***

The hour hand is just shy of reaching eleven when the receptionist buzzes to let me know my next patient is here, right on schedule. I go out to the waiting room to see Maria, and upon hearing her name, she sets aside the magazine she is reading and rises to greet me. As we walk to my office, we chat about the traffic, the weather, and how it has been a while since we last met. In my office, Maria tells me that things have been going well and her life is, finally, "back on track." Her cheeks are slightly red with the heat of excitement, and her voice is louder than usual, amped up by a mixture of extra confidence and happiness.

She spills the details of how the episodes of shaking and feeling suffocated have all but disappeared. She now sleeps soundly and does not need the sleep medication I prescribed for her. She is more aware of her trauma triggers, and they no longer have the power to send her into an emotional maelstrom. They provoke some anxiety, sadness, and the odd wave of anger or deep regret, but these are all emotions she accepts and can live with. Her memories are, once again, under her command. She tells me that she has been consistently taking the PTSD medication and that she is not having side effects. She wants to stay on it for now, but maybe in a few months, if things are still good, she will come off it. She has been offered a promotion at work, takes a weekly Zumba fitness class, and has joined a local book club.

As I listen to Maria, I think about what a difference a year can make. During those first several sessions she was barely able to make basic decisions regarding treatment. Instead, we took incremental steps: making the diagnosis, educating her about what was happening, starting her on PTSD medication, encouraging her to take it regularly, and titrating the dose up until it took effect. Only after that was she stable enough for me to refer her to a therapist who specialized in treating survivors of childhood sexual abuse. It took several sessions of therapy before Maria felt comfortable enough to talk about the sexual abuse, partly because of the painful nature of the subject and partly because of her reticent personality.

Things took a significant turn for the better after about six months. She was having fewer symptoms and growing healthier every day. Her improvement meant our appointments could be spaced out. We started out meeting weekly, then monthly, then every three months, and today we were meeting after four months. Again, awareness of time was providing me with invaluable data. The steady rhythm and predictability of our meetings served as a proxy of Maria's improved well-being.

Today I marvel at Maria's progress and ask her what she thinks helped her.

"I don't know . . . The therapy was huge. I had kept so much buried for so long, and I had no idea how much until I started talking. The meds helped, too. Once I could get some sleep, I could start to think straight, and the PTSD med, it acts like a kind of glue. It stopped me from falling apart, so I could get through some of the hard stuff in therapy."

Maria had come to realize that she had navigated her whole life thinking that it was okay for other people to use her in any way they wanted. That belief had started during her childhood, after the abuse, but had infiltrated many of her adult relationships, most notably her relationship with her ex-husband. She now saw that it was not the ideal marriage she once believed it to be. It was a one-sided relationship in which she moved heaven and earth to please him and he went out of his way to ridicule and mock her.

"It's probably for the best that we got divorced. I see that now . . ."

Today is such a contrast to that early appointment when Maria appeared to be drowning in a flood of her traumatic memories. I gently inquire if she recalls that session.

She looks at me, her brow furrows, and she seems puzzled. "Dr. Jain, if I'm honest, that whole time is a bit of a blur. I was a mess. I am just so relieved to have my life back."

Maria has little to no recollection of that appointment. The irony for me is that the memory of her reliving her abuse in my office is emblazoned in my mind.

"Never mind, I was just curious. Forget I asked," I say quickly. "I agree with you one hundred percent, Maria. You have your life back now, and that really is all that matters."

NIGHTMARES

My sleep wasn't peaceful, though. I have the sense of emerging from a world of dark, haunted places where I traveled alone.

—Suzanne Collins, *Mockingjay*

The classic PTSD nightmare involves a repetitive replay of the trauma, complete with related emotions, bodily responses, and movements. Many spouses of veterans with PTSD tell of frequently being awakened from a deep slumber by a thump, slap, or bloodcurdling scream as their spouses reenact a battle scene in their nightmares. PTSD nightmares may occur as frequently as six nights a week and can continue for up to five decades after the original trauma. The chronically disturbed sleep leads to depression and anxiety problems. Some turn to alcohol or illicit drugs to "escape" or simply do not function well—they lose jobs, are irritable and short tempered with their loved ones, and lack energy and verve.

Nightmares also have a way of catching one off guard, as was the case for my patient Michael. As a psychiatry resident required to rotate through a county clinic, I inherited Michael's case after his previous resident graduated. The departing doctor's careful chart entries summarized Michael's treatment thus far and indicated his to be a true success story. Michael, now in his late fifties, had suffered from PTSD and regularly abused alcohol throughout his twenties, thirties, and forties. His life had been chaotic, he had lost job after job, his marriage ended in divorce, and he had been absent from the lives of his children when they were young.

For the last decade, however, he had been treated for PTSD, was now sober, and was working more steadily. By the time I first met him, he needed only minimal treatment; an appointment with me every two to three months for a medication checkup and weekly Alcoholics Anonymous meetings. He was now semiretired, was spending more time with his grandchildren, and enjoyed gardening and watching the History Channel. Our visits were typically short and pleasant. He would muse about current affairs, the state of his roses, and things that irked him, such as the relationship with his daughter and her domestic partner: "If he really loved her, he would marry her, don't you think, Doc?"

To my ear, his meanderings were welcome. The range of his interests and the depth of his concerns were all encouraging indications that his recovery was strong. On occasion, as he was mostly symptom free, I would broach the option of tapering him off the medication. He would pause and then say, "Nah, Doc, I think we should leave things be."

But one day as he dined with his daughter and grandson at a local Bakers Square restaurant, Michael had a chance encounter with a server who bore a strong resemblance to his best friend, who had been killed over four decades before. Until this point, Michael had never talked much about his specific trauma history; he had never felt a need to. But now he had little choice.

"That server could have been his twin," he whispers. His throat seems to close, causing him to have difficulty speaking, and big tears roll down his cheeks.

Upon seeing the server, he instantly lost his appetite for the French silk pie sitting in front of him. His stomach churned, and he thought he was going to throw up. For a few seconds, he felt he was right back in that frigid Wisconsin winter night when his best friend had been killed in a car accident. The tragedy had occurred during his senior year of high school. Michael had been driving, and after the horrific collision, he had tried to stop the bleeding, but his friend was dead. The indelible image of his lifeless eyes was now haunting Michael in his dreams.

"I think maybe I was fooling myself to think I would ever be free of this thing, Doc."

Since seeing the server, Michael reported having had nightly nightmares. He would wake up in soaked sheets with his heart pounding. He would distract himself from the nightmares by getting out of bed and doing crossword puzzles. When he felt sleepy again, he would go back to bed, but he still woke up three or four times a night, only getting about two hours of sleep total. After the Bakers Square incident, the Michael I knew changed almost beyond recognition. An ex-smoker for a decade, he resumed his habit. His clothes were rumpled, dark circles appeared under his eyes, and deep creases lined his forehead. The nightmares destabilized him, and quick action was needed to restore his balance. Unfortunately, before his balance could be restored, he started to drink heavily again. He stopped refilling his medication and started missing his appointments.

One day, I received a message that Michael's daughter, Claire, wanted to talk with me. As I dialed her number, I braced myself for what I knew would be a difficult call. There was no doubt Michael's life was unraveling, and, for his loved ones, I knew this was heartbreaking to watch. Naturally, they would expect that I, as the doctor, would do something to intervene, but the reality was that I could not force Michael to come to appointments, stop drinking, or take his medications.

Claire's voice was panicked, and as I listened to her concerns, I scanned it for hints that Michael was a danger to himself or posing a threat to others, as these were the only circumstances under which I could consider taking legal steps to require treatment. Convinced that there was no such situation, I took a deep breath and explained that there was little we could do at this point. Claire went silent, and I waited for her to process what I said. After a few moments, she spoke, and this time her voice was shrill. "Dr. Jain, I basically grew up without a dad, do you know that? He was a drunk who was in and out of my life when I was a kid. The last ten years, I finally got to know my father, and my son got to have a grandfather. Are you telling me we are going to lose him again?"

"I'm so sorry, Claire. I don't know what to say. I can't force your dad into treatment. All we can do is be there for him when he is ready to come back . . . Please do call the clinic with updates . . . We want to know what is going on with your dad."

For a few moments I shifted uneasily in the silence that hung between my answer and her response. I heard Claire letting out a big sigh. "Okay, I'll call if things get worse," she said before abruptly hanging up the phone.

As I prepared to move on to my next rotation, I wrote a summary in Michael's chart for the next resident assigned to his case. Michael's case no longer qualified as a success story.

During the time when I was Michael's psychiatrist, clinical lore recommended that his nightmares be addressed by treating his PTSD. What I did not know at the time was that arguments were being hashed out in the pages of scientific journals and at international medical conferences to change this approach. Essentially the world's sleep experts were arguing that disturbed sleep should be viewed as a core feature of PTSD.

In the first decade of the twenty-first century, sleep researchers discovered many sleep-related problems in people with PTSD. In addition to the debilitating issue of nightmares, insomnia is a distinct problem for almost 50 percent of sufferers. A high incidence of sleep-disordered breathing and limb movements is also seen in sleeping PTSD patients. Moreover, PTSD sufferers do not sleep as deeply as healthy people. For example, a woman who has had PTSD from the time she was raped by an intruder may, twenty years later, fall asleep with ease, but any noise—a car screeching to a halt on the street, her child getting up to use the bathroom, the heating system kicking in—will awaken her more easily than it would the average person. Once awake, she may feel compelled to double-check that the doors and windows are locked or patrol the house with a chopping knife in search of intruders.

These findings raised some fascinating questions: Is the disturbed sleep causing or contributing to the development of PTSD? Are sleep disorders a risk factor for PTSD? Two decades of research have since coalesced in the following conclusion: In adults with PTSD, sleep disturbances often develop into independent sleep problems. These sleep disorders exacerbate the PTSD symptoms and require their own focused treatment.

If Michael were my patient today, along with his PTSD treatment I would offer him imagery rehearsal therapy (IRT), a talk treatment that specifically targets nightmares. The therapy involves recalling the nightmare, writing it down, and changing the theme into a more positive story line. Patients rehearse the rewritten dream scenario so that they can displace the traumatic content when the dream recurs (they do this by practicing ten to twenty minutes during the day). Instead of having nightmares of a deadly car crash, Michael could rehearse an alternate outcome in which the car ran into a tree that was actually made of paper. Michael and his best friend would go on with their lives, unharmed and happy. IRT has been shown to inhibit the original nightmare by providing a critical shift in thinking that challenges its very origins.

Moving away from the one-size-fits-all model that has dominated psychiatric practice to this point and finding newer ways to tailor PTSD treatments to specifically target nightmares would appear key to offering patients like Michael tangible relief from their symptoms.

FLASHBACKS

In the traumatic universe the basic laws of matter are suspended:
ceiling fans can be helicopters, car exhaust can be mustard gas.
—David J. Morris, *The Evil Hours: A Biography of Post-traumatic Stress Disorder*

Doug sits in my office. A Californian midday sun pours in through the windows, falling directly onto his bare forearms, which are tanned and heavily tattooed. His hair peeks out from under his Iraq War Marine Corps cap, and it occurs to me that I don't recall ever having seen him without the cap. He tells me what happened a few days prior, while he was sitting on his couch watching television.

"I heard the sound of a helicopter over the house, and I thought to myself: stay calm, it's just the emergency medical helicopter from the hospital."

His voice slows and croaks, and his normally placid demeanor gives way to an intense grimacing. "I hear those helicopters sometimes, you know, from living so close to the hospital, but for some reason this time it sounded loud. I thought to myself, what the heck is going on? That is when I made the mistake—I went to the window and BOOM! As soon as I saw those bright lights, I was back in Iraq."

Doug pauses. He bends his upper body forward so that his head hangs over his legs and his forearms rest on both thighs. All I can see is his profile: sun-damaged leathery skin, sharp nose, and overgrown sideburns. The rim of the cap hides his eyes, and he continues, talking to the floor between his feet. "I saw the helicopter that came to rescue us after the explosion. I could smell the burning flesh, hear the screams, and feel the heat of that sun, and all I could see was blood everywhere. I saw the bodies of those two kids I told you about. Seconds before, they were playing together, right in front of me. Then the explosion happened, and that was that."

Doug's voice chokes, and he looks up, staring into the distance, momentarily lost in thought. "I must have been out for a while, because next thing I know, the show I was watching was over. Then I just freaked out, my heart was racing, I was sweating like a pig. I felt irritable for the next few days, too. It was my weekend with the kids, but there is no point in me being with them when I am in a foul mood. I called my ex and told her I wasn't going to pick them up ..."

Doug's face shifts in a moment of recognition, as though he has seen a glimpse of his future. "I don't want to turn into a bitter old man. I really don't, Dr. Jain."

***

Flashbacks are triggered by trauma cues, are fragmented in nature, and involve an intense, vivid reliving of the event in the present. During a flashback people can feel sensations such as heat or pain, and they relive the emotions of fear or horror that accompanied the original trauma. There can be physical changes in the body, too. Blood pressure can rise, and the pulse can race out of control. People may find themselves fighting or running, just as they did during the original trauma. PTSD flashbacks are *involuntary* and distinctly different from taking a trip down memory lane, which, of course, involves a process of deliberate retrieval. For Doug, once the flashback was under way, he reexperienced the day when a bomb ripped through a crowded street, killing and maiming dozens of civilians, and the fact that he was standing in the living area of his apartment in California did nothing to ground his brain in reality.

What was happening in Doug's brain during that flashback? A recent functional magnetic resonance imaging (fMRI) study provides some promising insights. fMRI scans measure changes in blood flow in the brain to detect areas of activity. The computer images that result help decipher what is going on in the PTSD brain. The researchers compared scans from thirty-nine subjects; ten participants had been diagnosed with PTSD, fourteen with depression, and fifteen were control subjects (they had a history of trauma exposure but no PTSD and hence were considered healthy). The participants' brains were scanned as they were asked to perform tasks that would trigger memories related to their trauma.

When the study participants with PTSD had a flashback, their brains showed increased activity in the regions of the dorsal stream, a pathway of the brain that traverses the occipital lobe, primary motor cortex, and supplementary motor areas. The occipital lobe is tucked in the back of the skull and is the place where all visual sensations are processed. The primary motor cortex is part of the frontal lobe of the brain and with the supplementary motor areas is responsible for how humans perform physical movement. The fact that these areas are activated during a flashback offers clues that help explain the vivid visual nature of flashbacks and how a person can simulate the physical actions of the original trauma.

The researchers also found reduced activity in the inferior temporal cortex and parahippocampus, which are involved in processing spatial awareness, which is how we relate to our immediate surroundings and other objects in physical space. Decreased activity in these brain structures may help explain the feeling of disconnection from our immediate physical environment that occurs during a flashback.

AN UNLIVED LIFE

The Hidden Cost of Avoidance

The more unlived your life, the greater your death anxiety. The more you fail to experience your life fully, the more you will fear death.
—Irvin D. Yalom, *Staring at the Sun*

I think I have spotted my new patient even before I call his name. John is perched on the edge of his waiting room chair, which struggles to accommodate his large girth, and every few seconds, he wipes the palms of his hands on faded blue jeans that are stained and tearing at the knees. He is elderly and wears a black baseball cap with "KOREA VETERAN" stitched into the front in bright hues of red, yellow, and green. John is staring at the wall in front of him; his stare is not a daydream stare but more tunnel-like, almost as though he is challenging himself to look neither left nor right. He catches sight of me out of the corner of his eye, and when I call out his name, he is up in a flash. He offers me a cursory nod in exchange for my greeting and mutters under his breath, "Come on; let's get this over and done with."

John is seeing me at the insistence of his primary care doctor. He tells me that, a few months back, he suffered a small stroke and a mild heart attack and his recovery was complicated by bedsores that got infected and required operations. His doctor ordered a CAT scan, but John kept canceling the appointment with radiology.

"My nerves are out of control." John tells me how he cannot bear the prospect of being flat on his back in the scanner. He tells me that for decades he has hated any type of confined space, including waiting rooms, especially ones filled with people. Before his retirement twenty years ago, he worked in construction because it meant he could be outdoors. To avoid people, he also volunteered to work the night shifts, repairing the surfaces of deserted highways. He requested his primary care doctor to prescribe him diazepam to help him deal with his anxiety over the scan. For years, he had a regular prescription for diazepam, and as far as he is concerned, it worked well.

"After the service, I used to drink alcohol, probably much more than I should have. After my first heart attack, I quit the drinking, but then I needed something for the nerves. My old doctor gave me diazepam, and it did the trick. But this new doctor has some VA protocol he needs to follow. Told me he would not prescribe me diazepam until I saw a shrink!" John scoffs.

"Sir, have you ever seen a psychiatrist or other mental health professional before today?"

"No, never. My doctor tried, in the past, you know, to recommend that I see someone like you but I told you, the diazepam does the trick. I can't believe I have to put up with this bullshit just to get a prescription!"

I explain to John that I need to ask him several questions to know if there was something more to his anxiety about the scan. Perhaps there was some underlying problem that I could offer him better treatment for? I tell him about the medical research that shows medications like diazepam act more like a Band-Aid, providing temporary relief but not addressing what is really going on, and in the long run, might have serious side effects, too.

"Okay, whatever, let's get on with it, then!" He bristles, taking a handkerchief out of his trouser pocket and wiping the sweat from his forehead.

John tells me that he has always been independent but his recent health issues now challenge his autonomy. My inquiry about the presence of family or friends he might call upon to help him is met with a terse "No. No one."

I try to pinpoint when he first started to have anxiety, and his face tenses. "I don't know . . . probably after the service . . . there is only so much a man can take." Tears swell in his eyes, and he starts dabbing at them furiously with his handkerchief. "What's the point in thinking about the past like this? Why are you dredging this all up?"

Sensing his discomfort, I back off and turn instead to more benign topics. Do you have a family history of mental illness? Do you use nicotine? Caffeine? In parallel, I try to imagine what lies behind my patient's guarded responses. Did he witness something horrific in Korea? Maybe his life was endangered? Perhaps he was trapped somewhere? In a confined space?

John soldiers on, offering me curt phrases and one-word responses to my barrage of questions. I sense he is not being purposefully obstructive; rather, he is putting extraordinary effort into avoiding his feelings. In the sixty minutes we spend together, John does not smile or laugh; he becomes tearful (but does not cry) and is irritable but never angry. In short, he has a restricted range of emotions. As I wind up the interview, I can't help but wonder if underlying his anxiety is a fear that if he lets himself feel difficult emotions, they might overwhelm him. Is he afraid that if he starts to cry, he will not be able to stop? Or that if he allows himself to express the anger inside, he might explode?

My hunch was that John had suffered unnecessarily over the years and probably paid a heavy price for not heeding the advice of his doctors to visit a mental health professional. His story was peppered with features of avoidance, a core symptom of PTSD. But trying to help a PTSD patient with severe avoidant symptoms can be like trying to catch a cloud in a jar.

***

"Forget it ever happened," "It does not bear thinking about," and "Don't dwell on the past" are all suggestions commonly offered to those who have lived through a trauma. Humans are hardwired to engage in such avoidance tactics in the aftermath of trauma. Not only is it natural to avoid thinking about sad or tragic events in order to avoid intense emotions, but such a strategy can also restore normalcy to lives temporarily derailed by trauma. But if this coping strategy goes on for too long, it becomes a problem. It lulls the trauma survivor into a false sense of security—if I just avoid thinking about this or avoid doing that, everything will be okay. But it won't. As was the case for John, avoidance starts to subtly shape a person's being, rendering him or her a lesser version of his or her former self. In this way, avoidance becomes a secondary symptom of PTSD, one that emerges in the months and years that follow the traumatic event.

Studies following different groups of people, from those living in war zones to rape survivors and road accident victims, all point to an inverse relationship between the intrusive symptoms of PTSD and the phenomenon of avoidance. Avoidance occurs on two levels. On the first level, there is an *emotional* avoidance of all distressing memories, thoughts, and feelings about the trauma. On the second, there is a *behavioral* avoidance of the people, places, conversations, activities, objects, and situations that cause those distressing trauma-related memories, thoughts, or feelings. These two concentric layers of avoidance can envelop a life, constricting it so that the traumatized person is cut off from avenues for healing. This disabling aspect of avoidance has earned it a place as one of the symptoms that need to be present for someone to be diagnosed with PTSD.

Avoidance is integral to the pathology of PTSD, yet it presents a conundrum. Unlike the hallmark features of PTSD—nightmares, flashbacks, and hypervigilance—avoidance leaves its mark more insidiously and means that I rarely meet those who, like John, struggle with severe avoidance. I do, however, meet the adult children of trauma survivors who have shut down in this way. They are still reeling from the toll avoidance took on their parents' capacity to feel emotion and demonstrate love. "I feel like I never knew my father." "My mother *never* talked about *it*." "He was always so distant, cut off from us, as though it was painful for him to be with us."

What can neuroscience tell us about avoidance? In trauma survivors, there is a dynamic interplay between emotion and skills such as memory, attention, planning, and problem solving. In a 2012 article, neuroscientists reviewed several studies that show how the autobiographical memories of people with PTSD are often more vague than those of healthy control subjects. People with PTSD tend to recall personal memories with very few details. Neuroscientists refer to such memories as "overgeneral memory," and they are thought to arise because the individual avoids a thorough search when asked to recall the details of his or her past. It's akin to people jumping on hot coals; they don't stay in any one spot for too long for fear of getting burned.

***

After my first meeting with John, I wondered if his complaint about his "nerves" was actually PTSD that he had dealt with by white-knuckling it. In my world, "white-knuckling" refers to the way John had spent the years since his military service—full of anxiety and dread, using sheer willpower to keep himself going. Even though he did not divulge a trauma history to me, what caught my attention was the way he had organized his life over half a century after Korea. His tunnel-like stare in the waiting room made me wonder if he was avoiding the two wall-mounted televisions tuned in to coverage of a resurgence of violence in the Middle East. Were the images of soldiers in combat gear triggering John's memories in some way?

Another red flag was the years of heavy drinking he alluded to. Had he self-medicated intrusive symptoms of PTSD with alcohol and diazepam? Then there was the lifetime of working a night-shift job and a preference for being awake when the rest of the world was sleeping. Did he feel unsafe around other people? Was the feeling of being constantly on edge so exhausting that it was better to avoid people altogether?

I hypothesized that John had managed to create an elaborate illusion of control in his life: if he could just avoid this or that, he could stay safe. Of course, in some ways he was successful, but his need for control stripped his life of essentials such as love, passion, laughter, and joy. In the process he became divorced, estranged from his children, and isolated from friends. With the challenges of old age, his carefully constructed illusion was crashing down. His recent health problems meant more doctor visits, procedures, and tests. He had less control over how he could spend his day and the number of people he had to interact with. His old demons were catching up with him, and he was left with little choice but to face them.

At the end of that first session, I did not prescribe diazepam as he demanded. Instead I told him that it was actually making his anxiety symptoms worse in the long run and that its side effects were particularly hazardous for elderly patients. He was open to considering alternatives, so I suggested sertraline, a medication that could help address his symptoms and would not react with the other medications he was prescribed for his heart disease. I warned John that the sertraline would take time to build up in his system and that, unlike the diazepam, it would not knock out feelings of anxiety completely but just make them more manageable.

Over the course of our follow-up sessions, John started opening up about his past. We were able to broach some painful subjects, if not head-on, at least by skirting around the edges. His elder brother, whom he adored, had died in a bicycle accident when John was in middle school, and years later, in Korea, he had witnessed the death of a close army buddy. Not long after that, John had decided it was best not to get too close to people. He wore a prickly exterior that kept people at arm's length. He found solace in his solitude mostly because his fear of losing those he loved far outweighed what he felt he might gain by investing in such relationships.

With time, John was able to go for his CAT scan, was not feeling anxious all the time, and was managing all his hospital appointments. Of course it helped that he was feeling much stronger physically, too. He was on an antibiotic that helped his sores heal, and he was able to get back to his regular routine.

One day he told me that he was having insomnia. He tossed and turned, thinking about how he was sure he was going to die from a heart attack. But what was filling his nights with panic was the question "How long might it be before somebody finds my body?"

In his book *Staring at the Sun*, Irvin D. Yalom, a psychiatrist at Stanford University, wrote that he often asks his patients the following question: "What precisely do you fear about death?" In Yalom's experience, knowledge of our own mortality affects the unconscious mind of us all, and the answer to this question often cuts right through to the crux of many issues and accelerates the work of therapy. A common theme he encounters when doing such work with patients is "the positive correlation between the fear of death and the sense of unlived life."

I wondered if John's fear about how long it might be before somebody found his dead body was actually an expression of regret about how he had distanced himself from his loved ones.

One morning during a busy commute to work, it occurred to me that I had not seen John for a while. Later, I logged on to the electronic medical record and searched for his name, only for the screen to deliver a somber pop-up alert: "This patient died. Do you wish to continue?"

My heart sank, and I felt overwhelmed by sadness. I perused the chart entries and learned that John had suffered a massive heart attack. I clicked on the tab that revealed information about his next of kin and saw that it named a daughter, so I dialed her number to express my condolences. She told me that her father had refused to carry a cell phone and often let his home phone go unanswered, and for that reason, she had maintained close contact with his neighbors, who had called her when they saw two days' worth of newspapers lying on his driveway. She had driven over right away and found his body on the kitchen floor.

Part of John's premonition came true: he had died of a heart attack, but he had underestimated his daughter's attentiveness. The savagery of traumatic stress had made him keep an unnecessary distance from her.

"Thanks for your call, Doctor. But, you know, my father is in a better place now. He suffered for so long. He is with God. It is all for the better."

I paid my respects and hung up, feeling remorse about the whole situation. John was in his early eighties and had a serious heart condition, so the news of his death could hardly be considered surprising. Still, I could not help feeling he had died leaving behind important unfinished business, such as reconnecting with his children or friends. I thought of the insidious way avoidance can constrict and inhibit life and how the impact of John's early traumatic experiences might have ultimately rendered him impotent to fully consummate his life.

DENIAL LAND

When Trauma Memories Are
Deeply Buried

Everything was perfectly healthy and normal here in Denial Land.
—Jim Butcher, *Cold Days*

Take avoidance to an extreme, and you have denial: a deep burial of
the trauma. Most of us can summon up what denial feels like on a
cursory level. Think of a time when you received bad news: an abnormal test result during a routine checkup, a betrayal by a significant
other, or the sudden death of a loved one. For a few moments, you
refuse to accept the data your eyes and ears are feeding you. Your
brain rapidly searches for alternative explanations: "The doctor's
office must have made an error" or "It's not an affair; he's just been
working late at the office" or "I just talked to her last night; they
must be talking about someone else." Through this denial process,
the brain gently acclimates us to our new reality. In the minutes,
hours, and days that follow, the denial lifts, and we start to absorb
the shock of what has befallen us. But for those who have experienced the unspeakable, extreme denial stays fixed and unshakable
for months, years, and even decades.

Not long after I graduated from residency, I met Daniel when he
was hospitalized for severe depression. His outpatient psychiatrist
had admitted him because the treatment he offered Daniel was not
working. Daniel was a professor at a local college, and he had had no
mental health problems to speak of until this current episode. His

mother had died at the beginning of the year, and he had fallen into a deep depression. He was hardly eating or drinking and was pre-occupied with thoughts of suicide. He was in his late fifties, white, and divorced, all facts closely correlated with a higher chance of death by suicide, so when he started to make plans to shoot himself with his hunting rifle, he was fast-tracked for hospital admission. Inpatient treatment meant around-the-clock observation and options for more intensive treatments. The inpatient team recommended electroconvulsive therapy (ECT), and when I first met him, it was as the covering weekend doctor doing rounds on the day after one of the ECT sessions.

Daniel was a tall man with a gentle face, mostly covered by a thick mustache and beard. He was casually dressed in cargo pants and a Milwaukee Brewers T-shirt. We were both seated in comfy armchairs, which were thoughtfully positioned by a large arched window that looked out onto expansive gardens. The richness of the colors caught Daniel's eye, and he commented on their beauty. "I love this time of year, all the autumnal foliage—the reds, oranges, yellows, and browns. It feels comforting, somehow . . ."

Such spontaneous chitchat made me hopeful that the ECT was working, and I continued by asking him about the side effects of his latest treatment. Do you have a headache? How is your memory? Do you feel foggy or disorientated? How would you rate your level of depression? Do you feel suicidal? His answers indicated that things were improving and I did not need to make any further changes; he was set for the weekend, and his primary team could resume his care on Monday.

I was wrapping up our visit when Daniel leaned in toward me, his voice dropping almost to a whisper. "Doctor, I have never told anyone this before. Since the second ECT session, I have been having this memory that I can't get out of my head. It's from when

I was twelve or thirteen, and my mother is touching me below and massaging my private parts."

I was totally caught off guard by Daniel's disclosure.

"It happened, you know. It's all coming back to me now. It was awful."

There are moments in the life of a doctor that require you to abandon the best-laid plans, when the structure of a demanding day must cave to the importance of a particular moment. Daniel's disclosure was one such moment, but unfortunately, at the time I was unable to recognize it for what it was.

"Um . . . okay. Well, that is very important information. I will be sure to pass that along to your primary team," I managed to muster before getting up and ending our session.

Fortunately, Daniel did not suffer for my ineptitude in that crucial moment. Until that point the memories of sexual abuse perpetrated by his mother had been buried deep. Her death had triggered a deep depression, and as his default coping strategy of denial collapsed, the memories eventually surfaced. Acknowledging the abuse would prove to be the first step toward his making a full recovery, and in the weeks that followed, he worked closely with a therapist. He found new ways to deal with his thoughts and feelings about the abuse instead of fearing or denying them. Gradually his mood improved and the intensity of the suicidal ideation abated. A few months later, he was able to resume his normal life.

When I shared my disappointment in my reaction to Daniel's disclosure with a seasoned psychiatrist, he told me this: "Mastering our own reactions to the really hard things our patients have endured and then share with us is really tough . . . I think doctors underestimate just how tough it is."

Looking back at my younger self, I realize how my brain was also in denial about what Daniel was disclosing. I had heard stories about sexual abuse perpetrated by a stepfather, uncle, grandfather, father, or male family friend, but I could not accept that a mother could sexually abuse her child. There was something so taboo about that scenario that, like Daniel, I simply denied that it could ever have happened, and so I ended our session abruptly. Today I like to think I would have stayed, listened to Daniel speak for as long as he needed to, and at least been a better witness of what he was going through: the painful experience of having the fog of denial lift and the reality of what he endured emerge from the darkness.

CARRYING SORROWS
IN THE BLOOD

Cortisol, Epigenetics, and
Generational Trauma

> PTSD is a whole-body tragedy, an integral human event of enormous
> proportions with massive repercussions.
>
> —Susan Pease Banitt

When I was a chief resident, I spent several months rotating through a student health center at a local college. My patient Rimma was a freshman referred by her primary care doctor for worsening anxiety and trouble adjusting to college life. Rimma was petite with dark hair, strands of which were dyed with different hues of purple. She invariably wore black clothes with clunky army boots, her nose was pierced, and she wore dark, heavy makeup that made her green eyes pop in contrast to her ghostly pale skin. Her appearance always struck me as somber and served to distract me from the fact that underneath all the makeup and layers of clothing was a young girl.

Rimma was precocious and intelligent and had graduated from high school at sixteen, so was much younger than her freshman peers. She told me she felt like an outsider and was finding it hard to connect with other students. Her academic performance was suffering, which caused her much anxiety. She suffered from insomnia, had lost her appetite, and was having panic attacks two to three times a week.

Rimma viewed the entire college citizenry—teachers, administrators, and students—as incompetent Neanderthals. She would spend whole sessions engaged in biting commentary about everyone she encountered. Somewhat disturbingly, it soon became apparent that she was not actually engaging with those people; she was judging them from afar. Her pervasive mistrust of the world around her made her keep an emotional distance from almost everyone else on campus.

Rimma also spent a lot of time talking about her relationship with her mother. Her parents had come to America from the Soviet Union in the late 1980s, Orthodox Jews who had left to escape religious persecution in the communist Soviet Union. Rimma had been born in the United States and had never been to Russia, and from what I could gather, her parents rarely traveled back either. Rimma often engaged in vivid descriptions of the bitter battles she had with her mother. With contempt, she would mock her mother's Russian accent and complain that "she never talks about anything that *really* matters" and "she lives in her own world, freaks out about the littlest of things."

Rimma had initially celebrated leaving for college and relished the chance to be on her own, but her struggles with adjusting to campus life, combined with her parents' concerns about underage college drinking, meant she had since moved back home and now commuted to classes.

At the time, I viewed this as typical teenage rebellion. Intellectually Rimma was mature, but emotionally she was still a teenager struggling with classic issues of separation and identity. But now, more than a decade on, it occurs to me that I did not consider the possibility that her parents had a very significant trauma history. What had happened to her Jewish parents in the communist Soviet Union? What had it been like growing up in an environment where you had to be secretive about your faith? Under such circumstances does one simply live life with a basic loss of trust and confidence in the world? Does this undermine your passions and commitment to your loved ones? And the most important question: Were Rimma's symptoms directly related to her parents' traumatic experiences?

Centuries of case reports have contributed to a conventional wisdom that parents living with traumatic stress are more likely to have children who suffer from depression, anxiety, or traumatic stress. For decades this "psychological damage" was attributed to the way the children were parented. By this logic, Rimma learned behaviors in her home environment that led her to react to the larger world in a fearful, emotionally volatile, and aloof manner.

Another plausible explanation would be that such psychological issues simply "run in families" and Rimma had inherited a genetic profile from her parents that made her more vulnerable to such problems. Indeed, though PTSD is, by definition, linked to a traumatic event, research studies have consistently shown that PTSD, like depression, is highly heritable, and genetic influences explain a substantial proportion of one's vulnerability to developing PTSD after surviving trauma.

In the early part of the twenty-first century, Dr. Rachel Yehuda, a neuroscientist at the Mount Sinai School of Medicine, offered an intriguing new idea: that children of traumatized parents are at risk for similar problems because of epigenetic changes that occurred in the biology of their traumatized parents. Epigenetics refers to how PTSD may possibly alter the way genes express themselves in a trauma survivor and how such alterations can then be inherited by children on a cellular level and alter their neurons, brain molecules, neuroanatomy, and genes. These epigenetic changes are transmitted to children by a process called "intergenerational transmission" by having a negative impact on the parents' sperm or egg quality or impacting the mother while she is pregnant.

How can one disentangle the effects of environment from genetic and molecular factors, especially when parents and their children often share the same living environment and are exposed to the same social and psychological stressors? By focusing on the stress hormone cortisol, researchers have ventured into these murky waters and emerged with enticing new insights.

After trauma, the brain's central coordinator of our response to stress, the hypothalamic-pituitary-adrenal (HPA) axis mounts a chemical and hormonal reaction. The HPA axis directs a cascade of complex chemical reactions, and one of the end products, cortisol, appears to be crucial in helping the traumatized brain recover. The scientific community predicted that cortisol levels would be high in PTSD sufferers, yet over the last two decades, study after study has shown that patients with PTSD actually have lower-than-average cortisol levels than those who have been exposed to trauma but do not have PTSD and healthy controls. Indeed, the story of cortisol and PTSD has turned out to be complicated, moving beyond cortisol to encompass metabolites of cortisol, glucocorticoid receptors in the brain, and the genes and proteins involved in regulating the activity and sensitivity of those receptors.

To study the epigenetics of PTSD, Yehuda examined the impact of trauma exposure on the salivary cortisol of pregnant women. Researchers collected salivary cortisol samples from thirty-eight mothers who were pregnant when they evacuated the World Trade Center on 9/11 and from their one-year-old babies. When compared with mothers who did not develop PTSD after 9/11, lower cortisol levels were observed in both the mothers who did develop PTSD after 9/11 and their babies. Mothers who were in their third trimester during 9/11 had the lowest cortisol levels.

This trimester effect may have been related to the traumatic stress altering the expression of a specific enzyme in the placenta. This enzyme, which becomes active in the placenta only late in the second trimester, is supposed to break down cortisol into an inactive form. If the activity of the enzyme is altered, elevated levels of maternal cortisol hormones circulating in the placenta could have had a negative effect on the fetus's cortisol hormones.

When I asked Yehuda what the take-home message from this study was, she said:

> The message is simple: mothers who are traumatized during pregnancy can transmit defects to their offspring, in utero, because the offspring accommodates somehow to the level of stress hormone. . . . The offspring do not need to have actual (traumatic) experiences in their life for this to be true. We do not think about pregnancy as the very important developmental event that it really is. Otherwise, we would take much better care of traumatized pregnant women than we do.

Other studies showing that pregnant women with PTSD are more likely to have impaired uterine blood flow, low-birth-weight babies, and premature babies underscore the crucial relevance of in utero exposures to PTSD on the biology of the developing baby.

These novel ideas linking traumatic stress, epigenetics, and intergenerational transmission now come to my mind every time I meet a patient who comes from a community that has survived a group trauma. I can't help but wonder about how much of his or her suffering today is rooted in historical events and if what I am witnessing is, in part, the brunt of a much broader and deeper injury. Are the traumatic echoes of massive group-based oppression, forced relocation, or political subjugation also present in the room with us? Are these collective sorrows now carried in the blood of future generations? If future generations don't recognize these collective sorrows for what they are, will they become curses that permanently wound their souls?

Though the science of epigenetics remains in its infancy, what seems to be clear is that we humans are an accumulation of our traumatic experiences, that each trauma contributes to our biology, and that this biology determines, to some extent, how we respond to further traumatic events as they emerge in our lives.

A WILDNESS
IN THE BONES

Acute Awareness and Shady Moods

After a traumatic experience, the human system of self-preservation seems to go onto permanent alert, as if the danger might return at any moment.

—Judith Herman, *Trauma and Recovery: The Aftermath of Violence—From Domestic Abuse to Political Terror*

My patient Gregg was a senior executive whose job required regular car travel. One day a college student ran through a red light and smashed into the back of Gregg's SUV. Gregg was knocked unconscious and sustained fractures that required surgeries and extensive rehabilitation. When he was ready to return to work, he was filled with panic at the thought of getting behind the wheel, and any attempt to drive triggered flashbacks of the accident. Unable to meet the travel demands of his job, he ended up retiring early. With the passage of time, he started to drive again, usually local trips on familiar routes, but being on the road still presented challenges.

One day, he was driving on the highway. He avoided peak traffic at all costs, so he was surprised to find that the road was busier than usual and alarmed when he saw a truck that appeared too close behind him. "I could feel myself getting sweaty, and my heart was beating fast. Then I felt so mad! How dare he drive so close to me! I started yelling at him in my rearview mirror!"

Gregg then described how the truck had tried to overtake him and how he had swerved his SUV to block him. "I don't know what the heck got into me. I was just convinced I was not going to let him get past me. Somehow he overtook me on the right side and took an exit off the highway. I took off after him, chasing him up the exit ramp. I followed him all the way to a gas station and got out and went right up to him. I was yelling, and he was just staring at me. He told me to go to hell and turned his back on me. Thank God I finally came to my senses and got back into my car."

The problem was that Gregg was not alone in his car that afternoon. His wife was next to him, and their two-year-old granddaughter was in the back. They were taking her to the park and then for ice cream, the highlight of Gregg's week. Later, after his wife relayed to their daughter the events of that afternoon, his daughter called to tell him she would not be letting him take his granddaughter on weekly outings anymore.

Although individuals with PTSD lead a life of emotional restriction, their bodies continue to react to their environment as if they are under threat of annihilation. The PTSD brain assumes that danger is present and is stuck in a mode of overprotecting itself. This predicament explains the most disruptive dimension of PTSD: outbursts, reckless behavior, hypervigilance, and an exaggerated startle response.

Gregg's brain was out of balance. The neurocircuitry that controlled activation and the circuits that controlled relaxation were no longer working in sync. The delicate balance between these brain systems, a prerequisite for normal functioning, meant that his nervous system had a low threshold for sensing danger and reacting accordingly.

During his recent episode of road rage, Gregg's brain over-responded and went into fight mode. After he got back into his car, it took him more than thirty minutes to calm down. This heightened state of arousal tested his brain's resources, which become embroiled in this abnormal and excessive activity. His brain had crashed, and he needed that time to reboot.

Individuals with PTSD have abnormally high levels of noradrenaline. Noradrenaline is the main neurotransmitter of the body's sympathetic nervous system and is vital to mounting the body's response to a threat, the "fight-or-flight" reaction. It is produced in clusters of specialized cells that can be found not only in the brain but in the spinal cord, gut, and adrenal glands. When faced with a threat, the brain releases noradrenaline, which acts to increase anxiety and alertness to one's surroundings, enhances the formation and retrieval of memories, and focuses the brain's attention exclusively on the source of the threat. In the rest of the body, norepinephrine increases heart rate and blood pressure, triggers the release of glucose from energy stores, and increases blood flow to muscles. All of these actions prepare the human body to survive the threat. In the PTSD brain, however, this process has gone awry and become hyperreactive. It not only takes less to activate the "fight-or-flight" response, but when it is activated, the response is more pronounced. All of this leads to the hypervigilance and exaggerated fear states that are hallmark features of PTSD.

The amygdala, an almond-shaped set of neurons located in the temporal lobe of the brain, plays a key role in the processing of emotions such as fear and pleasure. A landmark study used fMRI technology to investigate the amygdala's response to threats. As the brain's blood flow and neuronal activity are coupled, the fMRI detects changes in its blood flow and uses those measurements to create a picture of amygdala brain activity. In this study, Dr. Scott Rauch and his colleagues at Harvard University studied eight men with PTSD and eight trauma-exposed but healthy men who served as the control group. The researchers measured how the amygdala responded to a threatening visual image (a fearsome human face). Comparisons of the fMRI images found that the men with PTSD had an exaggerated amygdala response to threatening visual images when compared to the control group.

Related to amygdala misfiring is inactivity of the frontal lobe of the PTSD brain, a region integral to our ability to make decisions, plan actions, control our impulses, and exercise judgment. In a 2004 study published in *Archives of General Psychiatry*, Dr. Lisa Shin and her colleagues at Tufts University used positron emission tomography (PET) scans to examine the frontal lobes of research subjects with PTSD. A PET scan detects gamma rays emitted by a tracer that is introduced into the body on a biologically active molecule. Using a special camera and computer, the researchers were able to generate images of the way the subjects' brains were functioning by monitoring the brain's metabolism. After carefully triggering some PTSD symptoms in the subjects, the researchers looked to see what happened in the amygdala and frontal regions of their brains. The results confirmed what earlier research findings had hinted at: in PTSD, the frontal lobe is more inactive than it should be and thus unable to exert control over an overly active amygdala. This means the PTSD brain overreacts to threats of danger and can even imagine danger where it does not exist.

***

Anger. Guilt. Horror. Fear. These are the mood states that dominate the daily lives of those living with PTSD. Driving these moods are self-denigrations that have become intertwined with the traumatic event: "It's all my fault." "If only I had done this instead." "I don't deserve to live." These denigrations are so powerful that they start to influence the sufferer's worldview, rendering it pessimistic: "I can't trust anyone." "This world is very dangerous."

These moods and thoughts infiltrate all personal relationships, stifling passion and stunting ambition.

Survivors feel emotionally estranged from their loved ones, viewing their entire world through the lens of trauma. Such loss of trust and confidence in the world can even result in survivors living with a sense of a foreshortened future. They live without expectation of reaching normal milestones or life span.

Such mood changes were apparent in my patient Leticia. Leticia lived in a rough neighborhood with her young twin boys. After her boyfriend, the father of her children, was arrested on larceny charges, she decided to go back to college to become a medical assistant. She would attend classes while her twins were in preschool, pick them up, make an early dinner, and then drop them off at her mother's home. From there she would go to her retail job at a local mall. One night, she volunteered to work late to earn extra cash for Christmas gifts for her children. When her shift ended, she headed to the quiet parking lot, where she was attacked and raped at gunpoint by two strangers.

It was months later when I first met Leticia. She was sitting with her back against the wall, scanning the waiting room and clutching her handbag on her lap. She looked ready to bolt. Leticia told me that since the rape she had seen danger everywhere, even at the grocery store. Navigating the crowded aisles from the produce section to the baked goods section would leave her drenched in sweat and in a heart-thumping panic. Leticia's brain and blood vessels were flooded with excess noradrenaline, and this was holding her petite frame hostage and in a perpetual state of fight or flight. Even on her commute to college she perceived a stranger offering a smile or a group gathered on a street corner as potential rapists. She ended up dropping out of school.

Of course, the human brain being tuned into potential sources of danger offers an important survival advantage. The problem comes when the brain is unable to properly regulate this process, which results in a lot of false alarms. In Leticia's case, she would often "overreact" for no reason.

One day at work, a customer engrossed in her shopping list swirled around too fast and knocked into Leticia. Leticia flew into a rage, showering the woman with all manner of verbal threats. She lost her job; her behavior was not compatible with good customer service.

"I am stuck! I wanted something more for my life, but I don't even dare to hope anymore." She shook her head as her eyes teared up again.

I was also struck by the intensity of Leticia's anger and irritability and could not help but think of the circuits of her brain and serotonin levels gone awry. Serotonin is a neurotransmitter made from the amino acid tryptophan that can be found all over the brain, including regions implicated in the neurobiology of PTSD such as the hippocampus, prefrontal cortex, and amygdala. People with PTSD have lower levels of serotonin in their blood, and for reasons unknown, their central nervous system does not mount as strong a response when challenged to produce this transmitter. These abnormal alterations in serotonin transmission likely contribute to the depression, anger, and aggression so often seen in PTSD sufferers and likely played a role in the symptoms Leticia was describing to me.

Unfortunately, Leticia came to see me for only a handful of visits. Like many of my patients with severe PTSD, she disappeared before we could complete treatment. The last time I saw her, she was frustrated that her symptoms were not responding as quickly as she had hoped and was doubtful that I could offer her relief.

Understanding exactly how the amygdala and prefrontal cortex communicate would appear to be vital to helping patients such as Gregg and Leticia. A 2016 study attempted to do just that by using a cutting-edge technique called magnetoencephalography (MEG). MEG measures the magnetic fields generated by brain cell activity and therefore is a direct measure of brain function. Brain-imaging technology such as MRI, fMRI, and PET scans provide indirect measures of brain structure and function, which means one has to factor in a host of other plausible possibilities that might explain the changes seen on such scans. One of the huge advantages of MEG is that it offers precise real-time data about what is happening in the human brain.

Researchers compared the brain activity in the amygdala and prefrontal cortex of PTSD participants as they were shown various images. They found that when participants were viewing threatening images, a large number of their brain regions appeared to become overconnected and hence launched an exaggerated response to perceived threats. Perhaps what is most enticing about this latest research is the promise of a new technology that can offer glimpses into real-time brain function. With this promise comes the hope of a future where physicians will be able to offer patients like Gregg and Leticia more effective ways to not only diagnose but treat PTSD.

DISSOCIATION

The Two-Thousand-Yard Stare

Traumas produce their disintegrating effects in proportion to their intensity, duration and repetition.

—Pierre Janet

When I was an intern, I met Melody, a young woman with a nasty compulsion to insert paper clips, thumbnails, and sewing needles into her bodily orifices and skin. She was famous in the hospital, as half the medical staff had, at one time or another, been awakened from a deep slumber to evaluate her on one of her multiple visits to the emergency room. Melody would sit in her hospital bed, her chestnut brown hair straggling over her broad shoulders, and pick at the dirt under her fingernails as the drama unfolded around her. Mysterious complications in her treatment, to which she reacted with a peculiar indifference, often lengthened her stays. Her condition demanded the attention of many specialists: one or more from urology; ear, nose, and throat; and gastroenterology, depending on which orifice (or orifices) she had assaulted; plastic surgery for the wounds caused by the repeated puncturing of her skin; infectious disease specialists to ponder over which antibiotic should be used to treat the superbugs making their home in the deeper layers of her skin; and, of course, psychiatry.

Munchausen syndrome, somatization, and borderline personality disorder were just a few of the many diagnoses that filled Melody's chart. What I did not know then, as an intern, was that we were missing a key diagnosis. Now, almost twenty years later, I realize that Melody's disturbed behavior, her "checked-out" expression, her lack of emotion and apparent desensitization toward having various body parts poked and prodded for tests all hinted at the possibility of a history of severe childhood trauma. Her memories of such traumas were likely deeply buried, and she was probably unaware of them, her mind having dissociated itself from those early horrors. Instead, the impact of her enduring the unspeakable was manifesting as this disturbing self-mutilation and the perverse relief she felt in the dramatic environs of a hospital.

***

Derealization (feeling as if the world around you is not real) and depersonalization (feeling as if you are not real) are symptoms of dissociation. These curious symptoms have an eerie quality. With derealization, other people and objects appear unreal, lifeless, or visually distorted. During depersonalization, individuals experience themselves as detached from the rest of the world or as an outside observer of their body, thoughts, and actions. They lose the ability to feel emotion and appreciate bodily sensations. They feel absent from themselves and lose all sense of time. These experiences are occasionally felt by healthy people during stressful periods such as a bereavement or sleep deprivation, but they become pathological when, as in Melody's case, they recur frequently, dominating day-to-day life.

Since Pierre Janet wrote about dissociation in the early 1900s, debates about the precise nature of the relationship between PTSD and dissociation have continued. Over the last two decades, converging lines of empirical evidence have led to the inclusion of a dissociative subtype of PTSD in the latest version of the *DSM*. According to Dr.

Matthew Friedman, a psychiatrist and PTSD expert at the Geisel School of Medicine at Dartmouth University, "Functional brain imaging studies show a distinctly different pattern of brain activity for people with the Dissociative Subtype, in contrast to non-dissociative PTSD. Studies to date indicate that among people with PTSD, 15–30% have the dissociative subtype."

When confronted with horrific events or reminders of such traumas, some people will detach from the world and dissolve into these dissociative symptoms of derealization and depersonalization in a process that neuroscientists call *emotional overmodulation*. So in addition to the more commonly known fight-or-flight response to experiencing a trauma, this third response of dissociation represents a "freeze" response on the part of the survivor.

What determines who will dissociate after facing a trauma? Several theories suggest that dissociating from reality represents a method of psychological escape when physical escape is not an option. This kind of response is more commonly found in survivors of severe childhood abuse perpetrated by a primary caregiver. One such theory, the betrayal trauma theory, argues that dissociating gives victims who are dependent on abusive caregivers for food, water, clothing, and shelter a way to maintain the attachments necessary for their physical survival. Dissociation also interferes with the coding, storage, and retrieval of trauma memories so that trauma survivors may not be able to acknowledge their trauma as the related information is kept out of their conscious awareness.

Though dissociation may have some immediate protective effect, there are serious long-term consequences. Survivors find it harder to function on a daily basis, can be suicidal, and may have other psychiatric problems. On top of this, trauma sufferers who dissociate are harder to treat because they shut down when dealing with their traumatic past, which renders many talk therapies ineffective.

Beyond Western research studies, data from the World Health Organization's World Mental Health Surveys that interviewed more than 25,000 people in sixteen countries found this dissociative form of PTSD present in 14 percent of the respondents with PTSD. It was more common among those who had suffered from PTSD as children and had experienced significant childhood adversity.

When I think back to Melody and her checked-out expression, self-mutilation, and emotional indifference, it now feels obvious to me that she was having symptoms of depersonalization and derealization. There was very little in her presentation that jibed with a conventional case of PTSD. She did not present a history of trauma, was not complaining of nightmares or flashbacks or hypervigilance—rather the opposite: she appeared absent from herself, detached from her body, and only loosely aware of her surroundings. The dissociative subtype of PTSD was the diagnosis that was missing from her chart.

PART 3

The Body

BODILY WOUNDS

Trauma may be one of the root causes of serious public health
concerns—both the behavioral risk factors that may lead to disease
and the diseases themselves.
—Paula Schnurr

Every freshly minted physician spends a grueling year as an intern.
My internship, twenty years ago, was a frenetic rotation through a
university hospital. By the end of that year, I was adept at diagnosing
failing hearts, livers, kidneys, and lungs. My nose, routinely flooded
by the smell of pus-filled wounds, was now desensitized, so I no
longer gagged at the odor of frothy urine, bloody stool samples,
or bile-streaked vomit. I was up at all hours of the night, for many
nights, boosting my patients' low potassium and magnesium levels,
catheterizing their stubborn bladders, culturing bugs responsible
for spiking fevers, and setting up morphine pumps for cancer patients and insulin drips for diabetics.

Through all such tasks my mind lingered on some of my patients'
more elusive backstories, which seemed crucial to understanding
their diseases. One such patient was Allan, who would come to the
hospital every few weeks to have the fluid drained that his failing
liver was no longer able to get rid of. My month-long immersion
on the liver unit meant I was now only too familiar with the toxic
effects of alcohol. There was the insurance salesman who, on the
way home from a boozy night with clients, had vomited blood on
the beige leather of his new BMW. The shock of that experience
and his diagnosis of peptic ulcer disease was enough to make him

drastically cut his weekly alcohol consumption. Then there was the housewife who, after her children left for school and her husband for work, had taken to drinking half a bottle of vodka while doing household chores. A painful bout of pancreatitis led her to quit drinking altogether and attend Alcoholics Anonymous meetings. Both had been teetering on the edge, but as soon as they experienced a health scare, they were able to bring themselves back from the brink.

Not Allan. Taking in his skin, daffodil yellow with jaundice, the ruby red palms of his hands, and his belly, so swollen with fluid that he looked seven months pregnant, I wondered how Bell's Scotch whisky had become so irresistible to him that he had chosen it over his marriage, children, and job. Why was he not shocked into making a lifestyle change as my other patients had been? Why did he opt to continue down this slippery slope of self-destruction?

Allan, with hollowed cheeks and a terse face, lay flat, stripped to the waist, waiting patiently for me to insert the drain. I organized the contents of my procedure tray: sterile gloves, antiseptic wash, local anesthetic drawn up in a 5 cc syringe, drapes to cover the rest of his tummy, a wide bore cannula, and a urinary bag roomy enough to collect the drainage. As I felt the tug from the needle puncturing his tummy and watched the straw-colored fluid gush out, I wondered what was so compelling about the amber-colored spirit that he had drunk more, year after year, till his liver was irreversibly destroyed.

Another patient, Dot, dreaded the winters, for they brought the threat of influenza, a danger for someone with chronic heart failure. Her failing heart meant that her lungs were overloaded with fluid, so with every breath she drew she felt as though she were drowning. On good days, even mild exertion rendered her gasping for air, but an infection was really bad news and often had her back in the hospital in need of intense oxygen treatments and antibiotics. During a particularly rough night, with nicotine-stained fingers and a face tight with worry, she whispered to me in a husky voice, "I'm not afraid of death, Dr. Jain, but the thought of *suffocating* to death terrifies me."

Unfortunately, those harrowing hospital stays did not serve to deter Allan from his daily liquid diet of whisky nor Dot from chain-smoking cigarettes. Somehow, they were both compelled to engage in those deadly habits despite the dramatic ways in which their bodies were signaling that enough was enough. Equally mystifying was the response of the hospital medical staff, which took two forms, either resigning themselves to the hopelessness of the situation or admonishing patients as though they were naughty children.

Once, on ward rounds, the attending liver specialist, while perusing Allan's medical chart, ran his forefinger down a page of liver test results. His finger paused momentarily at the gamma-glutamyltransferase (GGT) result, which was so high that the lab had highlighted it with an asterisk. The number was a telltale sign that Allan had been drinking heavily before his admission to the hospital. The attending physician looked up at the team and made sure we were aware of the result. We all stood for a moment, arching our eyebrows, tut-tutting under our breaths, or gently shaking our heads. Then, in a flash, the attending turned to Allan and in breezy tones told him that he was all set to be discharged from the hospital. In a form of surreal collusion, he never thought it necessary to address the elephant in the room.

Dot did not get off so lightly, as the pulmonologist attending, towering over her at the bedside, delivered a sermon on the perils of cigarette smoking. With dramatic hand gesticulations he told her that she would not survive another winter if she did not give up smoking and that it was, after all, a question of willpower. Dot simply nodded obediently and made affirmations at appropriate points: "Yes, Doctor" and "Of course, Doctor." To my astonishment, within minutes of rounds ending (and the attending's departure from the ward), she decoupled herself from the nasal cannula that connected her to an oxygen supply and tottered off to the smoking room to join the other patients sitting around in flimsy hospital gowns and puffing away.

As an intern it seemed obvious to me that for patients like Allan and Dot their brains were driving their behaviors and beliefs and that these were all intricately interwoven with the outcome of their illnesses. That brain backstory hinted at an undefined but nonetheless root cause of their problems, a cause that went beyond superficial notions of willpower and character and was most certainly worthy of serious examination. But twenty years ago such lines of inquiry were brushed off as "soft" or only marginally related to the issues at hand. Such matters were placed firmly in the separate domain of psychiatrists and other mental health practitioners, under topics often viewed as a patient's "personal business," subjects that other physicians typically had no interest, motivation, or skill set to inquire after.

***

Today the landscape is shifting in a favorable direction. Along with the battery of questions about abdominal pain, bowel habits, shortness of breath, and chest pain, patients are also being asked about symptoms of addiction, traumatic stress, depression, and anxiety. During their hospital stays, as they are tended to by physicians, nurses, physical therapists, respiratory therapists, dieticians, and phlebotomists, consultations with mental health specialists are also being requested.

Twenty years of scientific research have shown an unequivocal link between PTSD and poor physical health. What was once ambiguous intuition for many physicians has now been mapped. PTSD leads to an increase in one's use of medical care even after accounting for factors such as comorbid depression, chronic medical illness, and psychological distress. Indeed, compared with other mental disorders such as depression and anxiety, having PTSD is associated with the greatest increase in medical costs.

In 2004, Dr. Paula Schnurr and her team at the National Center for PTSD presented an elegant model to the scientific community. They described three ways (biological, psychological, and behavioral) in which exposure to trauma and having PTSD impact a person's physical health, course of chronic diseases (heart disease, diabetes, hypertension, etc.), and even death.

The biological pathway alludes to the disruption PTSD brings to hormone secretion, neurochemistry, and immune system functioning, all of which contribute to diseased cells, organs, and other bodily systems. Chromosomal studies have shown that PTSD patients have shorter telomeres—the segments on the ends of chromosomes that are a measure of cellular age—than their healthy counterparts do, suggesting a link between PTSD and accelerated aging, a biological process that leads to many physical illnesses. Indeed, national surveys of American adults show that having PTSD increases the odds of having a whole host of neurological, gastrointestinal, autoimmune, and joint conditions.

The psychological pathways in Schnurr's model emphasize the salience of factors such as depression, which medical science has known for some time increases the odds of developing conditions such as heart disease. When we consider the fact that depression often goes hand in hand with PTSD, it is not hard to imagine the combined toll they might take on one's heart health.

Finally, the behavioral pathways in Schnurr's model point out how abusing alcohol, cigarettes, illicit drugs, and food (which is more common among PTSD sufferers) either exacerbates poor health or leads directly to diseases. Beyond these obvious culprits there are other, subtler ways in which PTSD impacts lifestyle choices and physical health. Having PTSD means that you are less prone to take precautionary measures with your health (e.g., exercising regularly, eating healthfully, or practicing safe sex) and, when given medical advice, you are less likely to follow it.

Looking at the blunt relationship between PTSD and death, a recent study published in the *American Journal of Epidemiology* reported sobering findings about the long-term health effects of exposure to trauma. The researchers followed more than two thousand Vietnam veterans and gathered data about their risk factors for disease and death. They found that veterans with PTSD were nearly two times more likely to die over the study period than were combat veterans without PTSD, even after accounting for race, level of education, income, and marital status.

Researchers were already aware of the higher risk of death (typically from suicide, homicide, and accidents) for combat veterans in the first five years after their service, but what was alarming about these results was the sustained elevated risk for death for those with PTSD that persisted over decades. Cancer (in particular of the lungs and respiratory organs) and heart disease were the most common causes of death, hinting that the combination of having PTSD and being a cigarette smoker might be potently toxic.

The two decades since I was an intern have seen a radical shift in the way we think about the relationship between mental illness and physical disease. What was once viewed as separate and unrelated has been revealed to be intertwined and dependent. Specifically, for PTSD the message is now clear: assessing for trauma exposure and psychological consequences should be a routine part of *any* medical assessment. Indeed, there is increasing support for health care to become better trauma-informed across the board. In this approach, the health care team is mindful that many of their patients have experienced psychological trauma and that that trauma can influence the way they experience their health care. The aim is to ensure that patients feel safe and are not retraumatized, and their inner strengths are encouraged.

A SOLDIER'S HEART

PTSD and Cardiac Disease

He was too old. Not old in years . . . but in other ways he was old, old from too much life, old from seeing too much, old from knowing too much. He was tired and broken, walking with a cane and passing blood, and he knew it wouldn't be long for him.

—Gary Paulsen, *Soldier's Heart*

One crisp fall evening, my patient Richard asked his wife to drive him to the emergency room of his local VA hospital because he was having palpitations and felt pressure in his chest. Richard was in his sixties, a smoker with high blood pressure, so, as one might expect, the ER staff went straight to work ordering EKGs, chest X-rays, stat blood tests, and an urgent cardiology consult. Richard's EKG showed atrial fibrillation: instead of a smooth, steady beat, his cardiac rhythm was erratic and his heart muscle was pumping inefficiently. He was at risk of having a stroke or his heart failing altogether. The ER staff started him on medication to slow his heart, and he was soon feeling better. Buried in the documentation of his pulse rate, blood pressure, oxygen levels, and various tests was a note by the ER attending physician that Richard appeared highly anxious.

I had met Richard for the first time a few weeks before. Tall, with a slim build save for some extra pounds he carried around his midriff, he was dressed in beige khakis and a blue T-shirt. His face was round and pale, and his eyes, framed by designer eyeglasses, were rheumy. After settling into his chair, he drummed his fingers on the wooden arm. He was able to admit that he felt entirely out of his comfort zone.

"I'm not really sure I need to be *here*," he said with a nervous laugh.

When I asked him to elaborate, he told me that the previous year had been "the worst of my life." He was experiencing bankruptcy after his small business had failed. His wife had recently lost her job, which not only had worsened their financial predicament but was causing conflict in their thirty-year marriage.

Unemployed for the first time in his life, Richard found himself lost in memories of Vietnam. More than three decades earlier, after his discharge from the military, he had thrown himself into a career as an entrepreneur, creating profitable businesses from inspirational ideas. He had spent his life since Vietnam so busy that he had managed to avoid thinking about the war. He admitted to having spent his life in the office, micromanaging every tiny detail and garnering a reputation in the local community for his angry tirades and tough negotiation tactics. He also admitted, with sheepish bravado, that there had been years when he had drunk way too much scotch, chain-smoked cigarettes, and avoided sleep by guzzling strong black coffee.

His life had ground to a halt with the death of his business. As if the flood of Vietnam War memories was not enough, he was waking up every night in a cold sweat, his sleep ravaged by nightmares. His sex drive had plummeted, and he was finding it hard to concentrate. He felt as though his body were sucked of energy; he was irritable and felt "jumpy" for no reason. He had ended up in the ER on more than one occasion, thinking he was having a heart attack, only to be told that it was "just anxiety" and discharged home. His worsening finances had forced him to transfer his health care from his private doctor to a VA internist. When she had heard about the ER visits, she had immediately referred him to a psychologist.

The psychologist had diagnosed Richard as having PTSD and recommended group therapy, but Richard found himself overwhelmed with anxiety when others shared their stories. "I'm used to being the leader, telling people what to do," he said, "not having to listen so much or be told what to do." His therapist had referred Richard to my clinic for a medication evaluation, and I agreed that his symptoms were severe enough that medication was warranted.

Thankfully, Richard needed only a short hospital stay, after that fall visit to the ER, to settle his heart back into a regular rhythm. His hospital team did more tests to try to figure out why his heart suddenly went into atrial fibrillation but could find no obvious culprit other than his severe anxiety. Many months later, after Richard's PTSD was stabilized with the use of the medication paroxetine and the sleeping pill trazodone, he revealed to me that on that fall day, he had experienced, for the first time in his life, a full-blown flashback of his combat experiences in Vietnam. For hours afterward, he had felt petrified, and that was when the palpitations had started. The truly chilling thing is that Richard's untreated PTSD may have flipped his heart into chaos.

**

Several landmarked studies have highlighted the nuanced relationship between having PTSD and the risk of developing heart disease. Richard's uncontrolled PTSD meant his body's fight-or-flight response was constantly being triggered. Surges of noradrenaline gushed through his blood vessels, causing his pulse to race and his blood pressure to go through the roof. Abnormally high levels of noradrenaline alter a person's blood platelets, the disk-shaped cells that are key players in the formation of blood clots. These abnormal changes, in turn, make the person prone to arterial blood clots that can cause a heart attack or stroke.

Other PTSD-induced changes to Richard's stress hormones left him prone to gaining weight or developing diabetes, both of which elevate the risk of developing heart disease even further. Finally, his PTSD could lead to changes in his body's immune function and increase the levels of inflammatory chemicals in his blood. These increases fuel plaque buildup in the crucial blood vessels of the heart, causing heart disease. Though the research on immune system function in PTSD sufferers remains in early stages, many trauma scientists believe it to be the next critical frontier for PTSD research.

A research team led by Dr. Beth Cohen, a physician at the University of California, San Francisco, mined big data on more than 300,000 veterans of the wars in Afghanistan and Iraq, searching for a correlation between risk factors for heart disease (tobacco use, high blood pressure, high cholesterol levels, obesity, and diabetes) and PTSD. Though the medical establishment had been aware of studies with older veterans that had told of an unhealthy correlation between PTSD and heart health, Cohen's study was one of the first to examine the correlation in a younger veteran population. The results, which were published in *The Journal of the American Medical Association*, were startling. For the men in this study, the odds of their being a smoker, being obese, having high blood pressure, or having high cholesterol increased if they also had PTSD. The average age of the participants in the study was just thirty-one.

A similar pattern can be found in civilian populations. A 2014 joint study from Harvard and Columbia universities analyzed data from more than 50,000 women who had been followed over sixteen years and found that the women with PTSD were more prone to becoming overweight or obese. Follow-up studies found that the women with more severe PTSD symptoms had a nearly twofold increased risk of developing diabetes and were more likely to have a heart attack or stroke than the women who did not have PTSD.

Such studies are useful in that they illuminate correlations between PTSD and heart disease, but they do not prove that PTSD *causes* heart disease. A captivating 2013 prospective twin study published in the *Journal of the American College of Cardiology* overcame this limitation. The researchers followed male twins for thirteen years (studying twins allows for better control over genetic and environmental factors) and investigated whether the presence of PTSD increased their risk for coronary heart disease. Two hundred eighty-one pairs of twins were selected in which one of each pair had a history of PTSD. The researchers looked for whether or not participants had ever had a heart attack, been hospitalized for heart disease problems, or needed to undergo cardiac catheterization. They found that the incidence of heart disease was more than double in the twin with PTSD. The results were further adjusted to account for heart-unhealthy habits, such as being a smoker or not exercising enough, as well as other mental health conditions associated with heart disease, such as depression. By stripping away the other elements that might have explained their finding, they unearthed something stunning: PTSD appears to be an independent risk factor for heart disease.

As a new generation of scientists pushes for PTSD to be reconceptualized beyond the boundaries of mental illness and instead seen as a condition that impacts every cell, organ, and system in the human body, it is becoming harder to dismiss the urgent need to understand how this condition contributes to physical disease and suffering.

RUSSIAN ROULETTE

The Perilous Bond Between Traumatic Stress and Addiction

America's addiction to painkillers is as great a threat as terrorism.
—Barack Obama

My first job out of residency was in a century-old psychiatric hospital tucked away in a forestlike setting in the heart of a Milwaukee suburb. My job was to provide around-the-clock care to patients admitted to the inpatient unit, and not long after starting, I was assigned to be the on-call doctor over a long holiday weekend.

Tammy had been admitted on several occasions. Her thick medical chart suggested a complicated history: dysthymia, generalized anxiety, and bipolar disorder. Over the years, she had received group therapy, individual and couples therapy, and stints at the day hospital. She had been kept awash in antidepressants, sedatives, tranquilizers, and hypnotics. Buried in an old discharge summary was one sentence referencing her as being a survivor of severe sexual abuse, a tragic case of father-daughter incest.

I was doing rounds, making my way down the long list of patients who needed to be seen. Tammy was nowhere to be found. I checked the usual places—the dayroom, patio area, phone booths, and kitchen—but with no luck. I eventually found her fast asleep in her private room. I announced my entrance, and she stirred, muffling something inaudible from under the pillows. Tammy, barely forty, was a large woman with pale skin and a jet black bob haircut. She was dressed in a rumpled red lumberjack shirt and faded blue jeans. She roused, briefly, only to drift back off to sleep.

Despite her valiant attempts to engage with me, Tammy could barely keep her eyes open. This sleepiness was beyond a normal nap; she was in a medicated stupor. I persisted for a few minutes but then gave up, making a note on my list to return at the end of rounds, when I hoped she would be more alert. As I got up to leave, I crossed paths with the nurse, who was entering Tammy's room with a clear plastic cup filled with pills, capsules, and tablets.

Back in my office, I reviewed Tammy's chart, searching for why she was so overmedicated. I saw that over the last couple of years, OxyContin, a prescription opioid pain pill chemically similar to heroin, had been prescribed by her family doctor. He was using it to treat Tammy's chronic pain caused by fibromyalgia, a syndrome of widespread fatigue, muscle, and bone pain. I flicked through her discharge summaries, noting that her OxyContin doses had jumped higher and higher over time. Her current doses far exceeded what someone addicted to heroin might use in a day. Prescription opioids can slow down a person's breathing and heartbeat until he or she drifts off into a permanent sleep. I felt my face flush with heat. Under my watch, Tammy was getting pain pills at doses that made me nervous.

I raised my concern with Tammy's nurse, who shrugged her shoulders. "I've taken care of Tammy before, and she always looks this way. It's the depression; it has immobilized her. Besides, if she is in pain we have to help her, we can't deny her pain medication."

I took my qualms to the ward's internist, who did rounds on all the hospitalized patients. When I raised the suggestion that Tammy might be getting addicted to the pain pills, he looked uncomfortable. He did not think it would be professional to tread on the toes of his colleague and explained, "Her family doctor must have a reason to prescribe them. I don't think it is my job to interfere, especially when the patient has no complaints."

Frustrated, I went back to Tammy's chart and ran through the list of other medications she had been prescribed by her regular psychiatrist, circling the diazepam, quetiapine, and mirtazapine, all medications that have sedation as a side effect. I took a deep breath and started making cuts or reducing doses where I could safely do so. The staff nurse was not happy with my orders. It was clear she felt that I, as the temporary covering psychiatrist, was overstepping my bounds.

The next day, Tammy, a little less sedated, made it out of bed and was sitting in the dayroom. She was able to provide short answers to questions about her mood, anxiety levels, and appetite and listened while I explained my concerns and why I was making cuts to some of her psych meds. She expressed her support of the changes but then added, "Doctor, please don't change the dose to my pain meds. I've worked very hard with my family doctor to get the pain under control."

Later, I was doing some chart documentation at the nurses' station, where I had a clear view of the dayroom. It was visiting hours, and I looked on as Tammy's young daughters, accompanied by their father, came in to visit. Her children bounced in, calling "Mommy, Mommy." The youngest climbed on her lap, and the older one encircled her in her arms from behind, kissing her face and hugging her tightly. Tammy sat almost passed out, barely acknowledging their unabashed displays of affection.

I pulled up Tammy's medical record and saw that within minutes of my earlier interview with her, she had asked for pain meds. When the staff nurse had asked Tammy to rate her pain (before doling out the medication), Tammy had rated it a "nine"—excruciating pain. I felt irritation rise up in me. Tammy had *not* been in level-nine pain when I had interviewed her just minutes earlier. I paged the ward's internist, apologized for interrupting his dinner, shared my observations, and asked if he could make a modest reduction in the doses of Tammy's pain meds. He reluctantly agreed and told me he would make the changes and discuss them with Tammy during his rounds later that day.

When I arrived on the ward the next evening, I did a double take as Tammy walked right past me toward the phone booths. I looked at her; she was alert, her clothing was unrumpled, and her hair was styled. Her movements were no longer sluggish, and gone were her droopy eyes. She sat chatting animatedly on the phone, and as our eyes met, she mouthed a hello and gave me a hesitant wave. Moments later, I entered the nurses' station, to be greeted by the staff nurse.

"Dr. Jain, I was skeptical about what you were doing with Tammy's meds, but whatever you did, it worked like a charm! She is a totally different person. It's like I finally get to meet the real Tammy!"

***

In the early 1980s, American medicine started to undergo a radical shift in its attitude toward pain. Previously, the prevailing wisdom had been that physicians should be very cautious in prescribing strong and potentially addictive medications for pain. No doubt this had contributed to a neglect of patients' experience, and there was a massive compensatory shift that demanded physicians be more compassionate. Till that point, medical students all over the country had been taught about four vital signs: temperature, pulse rate, respiration rate, and blood pressure. Now the American Pain Society introduced "pain as the 5th vital sign," a term suggesting that physicians who were not taking their patients' pain seriously were being neglectful. So if your patients told you they were in pain, they were in pain, and it was your duty as a doctor to do something about it.

That shift in thinking meant that physicians now liberally began prescribing opioid pain pills, particularly for chronic, noncancer-related pain. That was precisely what happened in Tammy's case. By the turn of the twenty-first century, it became perfectly acceptable for Tammy's family doctor to prescribe OxyContin for her fibromyalgia. The liberal prescribing was further fueled by the expert marketing of the drugs to physicians. Indeed, when Purdue Pharma introduced OxyContin in 1996, it was aggressively promoted, with sales growing from $48 million to almost $1.1 billion over four years. All across the country health care professionals including nurses, hospital internists, and me were getting caught up in an awkward dance: a political correctness that demanded we validate our patients' complaints of pain, professional pressure not to question our colleagues' prescribing practices, yet a nagging feeling that something was awry.

Unfortunately, the consequences of American medicine's cultural shift toward pain management would morph into a public health tragedy that would unfold over the subsequent decades. The ready availability of OxyContin correlated with an increase in its abuse, diversion, and addiction, and by 2004 it became a leading drug of abuse in the United States. People were turning to street heroin when they ran out of prescription pills. Opioid deaths, whether caused by pain medicines or heroin, jumped 372 percent from 2000 to 2014, killing 28,000 Americans in 2014 alone. By 2016, President Barack Obama urged the nation to "recognize today we are seeing more people killed because of opioid overdose than traffic accidents."

Dr. Anna Lembke is a psychiatrist at Stanford University who specializes in addiction medicine. She told me that prescription pain pills such as OxyContin are particularly addictive because of the quantity and potency of opioid delivered with each dose. Each pill of OxyContin contains four hours of pain relief encapsulated by a hard shell that is intended to dissolve gradually and slowly release pain medication over the course of the day. She said, "What people discovered was that if they chewed the OxyContin and broke that hard shell then they got a whole day's worth of medication at once. With that came the typical rush that people who are addicted to heroin describe."

Tammy's story hints at an important subplot in this tragic national narrative: the perilous bond among traumatic stress, chronic pain, and opioid addiction. What has become obvious over the years since I first met Tammy is the significant overlap between chronic pain and PTSD. Indeed, 15 to 35 percent of all chronic pain patients also have PTSD. With regard to fibromyalgia, the plot only thickens, with one study reporting that almost 60 percent of fibromyalgia patients had significant levels of PTSD symptoms. As is so often the case, Tammy had never been screened for PTSD related to the childhood sex abuse she had suffered, much less offered treatment. The statistics now suggest that her trauma history, fibromyalgia, and subsequent opioid addiction were all linked.

On a national level, Tammy's story would eventually be echoed in big-data findings from a 2012 study led by Dr. Karen Seal, a physician at the University of California, San Francisco, that were published in *The Journal of the American Medical Association*. The study followed more than 141,000 Afghanistan War and Iraq War veterans diagnosed with noncancer pain over five years. The prevalence of PTSD among the group was 32 percent. Of the entire group, 11 percent had been prescribed opioid pain medication, but for the veterans with PTSD, that percentage jumped to a significantly higher 18 percent. The researchers also found that taking prescription opioids led to side effects such as having a fall, being in an accident, overdosing, getting into a physical fight, or attempting suicide. But those adverse effects were more pronounced in the veterans with PTSD. For the first time, the medical community had a bird's-eye view of the ominous linkages between traumatic stress and the misuse of prescription pain pills.

What is the precise nature of these linkages? While they have yet to be fully illuminated, hints can be gleaned by looking at the wider relationship between PTSD and addiction. Addiction has been called the tip of the addiction-PTSD iceberg, with some studies reporting that over 60 percent of addicted persons also have PTSD. Unfortunately, as was the case for Tammy, the addiction often masks the PTSD symptoms, leading to a delay in diagnosis and treatment. The situation is further complicated because mental health professionals have not quite figured out how to treat both parts of the iceberg at the same time.

Beyond prescription pain pills, I am constantly on the lookout for signs that my patients with PTSD are misusing, abusing, or getting addicted to anything from alcohol, street drugs, and gambling to sex, food, and nicotine. With alcohol and drug abuse, there is a two-way relationship with traumatic stress. On the one hand, having PTSD will increase patients' odds of developing alcohol or drug problems after trauma. On the other, some PTSD sufferers already have issues with drugs and alcohol *before* they develop PTSD. Being addicted, in and of itself, increases one's chances of being exposed to traumas. For instance, driving under the influence increases your likelihood of being involved in a serious traffic accident, and drug addiction can mean that you find yourself in unsafe situations where you might be sexually or physically assaulted.

It is not difficult to see why a propensity for addiction goes hand in hand with traumatic stress. Trust and faith are jarred, especially when someone has endured human-inflicted traumas, and a pervasive mistrust of people can then ensue. Rather than seek professional attention (which requires placing faith in another person) for trauma symptoms, sufferers choose to "self-medicate" with substances or activities that numb emotional pain, quell anxiety, or obliterate nightmares.

In the long run, though, the self-medication story rarely ends well. Often such indulgence escalates to problematic levels. DUIs, unemployment, depleted 401(k) accounts, wrecked marriages, and physical health problems such as obesity and diabetes start to compound the original problem of traumatic stress, morphing it into a more debilitating version. Collectively these problems seem insurmountable, and it becomes easier for hopelessness to set in. Indeed, one of the most frustrating problems I encounter when treating PTSD sufferers is when addiction enters their life.

Self-medicating has side effects, too. The human body often develops a tolerance to alcohol and drugs and requires greater amounts to achieve the same effects. Drugs and alcohol diminish the overall quality of sleep and exacerbate hypervigilance, anger, and irritability, and any relief gained is often short lived and, in the long run, impairs one's ability to be productive and fully enjoy life.

Another problem with self-medicating is that it feeds directly into the cycle of avoidance that is a core symptom of PTSD. By getting drunk or high, sufferers seek an altered state where they can escape from intrusive memories and nightmares, but this escape only serves to kick the proverbial can down the street, as the underlying trauma symptoms still plague sufferers when they become sober. So although people with PTSD may have full confidence in imbibing that nightly smidge of whisky, popping an extra pain pill because it helps them sleep better, or justifying their daily gambling as a well-deserved escape from their angst, the reality is that such behaviors will probably burgeon and, in the long run, make their PTSD worse.

Finally, when my patients self-medicate with alcohol and drugs, it ties my hands as to what treatment I can offer them. I'm reluctant to probe a patient's trauma history in a therapy session when I know that he or she may later go home and get intoxicated. I always tell my patients who are consuming unhealthy amounts of alcohol and street drugs that I don't feel comfortable prescribing them sleeping pills or PTSD medication. Unchecked addiction brings with it impulsivity and poor judgment, and those elements don't mix well with prescription medications. I remind them that the drug trials that test the safety of such medications often exclude research subjects who have substance abuse problems.

For these reasons, I often insist that they address their addiction issues, either themselves or with formal addiction treatment. Though I really wish to help them, the dangers of mixing prescription psychotropics with alcohol or street drugs are too high. As I tell them, "It's like playing Russian roulette; I have no way of predicting what may happen, and the consequences can be lethal."

BROKEN SMILES

The Toxicity of Childhood Adversity

If it takes a village to raise a child, it takes a village to abuse one.
—Mitchell Garabedian, a character in *Spotlight*

When I was in training to be a psychiatrist, I spent several months at a mental health complex with children who had been hospitalized. A sprawling one-story compound, it housed a crisis emergency service, outpatient programs, and several inpatient units for children, adults, and geriatric patients. When it was built, there had been a political appetite for making an investment in the mental health of the most disadvantaged. There had been a generosity of spirit, an acceptance of the importance of such an endeavor, and taxpayer dollars to back the effort.

The last two decades, though, had seen deep cuts to the county budget. Evidence of the cuts was apparent from the chipped tile floors, walls in need of new paint, and 1980s-style leather furniture that had seen better days. Below the surface was a more disturbing story. Talking to the doctors, nurses, and social workers there, I gleaned that every year they were being asked to do more with less. All of this threatened the quality of care they were trying to offer county patients whose needs were only growing.

Evie was a seven-year-old girl who was hospitalized because her behavior had been escalating dangerously. Evie's mother had conceived her when she was fifteen years old, and Evie had never met her father. Evie's mother was addicted to crack cocaine, and when she was using, she would disappear from home for long periods. Once her mother had left Evie in a playpen for hours. Neighbors had called 911, complaining that they could hear a baby crying nonstop. The police had found Evie in soiled diapers, bawling from hunger. Her mother was sent to rehab and Evie to foster care, and Child Protective Services had become a constant in their lives.

The time Evie spent in foster care came at a high price, as she was sexually abused by a foster sibling. For the last couple of years, her mother had been clean, but she was a surly woman with a sharp tongue who did not miss the opportunity to berate her daughter. She had also been involved in several relationships with partners who were violent, and Evie had been a frequent witness to the domestic disturbances that had resulted. At school, regular fistfights and name-calling were a routine part of Evie's behavior, but when she took a knife to school and threatened another pupil, the school psychologist, Evie's mother, and her CPS social worker insisted that Evie be hospitalized for an evaluation and adjustment of the medications she was prescribed.

I was in awe of the attending child psychiatrist, who led the children's inpatient unit. A dedicated county doctor who had spent his entire career caring for underserved and uninsured children, he somehow had weathered the whittled-down budget, county politics, and chronic staff shortages. As I was new to child psychiatry, he suggested I watch him interview Evie to get a sense of how his interview was different from a regular psychiatric interview with an adult.

I followed him as he entered the lunchroom where Evie sat alone, eating a snack of graham crackers and applesauce. I watched him sink down on his knees, so his face was at the same level as hers, and quietly ask her permission for him to pull up a chair and "chat" and also if she was cool with me, as the "trainee doctor," sitting in. Evie silently nodded her assent. The attending was kind and nonjudgmental, and there was nothing hurried about him. I watched how his body language and posture seamlessly shifted so he would not appear in any way threatening to the young girl.

He slipped into conversation with Evie the way a loving parent would at a family dinner. "Do you prefer Oreos to graham crackers?" "Are you still into Power Rangers?" "How's your day? . . . I hear things have been tough at school lately." Even his language shifted and he started to use lingo that resonated with a seven-year-old. I watched as Evie's defiance slipped away and her tightly bound armor started to unfurl. Over the course of the next thirty minutes, we heard about the teacher she liked who had left the school, the constant bullying in the schoolyard, and her mother's most recent boyfriend, who had a low threshold for punching or kicking Evie's mother.

Later, I sat at the nurses' station flicking through Evie's thick medical chart. Every few pages, I would catch myself gazing at Evie as she sat, legs curled up beside her, on the sofa, quietly watching TV in the communal living area. She was small for her age and chunky. Her eyes were big and brown, and her hair was braided with multicolored beads that rustled every time she moved. Something on the TV made her smile, a wide and beautiful smile, and the sight of her left me overcome with a deep sadness.

Evie's chart was littered with diagnoses: post-traumatic stress disorder, oppositional defiant disorder, mood disorder, and attention deficit/hyperactivity disorder. Then there were the medications: sertraline, risperidone, valproic acid, methylphenidate, and clonidine. With Evie's story of neglect, sexual abuse, and frequent exposure to domestic violence, I readily accepted her diagnosis of PTSD and even the medication sertraline that had been prescribed to treat it. To help bear the brunt of the trauma exposure her young brain had endured, Evie needed every possible advantage that medical science could offer. What I could not reconcile with the child who was sitting in front of me quietly watching TV were all the other diagnoses (and the heavy-hitting psychiatric medications that came with them). I felt that many of Evie's current behaviors were attributable to the toxic environment she lived in. What about the problematic "village" in which she was being raised? What was being done to treat that?

I knew about the neighborhood where Evie lived. It was famous for gun violence and often mentioned on the local news due to a robbery, homicide, or drug raid. Once I had accidentally taken the wrong exit off the highway and ended up driving the streets of that neighborhood looking for a place to do a U-turn: graffiti-sprayed walls, littered streets, clumps of young men hanging out on street corners, unaccompanied children roaming the streets during a school day, and house after house with boarded-up windows. For any child being raised in Evie's zip code, it was not a matter of *if* she might be exposed to a traumatic event but *when*.

Of course, Evie's zip code was only the beginning of her problems. Her mother's drug addiction had led to legal issues, and she had served jail time for prostitution and drug possession. Her relationship with Evie was toxic, and she fixated on blaming everything on the child: "She needs a pill that will fix her attitude!" "She needs to grow up; she ain't no baby no more!" Cuts to services that historically would have helped her mother meant less access to food stamps, health care, and educational resources.

What about Evie's school? I had never visited it, but from what I could tell it was overwhelmed by budget cuts and the demands of educating children with a variety of needs. Would the personnel in a school in that neighborhood even notice that Evie was in the psych hospital for a month? Would they have time to care?

And what of my profession? How were we helping Evie? There was the individual talk therapy with Evie, which was often followed by making some adjustments to her meds but not much more. I watched over days and weeks as the attending made valiant efforts to coordinate the arms of different agencies: the school, her mom's probation officer, and Child Protective Services—all fragmented agencies facing their own red tape, high demand, and low resources. To me it appeared nearly impossible to get those agencies (no matter how well intentioned) to align themselves effectively behind a child in need.

***

Along with exposure to trauma in the home, millions of children around the world are exposed to other traumatic experiences, such as living in a war zone or enduring natural disasters like hurricanes, earthquakes, or fires. Similar to trauma exposure and PTSD in adults, only a minority of these children will develop full-blown PTSD, but it is vital to note how children are uniquely vulnerable. A study done with more than eight thousand children in the New York City public schools six months after the September 11, 2001, World Trade Center attack, revealed a PTSD rate of almost 11 percent, a number that was more than double what the researchers had expected to see. Such findings were replicated in several other studies of children who had survived a severe earthquake in Taiwan, and a major bushfire in Australia, and who lived in war-torn Lebanon.

PTSD rates skyrocket in children who endure traumatic events that ravage their communities. How parents respond to the trauma and how close (geographically) the child is to the epicenter play a crucial role in determining outcome. Parents and caregivers who are able to be emotionally supportive and are not traumatized themselves exert a protective effect that reduces the odds that a child will develop PTSD.

Child psychiatrists will tell you that there are important differences in what PTSD looks like in children when compared to adults and that it also varies with the child's age. For example, a child younger than seven may not understand death as something that is irreversible, so in a situation where her life is threatened, she may not be as terrified as an older child or adult would be. Also, because children tend to be self-centered, which is a normal developmental drive that gets them the necessary attention they need from caregivers in order to survive; they take excessive responsibility and feel guilt, if something bad happens. This feeling of guilt is a strong predictor of whether a child will develop PTSD.

Children are also more likely to believe that there were signs or omens that predicted the traumatic event, and in an effort to protect against future traumas, they perpetually look out for such omens. Young children are less likely to experience flashbacks, but they will engage in traumatic play in which they act out some aspect of the traumatic experience. However, such traumatic play serves no therapeutic function and does little to alleviate the anxiety that consumes their post-trauma lives.

Dr. Victor Carrion, a child psychiatrist and PTSD expert at Stanford University, told me that the classic symptoms of intrusion, avoidance, mood problems, and hypervigilance are experienced by children with PTSD but are subtler than what is seen in adults:

> Kids may find themselves thinking or talking about the trauma when they do not want to. They may be playing basketball with friends, and all of a sudden traumatic images disrupt their enjoyment of the game. They might have a cognitive inability to talk about what happened and also a tendency to avoid trauma-related triggers. If something traumatic happened on a rainy day, on the next rainy day the child may feel anxious. We also see emotional numbing: kids say that they can no longer feel sad when something bad

happens. They may feel happy when something good happens but not as happy as they used to feel. The other type of symptom we see in kids is hyperarousal. That is what leads many kids, especially those who live in environments where they are surrounded by violence, to receive a misdiagnosis of attention deficit/hyperactivity disorder (ADHD).

Similarly to adult sufferers, children with PTSD have altered neurobiology. Using brain-imaging techniques and a simple memory test, Carrion and his team scanned the brains of sixteen children with PTSD along with a control group of children without PTSD. The children with PTSD made more errors on the recall part of a memory test and showed less hippocampus activity than the control subjects who were doing the same task. In a separate study, the team found that children with PTSD also had abnormalities in their frontal lobes, a part of the brain that helps us make decisions, think through a problem, and plan our day. It's easy to see how having PTSD could cast a shadow over a child's ability to learn and thrive in daily life.

In 2016, Carrion's team did MRI brain scans of fifty-nine youths; thirty of them—fourteen girls and sixteen boys—had trauma symptoms, and the rest of the sample acted as a control group. The researchers saw no differences in brain structure between boys and girls in the control group. However, among the traumatized boys and girls, they saw differences in an area of the brain known as the insula. The insula detects cues from the body and processes emotions and empathy. It helps to integrate one's feelings and actions and typically gets smaller as the brain matures with age. However, this region was already smaller in girls with trauma symptoms, hinting that traumatic stress contributed to an accelerated aging process. These findings highlight the different ways in which trauma manifests in boys than in girls and how treatment might be tailored to meet their specific needs. Such advances in neuroscience are giving us a better sense of how PTSD can leave a devastating imprint on the brains of developing children like Evie.

***

Just a few years before my stint on the child psychiatry service, Dr. Vincent Felitti, a physician with the Kaiser Permanente Health Maintenance Organization, and Dr. Robert Anda from the Centers for Disease Control and Prevention (CDC) started investigating the relationship between adverse childhood experiences (ACEs) and their long-term effects on physical and mental well-being in adulthood.

In the late 1990s, they surveyed 17,000 middle-class, middle-aged patients and asked them to recall whether as children they had experienced physical, sexual, and emotional abuse or neglect or witnessed domestic violence toward a parent. The surveys were unprecedented in not only asking about whether such events occurred but drilling down for further detail. "How often were you spanked?" "How severely were you spanked?" "How often didn't you have enough to eat?" "How often were your parents too drunk or high to take care of the family?" The patients were then followed over time to assess their health as they aged.

What was so significant about the ACE study (as it would come to be known) was the scale, rigor, and depth of the research. It would prove to be a landmark in epidemiological research, and it spawned a vast scientific literature that heralded a renewed public awareness about the devastating impact of childhood adversity on human well-being.

Contrary to what many people (including health care professionals) had previously assumed, the study participants commonly reported that they had kept their adverse childhood experiences hidden and that such experiences had often occurred together, referred to as "polyvictimization." For example, they reported not only being neglected as a child but witnessing a caregiver's alcohol addiction and family violence toward a parent. Of greatest significance was the finding that as the number of adverse experiences increased, the percentage of adults who had negative health outcomes also went up.

What the ACE study showed was that children exposed to adversity, in an attempt to deal with the associated psychological distress, take on risky behaviors such as smoking cigarettes, abusing alcohol or drugs, eating unhealthy food, having an inactive lifestyle, or being sexually promiscuous. Such high-risk behaviors correlate closely with diseases such as lung cancer, obesity, heart disease, diabetes, and HIV. The study also found a link between experiencing child adversity and ultimately experiencing an early death. Aside from these stark outcomes, childhood adversity also resulted in a reduced "life potential" by taking a toll on educational attainment and employment history.

The researchers ultimately concluded, "Adverse childhood experiences are the main determinant of the health and social well-being of the nation." This issue extends beyond the United States, with family violence increasingly recognized as a public health problem in low- and middle-income countries. In those countries, an estimated 250 million children younger than five years of age are at risk of falling short of their potential because of early childhood adversity.

If Evie, now an adult, were to enroll as a participant in the ACE study, I am sure she would check "yes" to every question about childhood adversity. She would be classified as someone who had experienced polyvictimization, and her ACE scores would be high enough to place her at elevated risk for many health problems. Though I will never know what happened to Evie, what is now clear is that the long-held notion that children are resilient just by virtue of being children is simply not true. Rather, childhood is a period of unique vulnerability when exposure to extreme adversity and traumatic events can have a potentially devastating long-term impact.

I can only hope that the ACE study heralds a new and, this time, permanent public commitment to tackling the mammoth problem of child abuse and adversity head-on. The ACE data prove what we as a society have to gain by not only devoting much-needed financial resources to affected children but combating the toxic environments in which they are being raised.

SENESCENCE

Traumatic Stress in Late Life

For as I draw closer and closer to the end, I travel in a circle nearer and nearer to the beginning. . . . My heart is touched now by many remembrances that had long fallen asleep.

—Charles Dickens, *A Tale of Two Cities*

I take in Estelle as she flits and fusses around Ronnie, her husband of almost fifty years. I have witnessed this scene, a caregiver in motion, hundreds of times before. The names of the patient and the caregiver and the details of each story are all unique, but the underlying narrative is universal. One member of the dyad (usually the woman) has been raised to prioritize the needs of others over her own; she lives to be of service, and she is often the undervalued reason for why my patient remains alive.

Ronnie had been treated for depression since his retirement, and over the last decade, he had also developed dementia. During recent visits, I had found it harder to communicate with him. He had been quiet, more passive. He had struggled to find words, and his answers had lost their richness. This had left me communicating more with Estelle: How is he sleeping? Does he eat enough? Does he wander? Does he get agitated when he forgets? Estelle always had a notebook with her, and from it she would share data from several weeks of caregiving.

Today, as she wheels Ronnie into my office, I can tell she is short of breath. As she adjusts his Korean War baseball cap and offers him a drink of bottled water, I notice that she has gained weight since the last time we met.

"Dr. Jain, these last few weeks have been very strange. I just find him staring into space for hours at a time, and when I ask him what he is thinking about, he can't stop talking about something that happened years ago."

To my surprise, Ronnie interjects with a level of assertion I have not seen in a while. "Hold on, Estelle. Let me speak with Dr. Jain. I have to tell her what has been on my mind."

Ronnie raises his frail right arm and motions with his forefinger for me to wait while he sips some water. I take in the flaky skin of his uncovered arm, skin that is loosely propped over his bones and mottled by the easy bruising of someone on blood thinners. Ronnie now looks at me with piercing blue eyes, forcing me to connect with him in a way that has been missing from our recent meetings. For the next fifteen minutes, he speaks with animated tones so propelled by surges of anger and fear that it feels as though the event he is describing occurred yesterday. But Ronnie is disclosing an event that happened more than half a century ago, when he was living in the Deep South and before he had ever laid eyes on Estelle. "I have not thought about that night for fifty years, and now it's all I can think about."

He tells me that as a young man he was working on a farm during the throes of the civil rights movement. One balmy summer evening, he and a group of his coworkers went straight from work to a local bar to get drunk. They all had their tools in tow and flung them into a corner as they crowded around the bar, flirting with the local girls and dancing to music blaring from the radio. As they spilled out onto the street after the bar closed, one of Ronnie's coworkers got into a fight with a young African American man who was alone.

"I think he picked a fight with that guy on purpose. He always had a mean streak in him." Ronnie shakes his head in disgust as he thinks about his coworker. His eyes move rapidly back and forth as he recalls what happened next.

"We all pulled him off the guy. Told him, leave it be, don't cause trouble. Then we carried on walking in the opposite direction, but next thing we know he had run back and in his right hand . . . I saw he had taken his ax from his tool bag. I remember thinking *This guy is crazy*, and then . . . I froze."

Ronnie looked on as his coworker took an ax and charged toward the young man, who let out a piercing scream at the sight of the ax. He dropped to his knees and started to pray, begging Ronnie's coworker for mercy.

Ronnie starts to weep. Estelle consoles him, as one would a small child. Through big sobs, he blurts out, "He was begging him for mercy. Why could he not just leave him alone?"

Instead, his coworker took the ax, raised it above his head, and slammed it down on the outstretched arms of the black man.

"I just cannot remember what happened after that, Dr. Jain. I am racking my brain, going over that night again and again in my head . . . I think I went to help him, but I can't be sure. Did he die? Did someone call for help? The next day, we were in a different town, that much I know . . . I don't know what happened to that kid, though."

Estelle, consumed with worry, says, "He spends hours just staring into space. He is thinking about this thing over and over. It's like he is stuck back fifty years ago. I am losing him, Dr. Jain. What can we do to help him?"

***

Decades of advances in medical technology, public health policy, and standards of living have culminated in a rapid increase in the numbers of adults who now live to an advanced age. With this shift, there has been an opportunity to witness how traumatic memories can emerge or reemerge in late life.

At first glance, the rate of PTSD appears to be substantially lower in older adults, but researchers have cautioned against taking such a statistic at face value.

Dr. Joan Cook is a psychologist at Yale University, and much of her research has focused on traumatic stress in older populations. She told me:

> I think events such as the September 11th terrorist attacks, the wars in Iraq and Afghanistan, and Hurricane Katrina have helped raise the national consciousness about trauma. But I still come across older adults who lack an understanding of the potential effects of traumatic experiences or don't accurately label such events as "traumatic." In addition, there are also cognitive, sensory, and functional impairments that may affect the experience, impact, or reporting of trauma-related symptoms.

Recent research advances that use sophisticated methodologies to specifically home in on older populations have highlighted some areas of concern. Partial PTSD (in which the patient does not meet the full criteria for a diagnosis but is still suffering) does appear to be common among older adults. Also, as they face a decline in their physical health and become more dependent on others for their day-to-day living, older adults become more vulnerable to being exposed to new traumas, such as elder abuse.

Another concern for older adults with trauma histories is the retirement phenomenon. Not long after I started my work as a research fellow at the National Center for PTSD, a social worker colleague shared with me something she had observed during her decades on the job: "There are so many veterans who went to war, came home, and went about their daily lives with apparently few problems, and then they retire and BANG! PTSD comes right to the forefront and is suddenly this major issue."

The retirement phenomenon has also been recognized in the wider medical literature. Along with advancing age comes a perfect storm of life changes that can thrust previously well contained (or well hidden) symptoms of traumatic stress to the forefront. Events such as retirement, a decline in health, and the death of loved ones are all major blows to one's resilience in dealing with traumatic stress. With such events protective walls come crumbling down and unmask PTSD. Also, many of the previous ways of coping with PTSD are no longer available.

Dr. Yael Danieli is a psychologist and director of the Group Project for Holocaust Survivors and Their Children. She studied Holocaust survivors and made important observations about the long-term effects of surviving that atrocity. Many survivors seemed to be at peace with themselves only as long as they continued to work. "I have to keep myself busy so I don't think," said one survivor. But as they grew older, Danieli found, traumatic symptoms resurfaced and intensified. She described how trauma renewed its hold as the aging brain diminished and the survivors faced other losses. Children leaving home and the death of spouses and friends were relived as traumas similar to the losses endured during the war.

Over the last decade, another story to emerge from big-data studies shows that PTSD sufferers are almost twice as likely to develop dementia in older age. Not only can having dementia unleash or exacerbate underlying PTSD symptoms, but PTSD may also be a risk factor for developing dementia later in life.

Cook told me that she found this data intriguing but stressed that there is still so much we don't know about the precise relationship between PTSD and dementia. What she feels is abundantly clear, though, is that older adults with PTSD do perform more poorly across a range of memory tests, particularly processing speed, learning, memory, and executive functioning, than do older adults without PTSD.

Late-onset stress symptomatology (LOSS) is a syndrome that appears to be a close cousin of PTSD. With LOSS, an older person has shown no trauma-related symptoms throughout life but suddenly becomes consumed with memories related to a significant trauma from his or her past. Recent research implies that LOSS may be a psychological mechanism through which older adults confront traumatic memories to find meaning in and build coherence into their life story. Indeed, if the effort is successful, they may experience positive personal growth and a resolution of the distress associated with the traumatic memories. In a way, LOSS is like taking care of unfinished business, an opportunity to make amends and put things right before it is too late. Though it is less severe than PTSD, LOSS still causes much distress to the person experiencing it.

Such was Ronnie's predicament. His dementia-ravaged brain could no longer suppress the violent memory that was deeply engraved into its neurocircuits. It made perfect sense that he wanted to come to terms with the brutality of that summer evening. Initially, I viewed his LOSS as an opportunity for him to do some important therapeutic work before the dementia vanquished all his memories, and over the next few weeks that was what we did. Ronnie and I went back to that night, revisiting the details, asking important questions, and exploring his emotions. All the while Estelle, a patient observer, sat next to him.

Therapy required Ronnie to be able to grasp concepts, rethink the situation, entertain various outcomes, and connect his cognitions to his emotions. His dementia was sabotaging any such efforts. Estelle told me that he seemed to be getting worse and was reliving that traumatic night over and over. He was barely eating, refusing to do any exercise or go for an evening stroll, and when he was not staring into space during the day, he just slept. At night, Estelle told me, he was having nightmares, which she knew because she could hear him crying out in his sleep. I could tell she was at her wits' end.

"I'm not sleeping either, Dr. Jain. He is not exercising, so I am not exercising. My doctor told me to lose twenty pounds, my cholesterol is out of control, and I am prediabetic. If something happens to me, who will take care of Ronnie? Is there something you can give him? A pill to keep him calm?"

I felt anxiety rising in my chest as I considered Estelle's request. What good could come of medicating away Ronnie's memories? He had to come to terms with the past, and I did not want to rob him of that chance. Yet his demented brain meant he probably no longer had the mental flexibility to complete the work of therapy. He was already maxed out on a medication that should have helped with the traumatic stress symptoms. I would have to consider something else. A mild sedative? Medicating an octogenarian was not something to take lightly. I followed the mantra "Start low, go slow," as the elderly have less ability to clear medications from their bodies and are more prone to developing side effects.

In the end I trusted my instincts about Estelle. If there was a way she could have helped Ronnie without medication, she would have. But Ronnie's symptoms were impacting her quality of life, too. What *would* happen to Ronnie if something happened to her? So I relented, prescribed Ronnie some low-dose quetiapine, and arranged for close follow-up. As they got ready to leave, I urged Estelle to keep up with her own health care appointments and take advantage of their thrice-a-week home help to get some fresh air and exercise.

"Don't worry about me, Dr. Jain," she said, shrugging off my concern. "As long as my Ronnie is fine, I will be fine."

PART 4

Quality of Life

COMPLEX TRAUMA

Self-respect and sense of self-worth, the innermost armament of the soul, lies at the heart of humanness; to be deprived of it is to be dehumanized, to be cleaved from, and cast below, mankind.
—Laura Hillenbrand, *Unbroken: A World War II Story of Survival, Resilience, and Redemption*

My duties as a resident meant that once or twice a week I would spend a fourteen-hour shift working in the emergency room. On call began at six in the evening and ended at eight the following morning. After the shift was over, I would leave the emergency room and head straight back to my day job.

During one such night on call, I was feeling particularly sorry for myself. A busy day in clinic meant I had had no chance to pick up dinner en route to the emergency room. Tired and starving, I had little choice but to munch on Doritos and Chips Ahoy, a hurried purchase from the battered hospital vending machine. As I waited for the elevator to take me to the emergency room, I fantasized about an alternative career in which I might indulge in the finer things of life, a job that would allow me to take bathroom breaks, have regular civilized meals, and finish a thought.

Moments later, I arrived to a bustling waiting room, and tense expressions on the faces of the staff signaled that we were in the throes of a busy shift. I got straight to work, grabbing the chart of the next patient.

Sharon, a young woman in her late twenties, had called 911 threatening to kill herself. The police had put her on an emergency psychiatric hold and brought her in for evaluation, the fifth time in as many months. Her previous visits had accrued a familiar cadence: she called 911 after an argument with her live-in boyfriend, she would be suicidal, and so the police would place her on an emergency detention and bring her to the emergency room. Within a couple of hours she would reconcile with her boyfriend, recant her statements, and then convince the doctors to let her go. She would promise to follow up in the mental health clinic but would then miss her appointments.

A deeper look at her chart revealed a history of teenage prostitution. Sharon was also HIV positive, and today her urine drug screen was positive for cocaine. As I headed out to the waiting room to meet her, I was troubled by her five crisis visits and felt that today something more should be done.

When no one responded to my calling out her name, the nurse pointed out that she was using the phone. Sharon was stick thin with mouse-colored brown hair and was talking intimately into the receiver, with a teenager's zeal. When I finally caught her attention, she came bounding over to the interview booth and announced, "Hi, Doctor. This has been a huge mistake. I got into an argument with my boyfriend. You know how that goes . . . I was upset, that's all. But all is good now. He wants me to come home now. When can I get out of here?"

Her voice was raspy and, as she spoke, I took in her pale arms with track marks and random bruises in various stages of healing. She looked washed-out, and her pretty hazel eyes were hardened, giving her an older appearance. I wondered why she had hijacked the interview and set the agenda so quickly. What was she hiding?

I introduced myself to her and reset the frame for how things would go down. First I would need answers to some questions.

Sharon flashed me a quick, saccharine smile. "Everything you need is in the chart; I have been here before."

I smiled back. "I know. But I'd like to hear your story straight from you. That way I get a real sense for who you are and what's been going on. Then I can come up with a plan of how best to help you. Okay?"

I watched Sharon's body tone relax. She became coy, almost childlike, and told me about her childhood. She had been sexually abused by her stepfather, and when she had told her mother, she asked the then twelve-year-old Sharon what she had done to "lead him on." By age fourteen, Sharon had run away from home and was living as a prostitute addicted to heroin. In her early twenties, after going to a family planning clinic for an abortion, she had found out she was HIV positive. She recalled her years as a prostitute and told me how she had lost count of the number of times she had been mugged or beaten up. Her current boyfriend was the best thing that had ever happened to her. Sure, they had their ups and downs, but they loved each other.

"Sharon, are you taking your HIV meds?" I was concerned that she was not staying on top of her long list of antiviral medications.

Sharon's face flickered with anger. She tossed her hands flippantly and rolled her eyes. "Doc, there are so many meds. It's very hard to keep track of them all . . . and I get side effects."

"Okay. I noticed your urine was positive for cocaine . . . how often do you use cocaine?"

My question was met with silence. Sharon made a big yawn and nestled her head on the interview desk, turning away from me and directing her gaze toward the side wall of the interview booth. I sat silently for a few seconds, wondering where to go next.

"Sharon, I'm very concerned about how chaotic your life is. I think underlying mental health issues are contributing. I see you are not getting treatment right now. I am recommending we keep you on the hold and admit you to the hospital, where we can observe you around the clock. Once the cocaine has left your system, we can see how you are sleeping and eating and monitor your mood. If you are having problems with your mood, we can treat that, get you into counseling and NA meetings. We can get you back on track with your HIV meds, too, and get you connected to the clinic again."

My sermon was received in silence. Then, in a flash, Sharon sprang up and turned on me. I recoiled, instinctively getting out of her reach. Before my eyes, she morphed into an entirely different person. Her eyes alight and glowing with anger, she spat, "Who the fuck do you think you are? Are you a student doctor? I want to see another doctor, a *real* doctor!"

Sharon now turned to the waiting room and started to advise other patients waiting to be seen, "Don't see this one! She will lock you away and throw away the key!"

Then she hollered over to the nurses' station, "NURSE, I DEMAND TO SEE A REAL DOCTOR RIGHT NOW!!! IT'S MY RIGHT TO GET A SECOND OPINION!"

The kerfuffle attracted the attention of the security guard and nurses. In an effort to deescalate the situation, they edged toward Sharon, encouraging her to calm down, all while exchanging awkward glances with me. A senior psychiatrist emerged from the doctor's office. He motioned for me to step away and told me he would handle the situation from there. I retreated to the doctor's office and slumped into a chair. I was exhausted, my eyes ached, and my ankles were swollen. I took some deep breaths, trying to lessen the sting of the bruising altercation.

***

Judith Herman has argued that PTSD, as it stands, does not fit the complicated symptoms seen in survivors of prolonged and repeated trauma. For those who have endured years of intimate partner violence (IPV),* grown up amid inner-city violence, been a prisoner of war, or survived harrowing childhood abuse, Herman offered the medical community the term *complex PTSD*. As she explained in *Trauma and Recovery*, "Survivors of prolonged abuse develop characteristic personality changes, including deformations of relatedness and identity."

Herman's diagnosis better explains the behaviors of patients such as Sharon, who have lived chronically traumatized lives. In contrast to survivors of a single trauma, such patients do not have a clear "before and after the trauma" narrative incorporated into their life stories. Remembering a good pretrauma life, even if only momentarily, can serve as a powerful anchor during troubled times. This serves as a beacon of hope, a place a person can aim to return to once the present storm has passed. In contrast, my patients who have spent years, even decades, in traumatizing situations are adrift with no such anchor. The boundary between before and after (if it ever existed) becomes blurred and faded until it disappears altogether.

At some point, they have been left with little other choice than to begin a perverse adaptation to their horrendous circumstances. This adaptation comes with a big price, for it requires them to block thoughts, stifle feelings, dissolve their sense of self, and alter the way

---

* Intimate partner violence (IPV) was previously called domestic violence. The use of the term *intimate partner* reflects the fact that violence can be caused by a husband, ex-husband, boyfriend, or ex-boyfriend. Women can also be abusers, but statistics show that they are more likely to be victims, bear the brunt of the most severe violence, and make up the majority of the victims of IPV-related homicides.

they interact with others. They live lives engulfed in clouds of help-lessness, shame, guilt, and despair. Denial, emotional numbing, and dissociation become powerful (and imperfect) ways to survive their day-to-day humiliations. They live at emotional extremes, either passively stifling their emotions or exploding in bouts of rage.

About patients who, like Sharon, have a history of severe child abuse, Herman wrote:

> The personality formed in an environment of coercive control is not well adapted to adult life. The survivor is left with fundamental problems in basic trust, autonomy, and initiative. She approaches the tasks of early adulthood—establishing independence and intimacy—burdened by major impairments in self-care, in cognition and memory, in identity, and in the capacity to form stable relationships.

In this way, complex trauma becomes entangled with character, chipping away at it and insidiously deforming it until it morphs into something bewildering.

The severely traumatized often have lives full of scenarios that are ripe for retraumatization. After being slapped and kicked down the stairs, a battered wife calls 911 and the police haul off her violent husband, only for her to drop the charges and let him back into the home. A college student who was sexually abused as a child shares explicit photos of herself online and receives sexual solicitations from strangers. A refugee, settled in a new life after being imprisoned and tortured for years, torments his young children, effectively making them prisoners in their own home. At first glance, such scenarios seem counterintuitive: surely if a man hit you, you would run for the hills and never look back. If you were abused as a child, why would you invite sexual attention from complete strangers? Or if you have firsthand experience of what it is like to be tortured, why would you ever inflict that heinous pain on another soul?

Integral to complex PTSD is a susceptibility to experience repeated harm, both self-inflicted and at the hands of others. Herman described this phenomenon of reenactment, and it explains how survivors of severe trauma become hardwired to exposing themselves (sometimes repeatedly) to situations reminiscent of the original trauma. On some level, they have come to view violence and abusive neglect as a way of life. Such reenactments can manifest in various ways. Survivors may engage in self-destructive acts such as mutilating their physical body by cutting or abusing alcohol and drugs. Or they may reenact traumatic situations by identifying with the original aggressor and becoming the victimizer who now traumatizes others.

Perhaps the most compelling evidence to illustrate this phenomenon of reenactment comes from the childhood sexual abuse literature. Being a victim of child sex abuse is a potent risk factor for future sexual revictimization. Research finds survivors to be eleven times more likely to experience sexual assault as an adult than assault survivors without a history of sexual abuse. Beyond revictimization, studies have also shown how child sex abuse survivors are more likely to engage in high-risk sexual behavior (e.g., having unprotected sex and engaging in sexual promiscuity or prostitution) as they get older, further perpetuating this cycle of victimization and reenactment.

Many factors exacerbate this cycle. For instance, it is harder to break the cycle of victimization and reenactment if the survivor comes from a dysfunctional family not equipped to deal with her plight, if she does not have access to financial or educational resources that could empower her, or if she belongs to a culture that blames her. Also, although studies show that nearly all prostitutes have a history of being sexually molested, assaulted, or physically abused *before* they became prostitutes, the reverse does *not* hold: not all child sex abuse survivors enter a cycle of victimization.

Patients with complex PTSD often come to doctors with vague complaints—intractable insomnia, unrelenting aches and pains, or stubborn depressive symptoms—so the link between their traumas and the present situation is not clearly identifiable. Such patients are often in search of a rescuer but are simultaneously mistrustful, especially of anyone in a position of authority. In treatment they often assume a posture of passivity yet sabotage any efforts made to help them. Their inability to regulate their emotions means they have a lower threshold for lashing out, which leads to harsh condemnation from those trying to help them. Their moral fiber is questioned, and their medical chart accrues damning language: "manipulative," "acting out," or "entitled behavior."

For me, this is where the concept of complex PTSD has value, as it helps me make sense of my own lapses in compassion and the intense reactions doctors can have when caring for patients such as Sharon. With complex PTSD, what we are often witnessing is a person who has been forced to spend every day in a quest for survival—no more and no less—and in that process the person's core character becomes the biggest casualty.

INTIMATE VIOLENCE

A Secret Pandemic

...If a woman cannot be safe in her own house then she cannot be expected to feel safe anywhere.
—Aysha Taryam

Geeta sits in the chair in my office nervously alternating between glances at the wristwatch that adorns her slim wrist and lightly fingering her 22-karat gold *mangalsutra* necklace. When she speaks, her voice is quiet, and though she has an excellent command of the English language, her Indian accent betrays her recent immigration to the United States. She is very pretty, thin, and in her mid-twenties, but in her casual dress of tight faded blue jeans and baggy deep turquoise *kurti* shirt she could easily pass for a teenager. She offers up a sweet demeanor, but something about her manner feels forced, as though she is trying hard to project a positive aura.

"So, Geeta, your internist referred you to me. She was concerned you might be depressed?"

Geeta clears her throat, then, in a voice that is almost a whisper, says, "I have a lot of family problems, Dr. Jain."

She tells me that she was born and raised in a small town in north India. Her marriage was arranged to an engineer named Akaash, who was from the same town but was currently working in Wisconsin. She first met him three years ago, during a visit he made to India. He came to her childhood home with his parents, and that was where she first laid eyes on him. Akaash was handsome, with fair skin and light brown eyes, and Geeta was instantly drawn to him. They met on two further occasions, once at a local restaurant and another time at his parents' home, and during both of their meetings they were accompanied by a gaggle of family chaperones. He seemed shy, but she did not mind that because she was a reserved person, too, and they had common interests: a love of Bollywood movies, classical music, drawing wildlife, and Sufi poetry.

When her parents asked her if she consented to the marriage, she said yes, and why not? Akaash was a well-educated engineer from a good family and was living in the United States. What an adventure her life would be! She had wanted to travel to America ever since her cousin had moved to Texas five years earlier. In the year that followed their formal engagement, Geeta and Akaash waited for her visa paperwork to be processed by the US Embassy in New Delhi. They Skyped regularly, and during those sessions she grew fonder of him and started to fantasize about the prospect of living abroad and seeing snow for the first time during the Wisconsin winters. They were married in India two years ago, and not long after, she arrived in Wisconsin on a dependent spouse visa to live with Akaash in his one-bedroom apartment.

Geeta tells her story with a surreal detachment, as though she is talking about a girl she once knew but has since lost touch with. She grows silent and appears lost in another world. To encourage her to keep talking, I interject with a disclosure of my own: "Geeta, it's not easy moving to a new country, starting over, being thousands of miles away from family and friends. I did the same when I moved from England to Wisconsin. I imagine Wisconsin must be very different from India . . ."

Geeta starts to cry hard. "I knew it would be difficult. I just did not know it would be this challenging."

She tells me that, on the weekends, Akaash drank heavily and then accused her of cheating on him during the week when he was at the office. "When am I going to cheat on him?" she asks me with a deeply pained look in her eyes.

She tells me that she has no access to money, no key to the apartment, and no cell phone. Akaash called her every thirty minutes from his office on their apartment landline to check that she was there, and after she said hello, he just hung up. She tells me how he drove her everywhere, for grocery shopping, hair appointments, and to shop for clothes; she could never go anywhere alone. During her weekly Skype call with her parents, he hovered in the corner and monitored her as she lied her way through the conversation: "Yes, Ma, I'm happy . . . Yes, Ma, I'm settled."

In the two years she has lived in Wisconsin, he has sabotaged almost every friendship she has made. She has one friend, a neighbor, also a young bride from India whom Akaash reluctantly allowed to drive Geeta to today's appointment. Geeta tells me the lengths she went to to make this appointment, how she lied and told him she had a gynecologist appointment for an urgent "women's problem" and of her plan to hide the health insurance statements that will arrive in the mail addressed to Akaash.

"If I told him the truth, he would never have let me come," she says. "I feel so trapped, Dr. Jain. In India, I had such a carefree life. My parents may have been from modest means, but I was raised in a loving home. I don't know what to do!"

"Geeta, does he hurt you physically?" I ask, half sensing the answer to my question.

She looks forlorn. "You cannot tell anyone, Dr. Jain. I am telling you this in complete confidence. No one else knows."

She tells me that Akaash frequently hits, slaps, and punches her. She rolls up her sleeve to reveal a scar on her arm from a gash she received when he pushed her onto broken glass. She had just served dinner, and he responded by telling her she was a lousy cook. He threw the dinner plates and glassware on the floor, spat food at her face, and then shoved her to the ground. Geeta tells me that her head swirls with the torrent of abuse he hurls at her: "You are ugly!" "You are a dimwit!" "Your family is trash, and you have rotten blood!"

Geeta is depressed, sleeps poorly, and has nightmares about Akaash's angry outbursts. She has lost so much weight that her periods have stopped, and she feels as though the joy has been sucked out of her life. Her days are spent feeling fearful, and frequently, as the time approaches for him to return home from work, her hands shake and go numb, her heart races, and she becomes drenched in sweat.

I tell Geeta that Akaash's violence is not acceptable, that she should call 911 the next time she feels threatened or he assaults her. I offer her a list of domestic violence shelters and other organizations that can help her. To my astonishment she waves away the list.

"No, Dr. Jain, you do not understand." She looks exasperated with me. "If I call the police, he will go to jail. He will lose his job and his visa and will have to return to India disgraced. Do you know how many people rely on Akaash's income? It pays for his brother's college tuition, his sister's marriage dowry, and his parents' doctor bills. What type of wife brings this misfortune on her husband? I will bring hardship to his entire family and shame upon my own parents, too. No, I would never call the police on him."

Now Geeta reveals her true intent behind coming to this appointment today: "Dr. Jain, tell me, how can I get Akaash to love me? How can I make our marriage work?"

* * *

For hundreds of millions of women all over the world, rape, battery, and other forms of violence are an everyday part of their lives. In the

United States, IPV (Intimate Partner Violence) is a public health threat. According to the CDC, nearly one in four women has been the victim of severe physical violence by an intimate partner in her lifetime. Despite these alarming statistics, until the turn of the twenty-first century, IPV was largely a secret pandemic. In 2002, Elaine Alpert, a physician and internationally respected scholar in family violence and sexual assault, wrote these words in an editorial in the *Journal of General Internal Medicine*:

> Over the course of human history, virtually no other public health problem has been as prevalent or as challenging to the health and well-being of humanity as intentional injury. Eclipsed only by war, domestic violence has remained at the forefront of violence-related human morbidity and mortality. . . . Although pandemic in scope, domestic violence until recently remained secret and undefined, in part because historically there was no common language to name the problem, describe its scope, garner the evidence, or take concerted action regarding intervention or prevention.

IPV leads to a whole host of conditions from chronic pain, unwanted pregnancies, and sexually transmitted diseases (including HIV) to psychological consequences such as depression, substance abuse, and suicide. PTSD[*] is a common consequence of IPV, with some studies showing rates as high as 64 percent, an alarming figure when one considers that lifetime estimates of PTSD generally lie somewhere in the 1 to 12 percent range.

IPV is a classic example of how social reality can negatively im-

---

[*] Historically, the psychological symptoms that occur as a consequence of IPV were called battered woman syndrome (BWS). BWS was previously identified as a subcategory of PTSD.

pact human biology. No doubt Geeta's traumatized state, dramatic weight loss, anxiety attacks, and nightmares were a direct result of her being abused. It's tempting to assume that if she could be extricated from the abusive situation, her symptoms would abate. But this is where the story gets complicated: severe IPV can contribute to biological changes, and Geeta's current traumatized state was impeding her ability to regain control over her life. The reality is that many victims of chronic IPV need some form of professional attention to help them take back their lives, and until they do, they are stuck in a vicious cycle.

Living in the aftermath of a disaster or in a war zone have a trickle-down effect, culminating in higher rates of IPV or other forms of societal violence. In other words, trauma begets trauma, and this observation extends to other adverse situations, too. In the case of Akaash and Geeta, their status as temporary legal aliens living an isolated existence in a foreign culture with uncertain employment opportunities and many family financial obligations likely set the stage.

When Geeta left India for the United States, rather than coming to the land of the free, she unwittingly walked into a preloaded scenario where the odds were not in her favor. Her lack of social capital (as a woman) and her dependency on Akaash for income and visa status further compounded the brutal impact of the IPV and rendered her more vulnerable to developing PTSD as a consequence. Her dangerous situation left no opportunity to recover and reset, zero access to social support, and no obvious way to escape.

To make matters worse, when survivors of IPV disclose their history, they are often met with a denial of their experience or misdirected anger or are shunned by people who do not consider it their business. Given the burden of IPV, it is stunning that there is not the same zeal or community effort one sees in the fight for breast cancer or heart disease prevention campaigns. The reason probably lies in the entrenched social stigma that still surrounds IPV.

***

Scattered among the weeks that followed my first meeting with Geeta were furtively arranged appointments, last-minute cancellations, and urgent rescheduling. During our sessions, she would have moments of scary optimism as she clung desperately to the rare instances when Akaash would be affectionate or show tenderness. On occasion, after hitting her, he would be remorseful, bang his head against the wall, apologize profusely, and promise that he would never do it again. Collectively, those incidents served to convince her that her marriage was fixable if she could just try hard enough.

I emphasized the positive things she did to protect herself from Akaash, reminding her that no matter what she may have done or said, no one deserves abuse. I tried to make my office a safe space and to create a rapport that empowered her. I told her she was not at fault or "crazy"; rather, her abusive marriage was eroding her physical well-being and breaking her psyche. In parallel, I listened to stories of Akaash throwing the remote control, empty beer bottles, and car keys at her head, yanking her hair, and screaming obscenities. I bit my lip, resisting the urge to beg her to call 911 and leave her marriage for fear she would not come back to see me. At some point she must have realized that I was not going to provide her with a magical playbook for how to make her marriage work, and she stopped coming.

Months later, she reappeared after requesting an urgent appointment. Since our last visit, she had aged beyond her years and lost more weight. Dark shadows encircled her eyes, and she now cast aside the charade of forced optimism. Her face was devoid of emotion as she relayed to me the event prompting her visit. The week before, when she had been Skyping with her parents, her mother had remarked how thin she was looking and that she was worried about her. After the call ended, Akaash went ballistic and accused Geeta of making him look like a bad husband. He went to the fridge, grabbed leftover food, and started shoving it into Geeta's mouth. When she gagged, he clamped her jaw shut in an effort to force her to swallow. Geeta threw up the forced food. Akaash then punched her in the stomach and she fell to her knees, howling in pain. She lay curled up on the hard linoleum floor for an hour.

Something snapped in Geeta that day, and later that week, after Akaash had left for work, she asked her neighbor friend if she could use her phone to make a long-distance call. "I called my mother-in-law," Geeta told me, "because I wanted to keep our problems in our family and not damage Akaash's reputation. I told her everything, about the punching, slapping, and yelling and how I tried to make the marriage work. I begged her for help and told her I could not take any more. My mother-in-law told me that it was my job to make Akaash happy, that I was failing him by making him angry, that I must learn to adjust to him."

Upon hearing her mother-in-law's response, I recognized it as "advice" that could only have come from the mouth of someone whose spirit had been destroyed by violence. I felt a chill run down my spine. Even though I would never meet Akaash or his mother, an image flashed in my mind of a boy raised in a household where he had routinely watched his mother being defiled and humiliated. My heart sank with the burden of vicious cycles of family violence.

Geeta told me how, after that phone call, her legs had started to tremble and she felt desperately hopeless. She found herself planning her own death, either by hanging or running out into rush-hour traffic, but just as those ideas started to take hold in her mind, she caught herself. In that moment, her lowest point in those two years of terror, she realized she needed to leave her marriage.

Days of covert activity followed as our clinic social worker helped me to formulate a plan of escape for Geeta. I learned that this time, when Geeta was planning on leaving Akaash, was a high-risk period. That fact caused a surge of my own fears. What if Akaash found out? What would happen to Geeta? Was he capable of murdering her? I grappled with all the factors of Geeta's case, trying to do a rough risk calculation, predict outcomes, and plan for all possible scenarios.

Geeta called her cousin in Texas from my office phone and told her about the abuse. Her cousin sent money to Geeta's neighbor so that she could purchase a cell phone and a plane ticket to Texas. Details of open spots at local shelters for abused women were communicated daily as discreet messages to Geeta's cell phone. She decided on a safety phrase, came up with several backup plans, and started gathering her most valuable belongings.

As the escape plan started to crystallize, Geeta got cold feet. How will I support myself financially? Where will I live? I can't drive. I don't know anything about America. Who can I trust? What will my parents say? My in-laws? What about Akaash? What might he do when he finds out I have left? Luckily, her self-defeating ruminations were quashed by a phone call. Her cousin in Texas, feeling overwhelmed and scared for Geeta, told Geeta's parents about their daughter's predicament. The next day, her parents called Geeta. "Leave, Geeta, at once. Just leave," they urged her. That was it, the push she needed to get out. The very next day, on a bright, crisp Wisconsin winter morning, immediately after Akaash left for work, she packed a single bag and asked her neighbor to drive her to a shelter. A few days later, she caught a flight to Texas to be with her cousin.

Three months later, I received a call from Geeta. She told me that she was safe in Texas and her mother had flown in from India and was helping her get back onto her feet. She was eating better and gaining weight. She told me about her daily feelings of anger, guilt, and shame over the failure of her marriage, that she was having nightmares about Akaash several times a week and truly believed she was incapable of trusting a man again.

Her parents were encouraging her to return to India, and as much as she wanted to, she was sticking to a promise she had made to herself: she would never allow herself to be dependent on others the way she had been dependent on Akaash for money, food, clothing, and shelter. She felt that her dependency had kept her hostage to the situation, and moving back to India would mean she would again become dependent. She got legal advice, had enrolled in school, and was seeing a therapist at a free clinic on campus. Her plan was to build an independent life, and if that meant she would be alone, then so be it. She ended the call by expressing her appreciation for our support and assuring me that she would stay in touch.

I never heard from her again.

A DANGER TO OTHERS

Hurt People Hurt Other People

I and the public know
What all school children learn,
Those to whom evil is done
Do evil in return.
—W. H. Auden, "September 1, 1939"

"You carry *what* in your car?" Mark's last sentence forces me to spin in my chair. His electronic medical record had been sucking up most of my attention; now I turn to face him.

"A baseball bat in the trunk, a machete under the driver's seat, and, oh, yeah, a dagger in the glove box," he answers.

I'm speechless. I raise both my hands and shake my head in dismay. My patient Mark is an Iraq War veteran with PTSD. At over six feet tall with a bodybuilder's frame, closely shaved head, and arms inscribed with an array of incendiary tattoos, he is an indomitable character. He has traveled all the way from the Central Valley region of northern California to see me. His medical record chronicles the day he walked into his local VA clinic, got angry, and threw over some tables and chairs in the waiting room. His record was then flagged with a behavioral warning that meant he could receive medical care only on VA campuses where there was a police presence.

The flag on his chart required Mark to check in with police upon arriving on campus and have an officer escort him to all his appointments. The officer would then wait outside the doctor's room for the duration of Mark's visits. Perhaps those measures helped Mark keep himself in check, because throughout the time I spent with him, he seemed cooperative, sincere, and even charming. Unfortunately, the same could not be said about his behavior outside my office. He was quite frank about disclosing the violent details of his day-to-day life because he very much wanted to change his ways. His biggest motivating force was his teenage sons. "I want to be a better role model for them." Still, our sessions often entered into difficult territory with Mark attempting to minimize his violence and persuade me that under his particular circumstances, his actions, though regrettable, were also justified.

"Have you ever visited my neighborhood, Dr. Jain?" was his response to my exasperation about the weapons stockpiled in his truck. "No, I didn't think so . . . lots of gang activity. I have to be prepared to defend myself and my family at all times. I tell you, you would do the same if you lived there."

"Okay, I take your point, Mark, but hear me out a second . . . You admit you have a short fuse, yes? My fear is having all these weapons at such close proximity will mean you end up doing something you regret. If that happens and you go to jail, then what will happen to your family?"

I was deliberately appealing to his sense of family because he was a devoted father and committed to providing his children with better options than what he had faced, growing up in a troubled home in a rough neighborhood riddled with gang violence.

Despite his efforts, his life remained steeped in violence and loss; every other month he told me of a longtime friend who had been murdered, shot, or stabbed. His family history was littered with first-degree relatives who had serious addictions to cocaine or methamphetamine, had been incarcerated for murder, or had died by overdose or suicide.

Against all expectations, Mark had signed up to join the military even before he graduated from high school. In many ways the military had been good for him, a place to channel his energies, and he had thrived under the rigorous structure military life demanded. Then came the Iraq War and his exposure to combat. Ever since, something seemed to have flipped, and he was permanently in fight mode: hypervigilant, paranoid, and ready to attack.

"I see your point, Dr. Jain . . . I'll think about putting the machete in my safe, maybe the dagger, too, because you are right, I do have a short fuse. The baseball bat stays, though . . ."

Mark's short fuse really was quite remarkable. In the few months I had been seeing him, he had relayed several stories of violent outbursts. Some of his stories were so brutal I found my mind drifting to scenes from a Martin Scorsese movie. There was the time when a driver had cut him off on the highway. Mark told me how he had "seen red" and gone chasing after him, darting and weaving through busy traffic, yelling and screaming and flailing his left fist at the offending driver through his open truck window. He had caught up with the driver, cornered him off an exit, hauled him out of his car, and started to pound him. His wife had pulled him off the terrified driver, who had taken that opportunity to scurry from the scene. Although he expressed remorse about his actions, part of him firmly believed that the other driver had "had it coming to him."

"I spent two years in Iraq dodging roadside bombs and IEDs. Of course I'm gonna lose it if you cut me off!"

Sometimes I would get the feeling that Mark was playing games with me. He claimed he did not want to be violent and was ashamed by his behavior. But my efforts to help him only stalled. When I

suggested therapy, I was often met with sly rebuttals and justifica-
tions for what he'd done. He found excuses to not take the pills I
prescribed for his PTSD and impulse control issues. "That Prozac
did zip for me," "That Buspar had me wired," and "The baby dose of
Seroquel knocked me out" were just a few of his complaints.

There were other issues that we skirted around but that held
more salience than Mark would admit to. His alcohol use for one
("Oh, just a few beers when I cook out on a Sunday"), but he had
a history of abusing alcohol and a DUI. Alcohol could dangerously
disinhibit him, loosen his tongue, and make him reckless, and I
often wondered if he had been under the influence during some of
his violent encounters.

Wanting to do more to ensure the safety of those who entered his
orbit, I spoke with his wife. I asked her if Mark was violent at home
with her or the kids or if he had immediate access to a firearm. She
answered no, Mark could be irritable, moody, and verbally abusive
but was not violent; she did not fear for her safety or the safety of her
children. His victims, along with his violent outbursts, appeared to
be totally random. He had never disclosed a plot to harm anybody,
nor was he fixated on or preoccupied with persistent violent thoughts
toward those nameless strangers. There was little I could do.

During a recent visit, Mark told me how he had been trying to
take an afternoon nap before picking up his sons from school.
Some construction workers in a neighbor's yard had been laughing
and joking over a cigarette break. Mark had been so enflamed by
their disturbing his nap that he had stormed out of the house and
threatened one of them with a dagger.

He flashed an impish grin. "That shut them all up!"

I started to entertain the notion that perhaps he was confabulating
just to get a reaction from me. Despite all the violent incidents, Mark
was not hauled to jail, and the police were never called. Why would

the road rage victim not press charges? What about the rest of the construction crew? Had their cell phones not been working when Mark took a dagger to their coworker's throat? Convinced that my theory held water, I pushed back on the latest story, challenging him about why the police had not been involved.

Mark's face flashed red, and he stammered, "I don't know . . . probably because it's the Central Valley?"

It took a few seconds for his words to register; then the truth hit me like a slap in the face: Mark's victims were all undocumented men who would never call 911, men with limited legal recourse, voice, or rights under which to defend or protect themselves. A feeling of nausea settled in the pit of my stomach. I felt a little light-headed but anchored myself with some conventional wisdom often spouted by PTSD specialists: "Trauma breeds further trauma . . . hurt people hurt other people."

***

Mark's dangerous volatility forced me to consider a fundamental question: Does having PTSD make one more prone to violence? Among American adults with no mental health issues, the prevalence of violence is about 2 percent. If you look at American adults with PTSD, that statistic jumps up to almost 8 percent, and at first glance, this figure certainly supports the notion that having PTSD makes a person more dangerous. But such numbers require careful interpretation. It turns out that abusing alcohol and drugs, having other psychiatric problems, and being younger (younger people are more likely to be violent) all contribute to making someone with PTSD more dangerous. The upshot is this: *Having PTSD is associated with a slightly increased risk of violence, but the reality is that the overwhelming majority of people with PTSD have never been violent.*

Research led by Dr. Nancy Wolff, an economist at Rutgers University, offers a more nuanced view of the relationship between violence and PTSD. Wolff and her colleagues investigated the rates of trauma exposure and PTSD in incarcerated men. They found that exposure to at least one severe traumatic event is a universal experience among this group and their rate of PTSD is tenfold higher than that found in the general male population. More than 50 percent of the incarcerated men involved in the research had been convicted of a violent crime, and those findings render it difficult to dismiss the notion of a tangible link among trauma exposure, behavioral problems, and violent criminality. Fifteen percent of the sample also reported a lifetime history of being raped, a rate several-fold higher than that reported by adult males in the general community. Moreover, the incarcerated men who reported a history of sexual trauma were much more likely to have PTSD, a finding that parallels other PTSD research and again speaks to the potently toxic effects of sexual violence on the human psyche.

Another finding to emerge from Wolff's work is the fact that prison itself is a hazardous place. People in prison experience sexual violence, and the consequences of these traumatic exposures follow them when they are released from prison back into the community. Inmates with a history of mental health problems appear to be at higher risk for becoming victims of both sexual and physical violence in the prison setting. The line between victim and perpetrator becomes blurred as both victim and perpetrator can come to reside in the same person. This research underscores the vicious cycle of violence and trauma. Wolff's contributions make a compelling case for why we need to use public funds to treat the traumatized, whether they be victims of trauma, perpetrators of trauma, or both.

ANGRY LOVING

The Stubborn Imprint of
Inner-City Poverty

Others noisily reenact their traumas by either retraumatizing
themselves or traumatizing other human beings, both inside and
outside their own families.

—Alexander C. McFarlane and Bessel A. van der Kolk, *Traumatic Stress: The
Effects of Overwhelming Experience on Mind, Body, and Society*

Many years ago, I had a patient named Rodney, an African American
man who was a retired city official. At well over six feet tall and
with a stocky build, he had the commanding presence befitting a
man who had spent four decades in city government. He had been
referred to me by his surgeon after he had suffered a life-threatening
reaction to anesthesia during a routine hernia operation. Although
he had made a full physical recovery, he remained traumatized by
the events of that day.

Rodney's early life had been very tough. He had grown up in
an impoverished part of Chicago, and by the time he was in middle
school, he had witnessed cold-blooded street murders, seen his
loved ones assaulted, and grown accustomed to the sound of gunfire
filling the night sky as he tried to sleep. A great-aunt who had a soft
spot for him had invited him to come and live with her in Wisconsin.
Rodney's mother, who was struggling to pay her bills, had readily
agreed, and just before he started high school, he moved. After he
graduated from high school, he had attended a local college and

married his college girlfriend. His first job out of university had been with the city, and that was where he had stayed for the next forty years, gradually ascending the ranks.

When I first met Rodney, he told me that he was having nightmares about the operation three to four nights per week. He would wake up in a sweat and be unable to return to sleep, and during the day, he was exhausted and irritable. He was also reliving memories, descending and ascending the steep slopes of his volatile childhood—vivid memories of violence that had occurred on streets and in parks long since displaced by gentrified housing. The memories triggered fits of rage.

"I feel like there is lava running in my veins!" he exclaimed.

Rodney told me that when he had moved to Wisconsin as a child, he had made a promise to himself that he would never return to Chicago and the violence in his past. He looked at me and in a cynical tone added, "But I suppose you would tell me that the past is not so easily forgotten?"

Rodney was correct. It would have been careless of me to dismiss the harsh realities of the zip code he had been born into. No doubt, his recent near-death medical experience had been harrowing, but I had a theory that the trauma had also triggered a reservoir of unresolved rage related to the violence he had been exposed to during his early childhood.

***

During my first few years of practicing medicine in the United States, I often worked in county-funded clinics and government programs set up to reach impoverished and uninsured communities. In those settings, I met hundreds of African American patients, and I was struck by how many of them lived in the poorest parts of the city, where death was a daily fact of life. Themes emerged from the stories I heard from these patients: poverty, violence, limited educational opportunities, and lack of access to high-quality health care were stubborn barriers to their fulfilling their dreams and ambitions.

Indeed, violent traumas such as homicide, physical assault, and rape are perpetuated more frequently against African Americans. With regard to PTSD, higher rates have been found in the following African American populations: combat veterans, low-income women, and teenagers living in high-crime inner-city areas. In fact, the rates of PTSD found in violent inner cities are comparable to the rates found in veterans of the wars in Iraq and Afghanistan.

PTSD in African Americans is complicated by several factors. First, as a group, they are more likely to minimize their symptoms in medical settings, which has probably led to an inaccurately lower "official" rate. Second, even if they are diagnosed with PTSD, they are less likely to use mental health services than their Caucasian counterparts. This difference can be explained, in part, by a general mistrust of medical institutions, but even those who wish to receive psychological help report other barriers to treatment, such as family disapproval of their decision.

The final (and biggest) wrinkle in understanding the rate of PTSD in African Americans is that it is more accurately explained by zip code rather than race. Living in an impoverished urban community is the strongest predictor of one's odds of experiencing violent trauma and trumps skin color. For African Americans with PTSD, if one factors in level of education and poverty, the contribution of skin color shrinks. You are more likely to have PTSD if you are poor, have a lower educational level, are unemployed, or are homeless, and in the United States, one is more likely to find oneself in those categories if one happens to be black.

***

Despite his unsettling symptoms, these were not Rodney's primary concern. The reason he had agreed to come see me was that he feared that his wife of nearly forty years "has probably had enough of me." When I asked for more clarification, he grew quiet and seemed at a loss for words. His voice croaked as he said, "It's not easy, living with me."

Unable to get more details from him, I invited him to bring his wife to our next session. He looked at me, his face full of doubt. "I will ask her, but I'm pretty sure she won't come."

A week later, when I went to greet Rodney in the waiting room, he appeared to be alone. As soon as he saw me, he called across the room to a Caucasian woman with her head buried in a magazine. I noted that there were at least five empty chairs between them. I introduced myself to Rodney's wife, Julia, who shook my hand and offered me a perfunctory smile. She looked tired, and her eyes were red as though she had been crying.

In my office, tension hung in the air between them as I struggled to get either of them to talk. It was clear that neither was comfortable airing their personal problems. I imagined what it must have been like for a biracial couple in Wisconsin in the 1970s: the resistance their union may have faced, unsolicited opinions, racist rhetoric, prophecies of doom and gloom from family and friends. Yet they had stayed married despite the odds.

Trapped in their frosty silence, I searched for a way in. "I could not help but notice that you were sitting on opposite sides of the waiting room . . . tough morning?" I offered, hoping to ease some of the palpable tension.

We all sat in silence for a few seconds. Rodney looked at Julia, who had her head down and was staring at the patterned fabric of her shift dress.

"Well, like I told you, Dr. Jain, I am not an easy man to live with . . . I can be a mean bastard sometimes. I put my wife through a lot, I know that. Actually, I don't blame her for not wanting to sit next to me."

Julia's pose shifted, and she sat upright. She seemed surprised, as though she was hearing something new. She spoke, guardedly but in a clear voice. "Rodney, you have been through a lot, I know. I suppose I am just glad you are getting help now. I hope you can help him, Dr. Jain."

"Julia, when Rodney says he can be a mean bastard, what does he mean?" I asked.

Julia told me that Rodney had always been an angry man: "He can walk into an empty room and start an argument." He was not only angry by nature but harbored and nursed his anger. Julia had come to view his "short fuse" as an essential part of his nature. In their earlier years, the anger had not been much of a problem. There had been outbursts where he would swear at her and say mean things, but after he calmed down, he had always been remorseful and would try to make it up to her.

She respected him as a self-made man who was not so different from her own father, a World War II veteran. She viewed Rodney as a pioneer, a black man who had accomplished so many firsts in a career where he was often the only person of color in the room. She had been willing to help him achieve his goals even if that meant she acted as a buffer for the various stresses that came with his ambition.

Over the years, she had become a master at predicting what could set him off and found creative ways to distract him. But everything had changed after his retirement and now the operation. He was home all day with nothing to do and seemed to spend his days in varying shades of anger—simmering, stewing, or going berserk. He showed her very little affection, and they were hardly ever intimate.

"That's when it became unbearable," Julia told me, and then, looking at her husband directly, "Rodney, I am walking on eggshells all day long. I can't live like this any longer."

"Do you fear for your safety? Has he ever harmed you physically?" I interrupted.

Julia was now crying. She shook her head no and between sobs said, "Sometimes I *think* he is going to hit me, he can become so threatening and gets this feral look in his eyes . . . it gets scary for me . . . but he never has."

Rodney's face fell, and he shook his head slowly. "Tell me what I need to do, Dr. Jain. I will do anything. I cannot bear to see my bride this way."

"Bride! Who are you calling bride, old man?" Julia laughed out loud.

All three of us burst into laughter, a much-needed respite from the tension dragging upon the session. By the end of that appointment, we had a plan in place for me to meet with Julia and Rodney together for several more sessions over the coming weeks. Rodney's primary reason for seeking help had been his acceptance that his anger was devastating his marriage, so it made sense for me to leverage this by involving Julia directly in his treatment. We said our good-byes, and the couple left my office. As I turned to my desk to prepare for the next patient, there was a quick knock on the door. Rodney reentered the room and surprised me with a big hug.

"THANK YOU," he mouthed. "I can't remember the last time I heard my wife laugh. I can't thank you enough for that," he whispered and exited the room with a big smile on his face.

Unfortunately, research suggests that the marriages of individuals with PTSD are generally not as resilient as Rodney and Julia's turned out to be. PTSD sufferers have higher rates of separation and divorce. They are less emotionally intimate with their partner and more likely to report problems in their sex life.

There is more violence in relationships in which one of the partners has PTSD. The more severe the PTSD symptoms, the more severe the violence perpetrated toward the spouse. Not surprisingly, spouses married to someone with PTSD are more likely to suffer from depression, anxiety, and social isolation. They are also overburdened as they take on a disproportionate load, from running the household to caring for dependent children and elderly family members.

A 2012 study published in *The Journal of the American Medical Association* described a clinical trial that randomly assigned couples to a fifteen-session couples therapy designed specifically for couples where one partner had PTSD or to be placed on a wait list. In addition to offering the couple education about the diagnosis and exploring some of the barriers to their emotional and physical intimacy, this specialized form of couples therapy homed in on an issue that is often at the core of such relationships: how one partner can sometimes, unknowingly, feed into the other partner's PTSD symptoms. For example, a sufferer who rages at the slightest of things may have his or her anger problem reinforced by a spouse who restricts his or her own life so as not to upset the sufferer. Such drastic accommodations are rarely effective; instead, much as with Julia and Rodney, it results in one spouse "walking on eggshells" while the spouse with PTSD continues to experience the symptoms. In this new therapy, couples are taught to cope with the symptoms together as opposed to reinforcing them.

The results of this study were encouraging in that the couples that received the specialized therapy showed significant improvement and were four times as satisfied with their relationship as the couples on the wait list. Furthermore, the partners with PTSD reported a 50 percent reduction in the severity of their symptoms, or about three times the improvement of those on the wait list. In fact, more than three-quarters of them no longer met the criteria for PTSD. In an interview, the lead author of the study, Dr. Candice Monson, a psychologist at Ryerson University, highlighted the importance of the partner's presence in the treatment: "PTSD patients don't do as well in individualized therapy. . . . Social support emerges as the most robust factor that encourages recovery."

THE FAIRER SEX?

Rape, Secondary Injuries, and
Postpartum PTSD

> I just want to sleep. A coma would be nice. Or amnesia. Anything,
> just to get rid of this, these thoughts, whispers in my mind. Did he
> rape my head, too?
>
> —Laurie Halse Anderson, *Speak*

"Are you sure my ten o'clock patient isn't here yet?" It is 10:15, and I
have called the clinic front desk in search of my patient Terry, who
is never late.

I listen as the receptionist covers her phone with her hand and
calls out Terry's name in the waiting room. A muffled exchange
follows. Moments later, she gets back on the line. "Sorry, Dr. Jain,
your patient has been sitting here since ten. I did not realize your
patient was a woman, I assumed she was a family member waiting
for a veteran..."

The VA health care system, hardwired to treat a purely male
clientele, is pivoting to meet the needs of an exponential increase
in women service members. I come out to the waiting room to greet
Terry and apologize for the oversight. Terry, dressed casually in
blue jeans and a white T-shirt, shrugs off the incident with an "I'm
used to it" sort of look. As we walk to my office, I note that there are
dark circles under her eyes and she does not seem to be her usual
breezy, confident self.

Terry has been my patient for a couple of years and comes to see me every four months for a check-in visit. I had been aware of her significant struggles since her discharge from the military, but by the time we first met any scars from those hard times were barely visible. Terry worked full-time as an executive, was happily married to her wife of three years, and together they were raising two children. During her spare hours she was a committed volunteer in local LGBT organizations.

During our previous visits, she had struck me as being an organized, smart, and energetic woman, and our conversations centered mostly on the challenges of balancing a career with motherhood and a stubborn insomnia that did not respond to anything but the sleeping pill zolpidem. I was loath to prescribe zolpidem in such a chronic way, but her insistence that it was effective for her—"It keeps the nightmares away, Dr. Jain"—the fact that she had minimal side effects, and the spectacular failure of all other treatments she had tried forced my hand.

Today I am seeing a different Terry. No sooner has she settled into the chair than her whole body crumples and she starts to cry. She tells me that over the last few weeks, she has been under much stress. An annual checkup with her internist had revealed an abnormal Pap smear result, and she was scheduled for more tests. Her family history was peppered with mothers, aunts, and sisters who had had various cancers of the breast, cervix, ovary, or uterus. The abnormal Pap result had been stressful, but she was managing to keep things together during her workday and in the evenings as she shuttled her children back and forth to soccer practice and school play rehearsals.

It was at night that her mind would start whirring with anxiety and dread, and sleep, even aided by a double dose of zolpidem, was starting to evade her. But the final straw had been the recent suicide of one of her army buddies. The tragic news had spread like wildfire among her tight-knit group of friends, all women who had served in the army and had stayed in regular contact since their discharge. Though dispersed over various time zones, state lines, and continents, news of the suicide was followed by a flurry of activity on social media, text messages, and phone calls.

Terry rocks gently back and forth in her chair, her eyes staring off into the distance and tears streaming down her cheeks. She tells me that, while deployed overseas, her buddy had been raped. "She never got over it . . . it got her in the end."

I felt a chill run down my spine as I knew that Terry herself was no stranger to sexual violence. She had been sexually molested by an uncle when she was a child and date-raped as a teenager. After she had joined the military, there had been several episodes of unwanted sexual attention from her male peers, and then one night, not long before her deployment ended, a senior male officer had raped her. After that, something snapped in Terry and she had struggled to reconcile the pride she felt for serving her country with the violation and betrayal she had experienced during her deployment. Unfortunately, when she had told her parents about the sexual assault, their response had been to blame her: "What did you do to lead him on?" When, years later, she had come out to her parents as a gay woman, they had disowned her. She had been estranged from them for the last several years.

Terry's military discharge had been followed by years of anger, especially if anyone asked about her deployment. She was often anxious, irritable, and hypervigilant and trusted very few people. Realizing her behavior was impacting her ability to mother her children, she had sought help and worked hard in therapy to deal with her experiences. Her other way of coping was by filling her life with a hectic schedule. "As long as I keep busy, it allows me not to think about it."

Terry utters a mantra under her breath: "This too shall pass . . . this too shall pass." I feel overcome by a wave of sorrow as, for the first time, I get a sense of the tremendous energy she put into presenting the composed version of herself that I had always known.

***

On the one hand, women are less likely to experience traumatic events than men. On the other, study after study shows that women experience PTSD at two to three times the rate that men do. Why is this? What about being a woman makes one more susceptible to PTSD? Though emerging evidence suggests that sex hormones, particularly estradiol and progesterone, play a role in these differences, answers can also be found by drilling down to the *types* of trauma that women are more likely to experience.

Women are *much* more likely than men to have been sexually abused as a child or sexually assaulted as an adult. Indeed, in the United States, nearly one in five women has been raped at some time in her life. A recent study in *The New England Journal of Medicine* reported, "Young women attending university face a substantial risk of being sexually assaulted. The incidence of sexual assault is estimated to be between 20% and 25% over a period of 4 years."

As in Terry's case, the issue of acquaintance rape, where the perpetrator is known to the victim, is emerging as a national problem. About 85 to 90 percent of sexual assaults reported by college women fall into this category. This statistic becomes even more sobering when one considers that rape is the type of trauma most likely to lead to PTSD.

What makes rape so difficult to heal from? The stigma that

shrouds this crime means that the traumatized survivor, who risks being shamed, is often forced into silence. This bolsters rape's power to wreak havoc on the life of the survivor.

When a woman does speak up about rape, she often faces "secondary injuries" caused by friends, family, and professionals who blame her (even if only by innuendo). Even when her account is believed, her character may be questioned, which can increase her odds of developing PTSD. Posttrauma social support is powerful in helping survivors recover. This support is especially powerful for women, which is why secondary injuries can be so damning for them. Secondary injuries can have an undesirable influence on whether she discloses her problems in the future, how severe her trauma symptoms become, and whether or not she decides to seek treatment.

When I first meet a patient, part of my standard evaluation involves asking if the patient has a personal history of childhood sexual abuse. Over the years, I have asked this question thousands of times, and I would estimate that 20 percent answer yes. When a patient answers yes, I always ask, "When the abuse was happening, did you tell anyone?" About a third will answer yes and recount how they told a parent or grandparent and the perpetrator was stopped cold by being banned from the home, reported to the police, and sometimes even prosecuted and sent to prison. Another third will also answer yes but explain, "She did not believe me" or "He said nothing," and for these patients, the sexual abuse often continued. When the answer is no, the assumption is usually that "no one would listen," that "they would not have believed me," or that "I didn't feel that I could." In my anecdotal experience, the first group overcomes the horror of sexual abuse and the effects do not linger into their adult lives. In contrast, those who were ignored or dismissed or who did not disclose the abuse in the first place live adult lives embittered by the trauma and, when it comes to any future intimate relationships, are often caught up in a web of ambiguity and psychological isolation.

***

Another type of experience that women are uniquely vulnerable to enduring is the psychological stress associated with giving birth. This experience has come to be referred to as "birth trauma."* Dr. Rebecca Moore, a psychiatrist at the Tower Hamlets Perinatal Mental Health service in London, works closely with pregnant women who have mental health problems through their pregnancy and up to a year after they give birth. She described what it means to experience birth trauma:

> When a woman has a traumatic birth, there was something subjective about the birth that was distressing. This does not have to be life-threatening or medically traumatic. We are thinking of the psychological impact of that birth experience on the mother.
>
> Birth Trauma definitions include "a negative and disempowering physiological and emotional response to a birth." Common themes include feeling unheard or not listened to, a lack of compassion from medical professionals, and feeling out of control or helpless.
>
> Around 25 percent of all births in the UK are identified by women as being traumatic. This really strikes me, as it is such a high rate. In fact, if we look at the annual birth rate

---

* The term *birth trauma* has arisen in recent years; the use of the word *trauma* here is more casual. It encompasses experiences that are psychologically stressful and is not limited to life-threatening traumas.

in the United Kingdom, this means around 173,000 women are traumatized after delivering per year.

For many women, these birth experiences will never be discussed or explored. Although women may not develop a diagnosable disorder, they will often experience significant levels of distress and symptoms may persist for many years without treatment. There is often a significant impact on women's future pregnancies and birth experiences, and I have met women who only have one child because their first birth experience was so negative and they cannot contemplate coping emotionally in another pregnancy.

Around 1 to 6 percent of women who experience birth trauma will go on to develop PTSD. Statistics on postpartum PTSD indicate a prevalence of 1 to 3 percent which, from an epidemiological standpoint, means it is quite common. Yet, in contrast to the more widely acknowledged phenomenon of postpartum depression, postpartum PTSD receives very little attention by medical professionals. A Google search for "birth trauma" or "postpartum PTSD," however, shows a large number of self-help organizations, patient advocacy groups, and online support forums. This finding suggests that medical practice may need to catch up with the stories evolving every day on the front lines.

The research that identifies social support as being powerful in helping traumatized women heal is echoed in studies that follow women who have postpartum PTSD. Women are more vulnerable to developing PTSD following a traumatic birth if there was a difference between the professional support they expected and the level of health care they actually received. As Moore added, "Women are not necessarily traumatized by the events of birth not happening as they expected, but are more affected when they do not receive the care they expect."

These findings bring us back to the difference between men and women when it comes to PTSD. Men and women experience trauma under different social circumstances, and this is vital to understanding why women are more susceptible to PTSD. In essence, women experience a boost in their ability to cope with a traumatic event if they can access positive social support, and the denial of such support is extra-devastating.

Another layer of complication arises when we consider how often a woman's social roles (e.g., mother, wife, or caregiver) compound the negative impact of her traumatic experience. Consider the following scenarios: a mother who is traumatized after giving birth is still required to nurse and care for her newborn; a wife who has a violent husband must still live, eat, and sleep with him; a daughter who was sexually abused by her father is now his primary caregiver in his old age. These scenarios showcase the daily bind that traumatized women face, a bind that strains their ability to recover from trauma because the very kernel of their day-to-day identity is intertwined with their traumatic experiences.

SHAME

The Cinderella Emotion

The difference between shame and guilt is the difference between "I am bad" and "I did something bad."
—Brené Brown

"I'm pregnant. We have been trying for almost three years, so I *should* be happy."

Eun is a heavyset woman of Korean descent who is in her early thirties. She has never been to see a psychiatrist before, and I catch her eyeing my office door as though she might get up and leave at any moment. She was referred to me by her infertility specialist for symptoms of depression that were worsening over the sixteen weeks of her IVF pregnancy.

She utters the phrase *"should* be happy" more than once. My guess is that congratulatory smiles are what she has received from everyone around her, and I need to offer something different.

"Eun, how do *you* feel about being pregnant?"

She tells me that at first she was over the moon but within a few weeks she was filled with fear and a deep sadness. She found she could not focus.

"I go into the kitchen to start dinner and then somehow ten minutes have passed and I have just been standing there, lost in my own head."

She has not shared this with her husband, who she tells me is loving and supportive. She fears he might not understand how she can be unhappy when they were trying for a baby for so long. She asks me for a pill, something that will make the depression and anxiety go away. I tell her I need to complete my evaluation before I can prescribe treatment and go on to ask the myriad questions that are the basic part of a psychiatric evaluation: Have you ever had symptoms of mania? Do you hear things other people don't hear? Is there a family history of suicide? Do you take any over-the-counter pills or herbal remedies? I also ask Eun how many times she has been pregnant and am surprised when she answers, "Twice. Now and once before, when I was twenty."

I wait for her to volunteer information about what happened with her first pregnancy. A miscarriage? Termination? Stillbirth?

Eun takes a deep breath. "I had a baby boy, Jerry, but he died when he was a few weeks old . . . SIDS."[*]

I feel my face fall. My patient has survived every mother's worst nightmare.

Eun tells me about her upbringing as the eldest child of Korean immigrant parents. She was raised, along with her brother, in a small apartment above the family's convenience store. She found it difficult growing up as a Korean American in 1980s Wisconsin and oscillated between desperately wanting to fit in at school and the expectations of her conservative Korean parents.

She told me how giddy she was when, as a freshman in high school, a classmate asked her out on a date. She kept the date a secret because the boy was Caucasian and her parents would not have approved. They were very religious, and the preacher in their church often warned his congregation about the perils of American dating. Then her brother heard rumors about Eun's dating and spilled the

---

[*] Sudden infant death syndrome (SIDS) refers to unexplained death in an infant under age one.

beans. Massive arguments erupted, and Eun's parents laid down the law. Eun could not accept how strict they were being about something that felt so natural, so she continued to date.

"That's when all the emotional drama started." Eun tears up as she revisits her teenage years.

One afternoon her mother held her hostage in the store until Eun vowed to stop dating "that American boy." At one point, when there were no customers in the store, her mother started banging her head on the countertop next to the cash register, shrieking "I'm better off dead than having a daughter like you!" Another time Eun came home one evening to find that she was locked out of the house. She tells me how she spent the night wandering the streets feeling scared, helpless, and in utter shock that her parents had done this to her.

Eun continued to rebel and got better at hiding the relationship by living two separate lives. In the first, she played the role of a dutiful Korean daughter, serving customers, doing her homework, and helping her mother in the kitchen. In the second, she dated and experimented with drugs and alcohol.

Before long, desperate for acceptance from her peers, she started to have casual sex with boys in her class. That was when the name-calling started: "whore," "Asian trash," "slut." That took its toll, and her grades dropped. She started to spend her days getting drunk and high with some of the older kids from her neighborhood. She tells me that she was sexually assaulted by a couple of boys in that group, an experience she had never told anyone about until that moment in my office. Not long after the assault, she dropped out of high school altogether.

Eun's parents were devastated that their firstborn was a high school dropout and turned all their attention to their son, hovering over his every grade and accomplishment and plowing all their aspirations into his success. They gave Eun an ultimatum: earn your keep by working in the family business, or get out of our house.

"Huh . . . I never actually realized this till now, but it was around that time I got this nasty habit." Eun waves her fingers in front of her face. I take in her stubby nails and the tips of her fingers: red, raw, swollen, with the skin around the nail bed peeling away in slim slithers.

Feeling defeated, she acquiesced to her parents' ultimatum and started working in their store. Within a year, they were coercing her to get married to a newly arrived Korean immigrant their church pastor introduced them to—"a nice boy from a good family . . . what more could a high school dropout expect?" By nineteen she was stuck in an awkward marriage with a man who could barely speak English. By twenty, she was pregnant and living with her husband in her childhood bedroom above her parents' shop.

"When I was pregnant with Jerry, I remember feeling trapped and unhappy. I thought about having the baby and then running away from home. But I swear, Dr. Jain, everything changed the second I saw my Jerry's face. He was an angel, a big face with rosy red cheeks . . . he was the most beautiful thing I had ever seen in my life."

After Jerry was born, she experienced a period of pure happiness. She found purpose in taking care of her baby and recalled that every cell of her body felt energized. Her marriage, on the other hand, was not going well. Her husband would disappear for long periods, was drinking heavily, and was neither working nor helping her with the baby.

One day, she awoke to the sound of her father calling her to help him open the store. She turned to see that her husband was not sleeping next to her and reasoned that he had probably never made it home from another night of carousing. She got up and quickly checked on Jerry, who was sleeping in the bassinet next to their bed. She threw on some sweats and rushed downstairs to help her father.

"I planned to come right back upstairs, but there was a rush of customers and I got busy. About an hour later, I ran upstairs to check on Jerry, and that was when I found him. He was blue in the face. I shook him . . . then I shook him harder, but there was nothing. I just screamed and screamed and screamed."

Eun relates her memory of Jerry's death in a trancelike state. Her face is devoid of emotion save for the tears that stream down her cheeks.

After that, Eun's life descended into a form of hell. Instead of sympathy, her husband rebuked her. Every day, he came up with a list of things Eun had done or not done and how this had caused the death of their son. Her parents blamed her for not living up to her duty of being a mother and for tainting their honor through her negligence. Eun tells me, "I felt like I wanted to crawl into a hole and die." She became consumed with thoughts of death and wanted to end her life so she could be with Jerry.

"I thought I might shoot myself with the gun my father kept under the shop counter or pour gas on my body and set myself on fire in the backyard . . . but it turned out I was too much of a coward. I did not even have the guts to kill myself even though my husband told me that would have been the honorable thing to do."

One day Eun just walked out of her family's life for good. Over the years, she got her GED, a divorce, and a job as a medical assistant. For the better part of a decade, she lived a hermit type of existence. She met her current husband at work, and after a long and hesitant courtship, they married. He was a good man and knew about her first marriage and Jerry, but they did not discuss her past much. Now that she was pregnant, she felt she could not share with him what she was going through. She felt winded all the time, as though her stomach had leapt into her throat. She would relive the moment she found her dead baby, over and over. The image of his face—swollen, blue, and lifeless—haunted her day and night.

Eun breaks down into sobs, and I let her cry without interruption. Her head is bowed, and she has turned her eyes away from me. Her body slumps, and she covers her face with her hands as though she wants to disappear, and her skin flushes red.

These are all the universal signs of shame.

***

Humans have long used shaming as a weapon to preserve social order and cohesion; indeed, our brains are hardwired to register shame. Benign forms of shaming serve an everyday function. If your spouse kicks you under the table for hogging the conversation at a dinner with friends or your boss glares at you when you are unprepared for an important meeting, you may feel embarrassed, but such experiences help us learn how to navigate the world. Shaming becomes dangerous when it leaves someone feeling degraded, humiliated, or disgraced.

The Harvard psychiatrist Dr. Judith Herman has long argued that in traumas in which a dominant perpetrator subordinates a victim, the emotion of shame becomes central to the survivor's experience. Shame has been nicknamed the "Cinderella of emotions" because it is often overlooked and draws much less attention than the fear, anger, and guilt that have come to be synonymous with traumatic stress. Part of the reason for this is that shame is a subtle emotion, much harder to identify by patients and clinicians alike.

How does shame relate to PTSD? Several studies with survivors of violent crime hint at a tight relationship between the level of shame experienced after the trauma and the survivor's developing PTSD. In a University of London study, researchers identified more than 150 recent survivors of violent stranger crime and asked about their symptoms of shame in interviews. Their results showed that a persistent feeling of shame predicted their developing PTSD symptoms in the six months following the assault.

In other studies, PTSD sufferers reporting higher levels of shame experienced a slower recovery from PTSD. Well over a half century ago, Carl Gustav Jung, the influential Swiss psychiatrist and analyst, went so far as to describe shame as "a soul eating emotion." His early observations hold chilling significance as modern researchers have found that PTSD patients who endorse shame are more likely to contemplate suicide.

***

Grieving the death of a loved one typically manifests as intense sadness, social withdrawal, and loss of joy in life. Normal grief, as thoroughly painful as it is, is transient, lifting gradually over the ensuing weeks, months, and years. But in a subset of individuals, grief can be traumatic, prolonged, and complicated. Jerry's tragic death, sudden and unexpected, left Eun traumatized. Her grief became complicated by other vulnerabilities in her life: her troubled relationship with her parents, her prior history of being traumatized through sexual violence, being unable to rely on her family of origin and first husband for support after her son's death, and, to make matters worse, their shaming her after Jerry's death. As I explained to Eun, part of her current depression was rooted in unresolved traumatic grief over Jerry's death.

I did not recommend medication for Eun but suggested we try talk therapy as her pregnant state increased the risks of taking medication. When I explained my rationale to her, she grasped it immediately.

Therapy would prove tasking; I explained that shame was a

normal reaction to the unjust ways she had been treated but Eun was a master at playing emotional whack-a-mole. Every time she felt a sensation of shame, her instinct was to shut it down. Feeling shame seemed like a weakness to her, something that in itself was shameful.

Gradually we took apart the buzzing confusion of her childhood and discovered how her feelings of shame seeped into every aspect of her identity. Deep down she viewed herself as a bad daughter, a stupid person, an immoral woman who deserved to have her baby die—his death was her punishment for dishonoring herself and her parents by her bad behavior as a teenager. And now, as a bad mother, she was unfit to have another child. She came to realize how, for much of the last decade, she had been living like a ghost: she walked around feeling numb and detached from the world and felt that a part of her had died with Jerry. What also became apparent during therapy was a deep reservoir of rage toward her parents, an anger so scary that she buried it deep.

After several weeks of therapy, I invited Eun to bring her husband to a few of our sessions. Jim had a rough idea about her earlier life, but he knew none of the details. At over six feet tall and with a burly frame, he towered over Eun. His face was kind, and he listened patiently as Eun and I updated him about our work together. He seemed to intuitively sense Eun's distress and welcomed the chance to be involved in her treatment. It was vital that my instincts about Jim and his connection to Eun be accurate, because if I was going to encourage Eun to fully disclose the details of her traumatic past, I needed to be sure she would be treated with the care that was long overdue.

On a hot summer's day, not long after Eun entered the final trimester of her pregnancy, I listened as she told Jim how she had been emotionally abused and shamed by her parents, sexually assaulted as a teenager, and blamed and ostracized after Jerry's death. Jim took Eun's hand and rubbed it gently back and forth as she narrated her story. After she was done, he sat in silence, his eyes moist and red. When he spoke, he looked directly into Eun's eyes and reassured her that she had never done anything to be treated that way, that she would be a wonderful mother, and that he would support her no matter what challenges life brought their way. His response was perfectly attuned to what Eun needed in that precise moment. As I watched them share tears and a long hug, I sensed the grip of shame loosen its tight hold over their future.

THE SCIENCE OF SUICIDE PREVENTION

As a nation, we should not be satisfied, will not be satisfied, until every man and woman in uniform, every veteran, gets the help that they need to stay strong and healthy.

—President Barack Obama, after signing the Clay Hunt Suicide Prevention for American Veterans Act in 2015

The alarm clock flashing 03:00 in green neon signals to me that I should be fast asleep. I close my eyes and take deep breaths, trying to lull myself back into a peaceful slumber; the day ahead holds a daunting schedule with no room for fatigue. Then it pops into my mind, a solitary question that has needled its way through my dreams, forcing me to deal with its implications: *Did you miss something with Dave?*

In the still darkness of my bedroom, I strain to recall the details of his clinic visit. My patient Dave, an Iraq War veteran, had been home for a few years, but the passage of time had not healed his psychological wounds. Through stifled tones he told me about his tormented nights—horrifying memories, so difficult to erase, now dangerously directing his life. Dave has a shock of overgrown hair, and tears welled in his honey-brown eyes dulled by the weight of war. Silence hung between us, and I shifted uneasily in my chair, hesitating to reach for the Kleenex. Then I asked the question "Have you had thoughts about killing yourself?" A pause, then "No, Doc, no."

I run through a mental checklist to make sure I had done all that was required. I had increased his paroxetine dosage (a medication to treat post-traumatic stress); prescribed a short course of sleep medication to help ease the agony of his insomnia; communicated my concerns to his therapist; and asked Dave to return to my clinic in two weeks (the time it would take for the extra paroxetine to kick in) instead of the usual month. As I walked him to the door, I made sure he had all the emergency numbers to call if things got worse.

It seemed, on paper at least, that I had done all I could do, so why am I tossing and turning?

My heart sinks as I realize what was missing from our visit: the "click." The click is a feeling beyond rational comprehension, and it can come and go in the blink of an eye. The presence of the click signals to me that my patient is telling me everything I need to know, that we are on the same page and share the same hope for recovery. Treating thousands of patients over two decades has taught me that the absence of the click invariably means that trouble is brewing.

I wait for dawn and a reasonable time for when I can call Dave to make sure he is okay.

***

More than 30,000 Americans die from suicide per year, and approximately 20 percent of them are veterans. An average of twenty veterans die from suicide each day, and six of the twenty deaths are among veterans who receive care in VA hospitals. The statistics are sobering and raise the question: What role does PTSD play in the tragedy of veteran suicide?

The "war is hell" camp cites data and an intuitive wisdom that the act of going to war itself *must* be a causal factor in the subsequent suicide of a service member. Yet an exhaustive 2015 study published in *JAMA Psychiatry* that investigated 5,000 suicides from a sample of almost 4 million service members failed to support such a theory: death by suicide occurred even among military members who had never been deployed to a war zone.

Having PTSD certainly puts veterans at a higher risk of death by suicide, particularly for sufferers who experience high levels of intrusive memories, anger, and impulsivity. Veterans with partial PTSD are three times as likely to report hopelessness and suicidal thoughts as their counterparts who do not have PTSD. The concern here is that some of the veterans who might not meet the textbook definition of having PTSD are nonetheless at higher risk for suicide and may be slipping through the cracks of treatment services.

Combat veterans who feel guilt about what they witnessed or did during war are also more likely to be preoccupied with thoughts of self-harm or attempt suicide. This relationship between guilt and suicide has prompted the recent emergence of a scholarly construct (independent of PTSD) known as *moral injury*. Moral injury occurs when someone experiences events that transgress his or her deeply held beliefs and shatter his or her expectations about life. In war, this might involve unintentional errors that result in the killing or harming of others, failing to prevent immoral acts, or giving or receiving orders that he or she perceives as moral violations.

Research has shown that moral injuries can send a person into a state of turmoil, marked by shame, guilt, anxiety, and anger. In a 2013 study of more than 500 veterans, researchers found that just over 10 percent of veterans acknowledged having been personally responsible for transgressions that could cause moral injuries, 25 percent had witnessed transgressions by others, and 25 percent reported having felt betrayed by fellow service members or leaders they had once trusted. Those who felt personally responsible for transgressions and those who felt betrayed were more likely to attempt suicide.

Also at higher risk of suicide are veterans who endured intense combat experiences, were wounded many times, or suffered traumatic brain injuries (TBIs). It is easy to see how PTSD and TBI can occur simultaneously in combat veterans. A soldier who survives a bomb blast sustains head injuries that result in a TBI. During that incident, he also witnessed the violent death of an army buddy. After the trauma, he is left to deal with those horrific memories with a brain that has been injured—a double whammy that is potentially lethal.

A disturbing trend has also emerged from research investigating cases of military sexual trauma, a VA term used to describe experiences of sexual assault or sexual harassment during military service. Though military sexual trauma is not a diagnosis, its occurrence often triggers mental health problems such as PTSD, depression, and substance abuse. By mining VA databases for veterans who screened positive for sexual trauma, a team of researchers led by Dr. Rachel Kimerling from the National Center for PTSD found a strong correlation between having endured military sexual trauma and subsequently committing suicide or other acts of self-harm.

Somewhat related to this are findings that the suicide rate of women veterans is six times higher than their civilian peers. Of particular concern is the dramatically greater risk of suicide among the youngest women veterans; those eighteen to twenty-nine years old have nearly twelve times the suicide risk of their civilian peers. One reason may be easier access to firearms, but having experienced military sexual trauma also appears to play a contributing role.

LGBT veterans who experience victimization related to their LGBT status are also at risk for committing suicide. Indeed, a recent cross-sectional national survey of more than 200 transgender veterans hinted that those who reported having experienced transgender-related stigma during their military service and had current symptoms of PTSD were at higher risk of suicidal behaviors.

The key to suicide prevention in veterans with PTSD is to provide high-quality treatment. This treatment includes a sufficient dose of talk therapy, and, if medication is warranted, the patient's taking the medication for long enough and at a high enough dosage to have the full effect. Yet clinicians cannot coerce people into accepting treatment. The reality is that suicidal patients may deny their suicidal thoughts for fear that they will be forced into treatment or that the disclosure will result in their plans being challenged.

Over the better part of the last two decades, the VA has undergone a dramatic shift in its approach to suicide. In 2004, it developed a Comprehensive Mental Health Strategic Plan and added a 24/7 suicide prevention hotline and an instant messaging and texting service that connects those in crisis directly to mental health professionals. In addition, screening and assessments have been set up through the system to assist in the identification of high-risk patients. Each VA medical center has a suicide prevention coordinator whose job is to ensure that a veteran at risk is connected to the right services and receives adequate follow-up. Those identified as high risk receive an enhanced level of care, including weekly appointments and focused follow-up for missed appointments.

***

Faced with the uncertainties surrounding the issue of veteran suicide, I find myself relying on a time-honored tradition of medicine: the power of a strong relationship with my patients and the importance of creating an environment in which they feel they can say whatever is on their mind. Creating such an environment is no easy feat as twenty-first-century medical practice offers endless distractions

to the practicing physician: back-to-back clinic schedules; an electronic medical record that dishes up a steady stream of alerts, notifications, and orders that demand continued visual attention; instant
messages, emails, texts, and phone calls that ask the physician to
make immediate decisions and judgments; and, of course, mounds
and mounds of paperwork.

In such an environment, I find that listening to my patients has
become one of the most powerful services I can offer. Listening
creates silent spaces that can be filled with a patient's expressions
of his or her worst fears and deepest secrets.

In my office, I watch the clock ticking on the wall. The second it
hits 8 a.m., I pick up the phone and call Dave's cell phone. The phone
rings and rings. My heart sinks as I fear the call is heading for voice
mail, then skips a beat as it is picked up.

"Hello?"

"Hi, Dave, it's Dr. Jain from the VA."

"Oh, hi, Doc."

"I know yesterday was a bad day for you, so I thought I would just
check in."

Silence.

"I am thinking you should come back to clinic this week instead
of next week; how does that sound?"

Silence. Then: "Yes, I think that would be a good idea."

There it is in his voice, what was missing in our previous visit, an
inflection in his tone, a change that is subtle but somehow reassuring:
the click. He is listening to me, and, perhaps more important, he
knows I am listening to him—we are working as a team toward a
mutually agreed-upon goal. I know this does not guarantee that
there will not be troubled times ahead, but for now this is enough.

PART 5

Treating Traumatic Stress

TALKING CURES
AND BEYOND

Look, you must speak.
As poorly as we can express our feelings, our memories, but
  we must try.
We have to tell the story as best we can.
In truth, I have learned something:
Silence never helps the victim. It only helps the victimizer . . .
If I remain silent, I poison my soul.

—Elie Wiesel (1996)

There have never been so many effective treatments for PTSD sufferers. Today, someone with PTSD can benefit from four decades of research and development that has produced a wide array of treatments. The zeal to advance further remains in full swing as all over the world clinicians and scientists explore new approaches and experiment with how best to tailor existing treatments so that they will have maximum impact and reach as many people as possible.

The gold standard in PTSD treatment is cognitive behavioral therapy (CBT). CBT typically involves a patient meeting with a mental health professional on a weekly basis for up to four months, with each session lasting anywhere from sixty to ninety minutes. In what has become a landmark paper, researchers Dr. Anke Ehlers and Dr. David M. Clark proposed a cognitive theory of PTSD including three crucial features: persistent negative cognitions (or thoughts) about the trauma, a distortion in the memories surrounding it, and the adoption of problematic behaviors and thoughts in an attempt to cope. It is this third feature that fuels the PTSD symptoms further. Effective CBT targets all three features, aiming to undo them and thus provide relief from the psychological suffering. CBT for PTSD is an overarching banner term that encompasses many therapies. The most effective are cognitive processing therapy (CPT) and prolonged exposure (PE).

Developed by Drs. Patricia Resick, Candice Monson, and Kathleen Chard, CPT involves a careful dissection of all the cognitions related to the patient's trauma. Trauma survivors typically have inaccurate cognitions that take control of their lives. For example, "If only I had not worn that dress, the rape would not have happened" or "If I had gotten there just two minutes earlier, I would have saved his life." Such faulty cognitions fuel PTSD symptoms, and CPT systematically challenges them. Guided by the therapist, the patient writes a detailed trauma account, reads it in session, and together they identify which thoughts are accurate and which are not. Through therapy, the patient undergoes a restructuring of the cognitions. Although CPT is most effective when offered to patients on an individual basis, it can also work well as a group therapy.

CPT also focuses on the experience of cognitive dissonance commonly found in PTSD sufferers, whose experience of trauma does not mesh with their pretrauma belief system. For example, prior to experiencing trauma, it is common for people to believe that "bad things happen only to bad people," that they can competently handle their lives, and that the world is a predictable place. Experiencing a traumatic event often shatters these beliefs, causing great psychological distress. CPT helps the sufferer reevaluate his or her core belief system and adjust it to fit the new reality.

PE, which was developed by Dr. Edna Foa, a psychologist at the University of Pennsylvania, remains one of the most effective treatments for PTSD. In PE, the therapist guides the patient through a repeated replay of the trauma. This process, called exposure, essentially encourages the patient to confront memories, objects, activities, and situations that trigger the trauma symptoms so that he or she gradually becomes desensitized to the anxiety and stress associated with these triggers. The triggers can involve trauma memories (internal cues) or factors in the environment (external cues).

For internal cues, the therapist asks the patient to vividly describe the memories of the trauma and include as much sensory detail as possible. The veteran who survived a deadly bombing in a crowded market, for example, might recall an image of people running around in chaos, the sound of screams, the smell of burning flesh, thinking that he was going to die, and feeling terrified.

For external cues, therapists encourage patients to expose themselves to environmental cues that trigger their PTSD symptoms. This same veteran, who might have hypervigilance and avoid crowds, will be encouraged to expose himself to a series of situations to help him overcome his fear of being around large groups of people. He might start with a trip to Walmart during a quiet weekday. If this outing is successful, the next week he may be challenged further and visit a mall on a busier weekend. Engaging in such exposure exercises helps the patient by diminishing the power of triggers to hijack his body and brain in the way they did prior to treatment.

Dr. Craig Rosen, a psychologist and researcher at the National Center for PTSD, described some of the overarching principles of how talk therapy helps:

> Trauma thoughts and memories are often "unspeakable" and "unthinkable" and it is because of this that the normal processes of recovery, after trauma, are impeded. They are like a dramatic movie trailer, so immediate and vivid

to experience, but by themselves they do not tell the whole story. These unspeakable trauma memories or thoughts become stuck points that inhibit the mental reintegration that is needed for healing. . . . These fragmented memories need to be integrated into a larger narrative, new learning needs to be added to old memory cues, and pre-trauma-related beliefs all need to be re-assessed.

Another important point Rosen reminded me of was that there is a misperception that having a survivor simply tell the trauma story is enough: "When someone has PTSD, a one-time telling is simply an opening and not a cure. The trauma story needs to be told over and over, with the assistance of a skilled professional, for it to be properly worked through."

Contrary to popular belief, deliberately exposing oneself to trauma memories in this fashion does not make symptoms worse; indeed, when it is done with the help of a skilled therapist, PTSD symptoms improve.

All these CBT therapies also include, as part of their protocols, education about the nature of trauma exposure, traumatic stress, and anxiety management skills such as breathing and muscle relaxation exercises. Grounding techniques are also taught in which patients learn strategies to help them detach from emotional pain and regain control over their feelings. A patient might learn to clench and release her fists when she is bombarded with intrusive memories or to self-soothe by remembering the words of an inspiring quote.

A promising technological advance currently being tested is virtual reality exposure therapy. This therapy uses real-time computer graphics, body-tracking devices, visual displays, and other sensory input devices to create a virtual world of exposure. A variant of the imaginal exposure typically used in PTSD therapies, virtual reality exposure is being actively investigated to see how effective it can be in reducing PTSD symptoms. Another way in which therapy is being reengineered is by offering it in a more intensive package. British researchers compressed versions of trauma-focused psychotherapies into a seven-day intensive treatment. This was found to work as well as the original therapy, which was offered once a week over twelve weeks. In another British study almost 250 veterans with PTSD were offered an intensive six-week residential treatment program consisting of a mixture of individual and group sessions. The researchers noted a significant reduction in PTSD symptoms that were maintained at a six-month follow-up.

Eye movement desensitization and reprocessing (EMDR) and brief eclectic psychotherapy are also considered first-line therapies for PTSD. Developed by Dr. Francine Shapiro in 1990, EMDR engages patients in a trauma memory in brief sequential doses while they simultaneously focus on an external stimulus. The external stimulus may be the therapist directing the patient in performing lateral eye movements, tapping a hand, or listening to audio stimulation. One of the touted benefits of EMDR over other therapies is that results can be achieved in just a few sessions, so the therapy is less intense than CPT or PE, which often require the patients to do homework exercises in addition to attending sessions.

Brief eclectic psychotherapy was developed by Dr. Berthold Gersons in the 1980s and, as the name suggests, combines elements of different psychotherapies with an emphasis on the fear and the horror associated with the traumatic event. More attention is given to patients' personal background, such as experiences in childhood, and their unique personality style.

On the global front, finding effective ways to treat large swaths of traumatized people who live in conflict-ridden low-resource settings is an important challenge. Clinicians working with such populations have long recognized the importance of acknowledging societal trauma as part of treatment. In recent years, a group of German psychologists combined the testimony therapy developed in Latin America in the 1980s with exposure to create narrative exposure therapy (NET). Along with exposure exercises, NET's protocol specifies that, upon the request of patients, their anonymous testimony can be passed on to humanitarian organizations to document human rights abuses, thus enabling survivors to place their traumatic experiences in a vital wider social and historical context.

What impact do all these trauma-focused psychotherapies have on the PTSD brain and body? The hippocampus (a part of the brain crucial to memory formation) is smaller in people who have PTSD. The PTSD brain also has an exaggerated amygdala response and a frontal lobe that is more inactive than it should be and thus unable to exert control over the misfiring amygdala. Psychotherapy appears to decrease amygdala activity and increase activity in the frontal and hippocampal regions. On the molecular level, early studies suggest that DNA breakages in the cells of PTSD sufferers heal after psychotherapy, and exposure therapy has been found to boost the immune systems of PTSD sufferers.

It is important to recognize that although the therapies discussed here have been scientifically proved to be effective for many people, they may not help every PTSD sufferer. Moreover, it is often hard to predict which therapy might work for whom, so there is often a trial-and-error process as the therapist figures out what the best approach is for a given sufferer.

***

Despite the fact that we have effective talk therapies for PTSD, it is widely recognized that many sufferers are not seeking these treatments and when they do, the dropout rate is high. This reluctance is likely related to the daunting nature of revisiting the traumatic event. For many who live with PTSD, the prospect of engaging in cognitive restructuring or exposure exercises may be simply too much to deal with.

In response to problems with dropout and engagement, approaches that focus less on the trauma have been used with encouraging results. Dr. Marylene Cloitre, a psychologist at New York University and the National Center for PTSD, developed Skills Training in Affective and Interpersonal Regulation (STAIR). STAIR focuses on the practical consequences of living with PTSD every day. It teaches sufferers simple skills to manage their negative emotions and improve their personal relationships and has proved to be a powerful alternative to trauma-focused therapies in sufferers with severe PTSD.

Acceptance and commitment therapy (ACT) is another treatment that can be helpful to PTSD sufferers. It combines mindfulness with encouraging patients to approach life and reengage in activities in a manner that is consistent with their personal values. Integrating spiritual approaches into the treatment of combat-related PTSD is also another area of intense interest. The results of one study hinted that veterans with PTSD who scored higher on dimensions of spirituality seem to fare better in treatment, and incorporating the spiritual dimensions of trauma-related issues offers the promise of making treatment more effective.

Talk therapy approaches work well for patients who are psychologically minded, accustomed to solving their problems by using reason and logic, and comfortable with reading, writing, and doing homework exercises. Of course, not everyone approaches life from this perspective, and alternative approaches that tap into dimensions beyond the cognitive have become increasingly popular.

Mind-body treatments such as mindfulness, relaxation (which includes biofeedback training, imagery, visualization, and progressive muscle relaxation), meditation, yoga, tai chi, massage, acupuncture, and hypnosis are widely used by patients with PTSD. There is some promising evidence to support the effectiveness of approaches such as yoga and acupuncture.

Preliminary evidence also supports approaches such as electro-encephalographic (EEG) biofeedback and mindfulness training. EEG biofeedback, also known as neurofeedback, has been in use as a treatment for more than thirty years and is now being studied in relation to PTSD. It is a behavioral therapy technique that iden-tifies the patient's abnormal brain electrical activity by connecting the patient to an electroencephalograph. The therapist then engages the patient in cognitive exercises to retrain the brain and change abnormal EEG patterns. A recent pilot study used neurofeedback for individuals with treatment-resistant PTSD, and the participants who completed forty sessions of neurofeedback training reported significantly reduced symptoms.

Mindfulness-based practices aim to cultivate patients' awareness of their thoughts, emotions, and behaviors on a moment-to-moment basis with the hope that this awareness will lead them to approach life in a nonjudgmental, kind, and curious manner. It challenges the traditional basis of many psychological therapies that require patients to "fake it till you make it" when they are retraining their behaviors. Instead, mindfulness aims to evoke curiosity and invites the patient to step out of older behaviors and let go of them naturally. A four-session mindfulness training program was offered to sixty-two veterans with PTSD in a randomized controlled study. The veterans who completed the program reported significant decreases in PTSD and depression symptoms, results that were maintained eight weeks later.

Art therapy can leverage artistic expression as a channel for sufferers to express their values, goals, thoughts, and emotions. Sports activities such as group cycling programs can target PTSD symptoms such as social isolation and avoidance. Programs that harness the power of nature, such as hiking, fishing, farming, surfing, gardening, and building relationships with animals including horses are also garnering increasing attention. Dance programs have been offered as complementary health approaches for veterans with chronic and severe PTSD, and many participants are overwhelmingly positive about their experiences. Perhaps one of the most talked about activities has been the use of dogs as service or emotional support animals for PTSD sufferers. Though all these alternative approaches hold appeal for many PTSD sufferers, it is important to note that they remain largely untested.

The shortage of mental health professionals in the United States, particularly in inner cities and rural towns, often limits the availability of effective talk therapies. Moreover, making the commitment to attend weekly sessions over a three- to four-month period may feel like a luxury for many. Lack of child care options, insurance co-pays, having to lay out gas money for every visit, and not having paid leave from a job are all common obstacles that patients tell me prevent them from committing to therapy. Then there are, of course, those whose symptoms are too severe, who are unable to tolerate the process of therapy, or who may have tried therapy but not found it helpful. For all these reasons, the default treatment for PTSD is often psychotropic medication.

PSYCH MEDS

Everything was numbered: the lenses, the painterly sky, the milligrams of my panic pills. I had prescription eyes that allowed me to see better, and prescription pills that allowed me to play blind.

—Jalina Mhyana, *Dreaming in Night Vision: A Story in Vignettes*

SESSION 1

Susan is a 50-year-old Caucasian female. Works as a teacher and lives with her teenage children. Recently moved to the area after an acrimonious divorce.

She reports a 20-year history of traumatic symptoms related to extensive childhood sexual abuse and then marital rape.

Recent worsening of symptoms because of the stress of the move, new job, and divorce.

Is currently depressed and has insomnia and trauma-related nightmares. Experiences no enjoyment in life and is socially isolated.

Poor motivation and concentration (intrusive memories of abuse) are interfering with her work performance. She is still on probation and fears being fired and losing housing and access to good schools for her children.

Main concern, "I spend 50% of my life feeling fearful." Fears she will be sexually assaulted again.

Is scared at home, jumps at the slightest noise, won't stand near the windows or go out after dark. Takes a knife with her if she gets up to use the bathroom at night.

Has had some therapy (not trauma focused, "too daunting"). She has never tried medication before and is ambivalent, "I would feel like a failure."

IMPRESSION:
PTSD

PLAN:
   1. Recommend a trial of low-dose daily
      sertraline 25 mg with plan to titrate up
      dosage over the next several weeks.
   2. Return to clinic in 2 weeks.

SESSION 2

Susan reports that her coworkers have noticed a change. She is feeling more energetic and less afraid. Daily adherence with sertraline and no acute side effects.

Depressive and other traumatic stress symptoms remain.

IMPRESSION:
PTSD

PLAN:
   1. Increase daily sertraline to 50 mg.
   2. Return to clinic in 2 weeks.

SESSION 3

Susan reports improvement. Less anxiety, hyper-vigilance, and fear. More relaxed than she has felt in years. Daily adherence with sertraline and no acute side effects.

Remains socially isolated and with nightly insomnia.

IMPRESSION:
PTSD

PLAN:
1. Increase daily sertraline to 100 mg.
2. Return to clinic in 4 weeks.

SESSION 4

Susan reports that the medicine has been helpful. Noticeably less hypervigilance and anxiety. She has more energy, able to juggle more with the kids, getting more enjoyment out of day-to-day life. Daily adherence with sertraline and no side effects.

Insomnia, nocturnal anxiety, and nightmares are still a significant issue.

IMPRESSION:
PTSD

PLAN:
1. Increase daily sertraline to 150 mg.
2. Return to clinic in 4 weeks.

SESSION 5

Susan reports she met with her sister, who tells her she is "a different person." Reports an almost 100% improvement in symptoms. Anxiety, fear, and hypervigilance have dissipated. She has even noticed fewer migraines and therefore takes fewer sick days from work. Was able to enjoy the holidays and visit with some friends and family, has not done this in years. Feels able to relax in her own home. Insomnia and nightmares have also improved; patient has more energy and better work performance. Daily adherence with sertraline and no side effects.

IMPRESSION:
PTSD

PLAN:
  1. Continue sertraline 150 mg.
  2. Return to clinic in 3 months.

SESSION 6

Susan reports she feels great. Sustained 100% improvement in symptoms with current dose of sertraline. She reports feeling physically different as the tension from the constant fear is gone. Has been more active, able to drive after dark, took the children out for dinner to celebrate their good grades.

These experiences further reinforce her confidence. Daily adherence with sertraline and no side effects.

IMPRESSION:
PTSD

PLAN:
1. Continue sertraline 150 mg.
2. Strongly recommended the patient consider
   a course of trauma-focused psychotherapy
   as an additional nonpharmacological way
   of treating her PTSD that can provide
   additional benefits. She is agreeable to
   this.
3. Return to clinic in 6 months. If patient
   remains symptom free will consider tapering
   off sertraline.

***

Antidepressant medications are effective treatments for many PTSD sufferers. The label "antidepressants" is misleading because these medications are helpful for a variety of mental health issues beyond depression with PTSD, anxiety disorder, obsessive compulsive disorder, and impulse control disorder being just a few examples. Several medications fall under the banner term of antidepressants, but the selective serotonin reuptake inhibitors (SSRIs) are the medications that have been most thoroughly investigated in PTSD.

The SSRIs fluoxetine, paroxetine, and sertraline, which have been studied in trials with more than 3,000 PTSD sufferers, have been found to reduce levels of intrusion, emotional numbing, and hypervigilance. Precisely how they work remains unknown, but it has been hypothesized that they target the serotonergic dysfunctions that belie many PTSD symptoms. One of the benefits of using this class of medications is that they are tried and tested. Many of them have been on the market for decades and prescribed to millions of people.

The decision as to which antidepressant to prescribe is often determined by factors specific to the individual patient. If my patient complains bitterly of insomnia, then mirtazapine can be useful; it is thought to target the brain's histamine receptors and cause sedation, which helps ease insomnia when the medication is taken at bedtime. The antidepressant venlafaxine is a serious contender for patients who also suffer from chronic pain because not only is there excellent evidence that it is effective for PTSD but it has analgesic properties, too. It always makes sense to use one medication to target many problems because this lean approach results in fewer side effects and harmful drug-drug reactions.

Medical genetics is not currently able to predict which patient is best suited to which antidepressant, so I often ask crude, but nonetheless useful, questions: Do you have any biological relatives who suffer from traumatic stress, anxiety, or depression? If so, do you know what medications worked for them? Did they have side effects? The answers to these questions help me decide which medication to choose for my patient.

The good news is that up to 60 percent of sufferers will have a good response to SSRI medications. Beyond contributing to overall patient well-being and symptom improvement, medications also lead to changes in the PTSD brain. A recent series of small neuro-imaging studies has shown that medications increase hippocampal volume, reduce amygdala firing, and increase prefrontal activation in the brains of treated PTSD patients.

Susan's case is just one of the many I have seen in which a PTSD sufferer experiences a life-altering transformation on medication.

In Susan's favor was that despite her initial ambivalence, she was committed to the treatment process and took the medication as instructed, did not skip doses, and came for her follow-up appointments. The fact that Susan did not abuse alcohol or use illicit drugs and consumed minimal amounts of caffeine likely contributed to her experiencing the full benefits the medication had to offer. Patients like Susan often express regret that they did not try medication sooner and that they suffered unnecessarily for too long.

Patients often come to me with erroneous beliefs about what psychiatric medications can and cannot do. They fear that they will become a zombie or get hooked on the pills or the medications will change the very essence of who they are. I tell patients that these medications are not magic bullets or happy pills but an opportunity for them to become the best version of themselves again. The pills require weeks to take effect, and patients must make a commitment to take them every day. I stress the importance of keeping follow-up visits because, over time, I can fine-tune their dose so they will experience maximum benefits with minimal side effects.

One should be able to live a full and active life while taking these medications. They must be taken as prescribed, not mixed with alcohol and street drugs, and doses should never be self-adjusted on a whim. I don't intend for my patients to stay on these medications forever; rather, I view them as a crutch, something to lean on while the brain and body are given a proper chance to heal. If a patient is symptom free for six months, I will always float the option of tapering off the medication altogether. Visits can be spaced out once my patients are stable, but until that time comes, I keep a close eye on them, preferring to see them every few weeks.

***

For those with severe or chronic PTSD, antidepressant medications may not be helpful enough. My own research has shown that classes of psychotropics such as mood stabilizers and second-generation antipsychotics (SGAs) are commonly prescribed for PTSD despite the fact that the science supporting such prescribing remains sketchy.

Mood stabilizers such as carbamazepine, divalproex, lamotrigine, and topiramate have been studied in PTSD research trials. These medications affect the balance between the brain chemicals glutamate, which excites nerve cells, and gamma-aminobutyric acid (GABA), which dampens the activity of nerve cells. It is thought that the restoration of balance has a favorable impact on the PTSD symptoms of irritability, anger, and aggression. Some studies suggest that topiramate has value for patients who fail first-line PTSD treatments. Other than this, research with other mood stabilizers has yielded mixed or negative results, and the value of this class of medications for PTSD sufferers remains questionable.

The use of SGAs such as olanzapine, quetiapine, and risperidone for PTSD patients is controversial. SGAs came onto the market in the late 1990s and were originally designed to treat severe mental illnesses such as schizophrenia and bipolar disorder, but a series of small controlled trials hinted that they might also be beneficial for PTSD sufferers. SGAs act on the balance between dopaminergic and serotonergic neurotransmitter systems and therefore impact mood stability and anxiety levels. Dopamine has been implicated in the abnormalities in emotional reactivity, executive functioning, and stress responses found in PTSD sufferers, so it makes sense that SGAs may be helpful.

Early studies found that SGAs helped dampen the intrusive memories and hypervigilance so frequently associated with chronic PTSD, and clinicians started offering baby doses of SGAs to PTSD patients who had these problems. To be clear, SGAs had not been officially approved for use in PTSD, but frontline clinicians, disenchanted by their patients' poor response to antidepressants, were searching for ways to help relieve their patients' suffering. The prescribing of SGAs was justified mainly because the doses being used were nowhere near the doses needed to treat patients with severe mental illness.

But then came mounting concerns that SGAs were causing patients to gain weight and develop high cholesterol levels and diabetes. At the same time, the United States was in the throes of an obesity epidemic. Psychiatrists were therefore duty bound to rethink the use of these medications for patients. In 2007, researchers from the National Center for PTSD and Yale University embarked upon a three-year trial investigating if the SGA risperidone was an effective adjunctive treatment for PTSD patients who did not respond to antidepressants alone. The results were disappointing. Patients who received risperidone showed little improvement in their PTSD symptoms. Furthermore, they reported more side effects in the form of weight gain, fatigue, and sleepiness. The study results, which were published in *The Journal of the American Medical Association*, were clear: using risperidone as an adjunctive treatment for PTSD was *not* an effective treatment strategy.

I now stay clear of this class of medications for my PTSD patients and prescribe them only for those who have exhausted all other avenues or if their symptoms are so severe that they are rendering them a danger to themselves or other people. Even then, my prescription is accompanied by careful counseling about the risks and benefits of the medication and my keeping a close eye on their weight and cholesterol and glucose levels. At every appointment, I revisit the decision to use SGAs and see if the time has come when we can start to taper off.

Recent studies indicate that the pendulum may be swinging back in favor of SGAs. The pain point spurring these studies remains the fact that not all PTSD patients respond to antidepressants, and doctors are eager to learn what other options might be available to them. In a study of eighty veterans with chronic PTSD, scientists investigated whether the SGA quetiapine would be effective as a stand-alone agent when compared with a placebo. Patients in the quetiapine group experienced improvement in their PTSD intrusive thinking and hyperarousal scores, and researchers found no adverse impact on weight. These early results suggest that quetiapine may have value as a stand-alone treatment for PTSD.

Some experimental approaches that use medications to boost the beneficial effects of talk therapies have also yielded encouraging results. D-cycloserine is a medication that is a partial agonist of the N-methyl-D-aspartate (NMDA) receptor, a brain receptor that plays an essential role in learning and memory. Preliminary data suggest that D-cycloserine can be useful in enhancing the effect of psychotherapy provided to patients with severe PTSD. A study at the Bronx, New York, VA hospital examined whether hydrocortisone pills can improve the effectiveness of prolonged exposure (PE) for PTSD. Veterans who received hydrocortisone showed greater reductions in their symptoms after a ten-week course of PE and also a lower dropout rate from therapy. More recently, similar results have been reported with the alpha 2 adrenergic receptor antagonist Yohimbine. Transcranial magnetic stimulation, a procedure which uses a magnetic coil to stimulate the prefrontal cortex, offered prior to Cognitive Processing Therapy (CPT) may also enhance a person's response to the therapy.

One class of medications that has emerged as a clear villain in the story of PTSD treatments is benzodiazepines, which include medications such as lorazepam, clonazepam, alprazolam, temazepam, and diazepam. These pills are popular among patients for the simple reason that they offer rapid relief from the anxiety and insomnia symptoms that are common PTSD complaints. The problem is that this short-term relief comes at a long-term cost. Not only is there a lack of evidence supporting their effectiveness in reducing symptoms, but data suggest that these medications actually make the symptoms worse.

A massive problem with benzodiazepines is their side effects. Researchers have carefully documented their abuse potential, something to be taken seriously when we consider how addiction and traumatic stress often go hand in hand. For older patients, the side effects are particularly hazardous: memory difficulties, confusion, impaired driving, and increased odds of falling and sustaining a hip fracture.

Benzodiazepines fell seriously out of favor with the publication of a 2012 big-data study in the *British Medical Journal*. The authors followed more than 10,000 patients who were prescribed these medications, mostly to treat insomnia, and found a 50 percent increase in overall mortality rates associated with their long-term use. Today, if I prescribe benzodiazepines to my patients, it is usually a supply for no more than a few days, something to keep in their medicine cabinet for emergency use only.

MEDICATION MANAGEMENT

In my early professional years I was asking the question, How can I treat, or cure, or change this person? Now I would phrase the question in this way: How can I provide a relationship which this person may use for his own personal growth?

—Carl R. Rogers, *On Becoming a Person: A Therapist's View of Psychotherapy*

For a long time, I understood "medication management" as an insurance term with little clinical value. Today, I have come to view it as embodying fundamental principles of good psychiatric practice. In our increasingly fragmented health care systems, in which we are all being required to do more with less, the fundamentals of treatment often get pushed aside. What does high-quality medication management look like? If you are seeking help for PTSD or help for a loved one, how can you tell you are getting the best care?

Honoring the Journey

It is not unusual, when I first meet patients, for them to minimize their distress. They try to present their best self and often try to talk themselves out of the need to see me. Sometimes it's tempting to collude with my patients, but then I remind myself to honor their journey to my office. Most people, if they could alleviate their trauma symptoms themselves, would do so. If taking a vacation;

spending more time in nature; having regular heart-to-hearts with their spouse, mother, father, or priest; taking a spinning class; training for a marathon; or consuming herbal teas could bring them real and sustained relief, then of course they would never reach out for professional attention.

More often than not, by the time patients make it to my office they have hit their version of rock bottom and are facing one or many of the following: marital tension; poor job performance; legal repercussions of their behaviors, such as driving under the influence of alcohol or domestic violence; homelessness; or having thoughts of suicide. Many have tried or at least dabbled in talk therapies but have experienced little relief. Reminding myself and my patients of the gravity of the situation is a fundamental of good treatment.

Therapeutic Alliance

Perhaps one of the biggest challenges to physicians is how to preserve our relationship with our patients. Today, many of us operate in settings in which we are pushed for time and bombarded by a constant stream of interruptions that have us focusing more on computer screens, pagers, voice mails, and instant messages than on the patient sitting in front of us. Not only is this frustrating for us as doctors, it is hazardous for our patients. Such an environment inhibits trust, rapport building, and the development of what, in my field, we call alliance.

Forming a therapeutic alliance with our patients is a fundamental of good psychiatric practice; it promotes collaboration, trust, and mutual respect. It can take years to build with false starts and setbacks, but the physician's commitment to maintaining it must be unwavering. Any factors that interfere with this dynamic thwart patients' inclination to disclose what is on their minds, share their fears and darkest thoughts, and be truthful in their communication with us. My job, as the treating clinician, is to preserve the sanctity of this relationship. It's important not to confuse creating a therapeutic alliance with having a warm and fuzzy relationship with one's psychiatrist. As I often tell my patients, "My job is *not* to be your friend, but it is my job to be your well-wisher, and sometimes that involves my saying things you might not want to hear."

A Thorough Psychiatric Evaluation

It's hard to imagine how any clinician could effectively treat traumatic stress without having done a thorough evaluation of the patient. This fundamental principle can get shortchanged in large health care organizations where dozens of professionals are asking patients a variety of questions and documenting all the answers in one electronic medical record. Though it's true that it does not make sense to repeatedly ask the same questions of my patients, I find that the act of my engaging them in providing this personal data builds their alliance with me. Furthermore, this one-on-one, live, real-time conversation leaves an imprint of their life story in my mind that reading an electronic medical record will never do.

Treatment Setting

In an ideal world, psychiatrists should have available to them a variety of options for where their patients can receive treatment. Patients who pose a serious threat of harm to themselves or others should have the option of hospitalization. Someone whose drinking is out of control should be offered a stay in rehab. Unfortunately, because of inadequate access to mental health care for many, psychiatrists are often put into the very difficult position of caring for PTSD patients in subpar settings. We are often required to defend our medical decisions in a way our colleagues in other medical specialties are not for the simple reason that societal stigma toward mental illness remains rampant.

Several years ago, I was talking to the relative of a patient and explaining to her that the insurance company had denied the patient coverage for a thirty-day stay at a residential program for his severe alcohol addiction. This relative was quite incredulous about the insurance company's decision. Don't they understand how sick he is? He has lost his job and his marriage. If he gets discharged this early, he will just start drinking again! After a few moments of silence, she admitted to me that she was a senior executive at a health insurance company, but she was so far removed from the consequences of her decisions that she had had no idea of their impact on real lives until it hit close to home.

Medication management needs to be supported with organizational scaffolding. Pills, by themselves, will never be enough.

Communication

US health care is famous for being fragmented. With so many different medical specialties, multidisciplinary teams, health care systems, and insurance providers involved, the simple task of talking to one another becomes daunting and thus a low priority for busy clinicians. This lack of communication can have disastrous consequences for patients. At minimum, before prescribing medication for patients with PTSD, I like to know the results of their last physical examination, what their vital signs are, and the results of any basic laboratory tests. An accurate list of all their current medications is vital to avoiding bad reactions between the pills they are already taking and the ones I will be prescribing. If they are seeing a therapist in parallel with seeing me, it's important that the therapist and I communicate about our mutual patient.

The power of supportive family or friends cannot be over-emphasized. Attentive children who call me when they sense their parent is struggling, spouses who nudge their loved ones to refill their medication, a good friend who offers to accompany a patient to an AA meeting, or a sibling who offers to drive a patient to appointments—all these acts and gestures have a significant impact on a patient's prognosis.

Quality of Life

PTSD impacts many spheres of a person's life, including work, school, family, and social relationships. Having stable housing, employment, and financial security is crucial for many sufferers. Unfortunately, it has become easier for psychiatrists to pull out a prescription pad than to take the time to advocate for their patients, make phone calls, write letters, nag colleagues, or insist that these services be provided within our health care systems.

Wellness

Living a healthy lifestyle is inextricably linked to mental well-being. I tell patients that any steps taken toward improving their wellness will augment and reinforce the positive effects of their medication. Eating a well-balanced, nutritious diet and exercising regularly are integral to good mental health.

One area of wellness I find myself talking about more and more with my patients is sleep. As a culture, we seem to be forgetting how to sleep. It started with irregular work schedules and shift work that messed up our body clocks, and then came a wave of popularity of heavily caffeinated beverages and energy supplements that kept people too wired to sleep. Cheap large-screen TVs found their way into bedrooms and primed our brains to equate bedtime with channel surfing as opposed to falling asleep. The arrival of smartphones and tablets brought to our bedrooms a never-ending stream of alerts, notifications, and messages.

It boils down to a basic matter of biology: sleep offers the brain an abundance of restorative functions that we are still in our infancy of understanding. I always recommend having a regular sleep routine, avoiding caffeine and daytime naps, and making the bedroom a screen-free zone as essentials for anyone living with PTSD.

Medication Adherence

Not a month goes by without my meeting a patient who has decided to stop taking a medication or never filled the prescription in the first place. Patients' stopping medication prematurely is a fact of life in PTSD treatment. Moreover, if physicians don't talk about the obstacles that are contributing to treatment adherence, then patients are erroneously labeled as treatment resistant and prescribed more medications under the false assumption that the original medications did not work.

Why do people suddenly stop taking their prescription medication? Some feel better and so assume they no longer need medication; some view having to take medication as a personal failure, and taking the pill every day reminds them of this. Others can't afford their co-pay or are frustrated by their lack of progress or side effects, and a few have a change of heart after talking to friends or reading something unfavorable about their medicine on the Internet.

Another reason is a deep-rooted mistrust of the medical profession, especially psychiatry. Though I am aware of (and sympathetic to) the historical antecedents of such mistrust, I am also saddened when patients stigmatize psychiatry on the basis of perceptions that are grossly misinformed. Good psychiatrists don't push pills; neither do they have the power to whimsically lock up their patients for prolonged hospitalizations. Today's psychiatrists have such extensive medical training that they emerge from residency uniquely equipped to treat their patients in a way that integrates both brain and body.

Rather than working in isolation, psychiatry has long valued the benefits of a multidisciplinary approach to care, and we are now primed to advocate for tried and tested treatments over fads and unproven remedies. As a group we are more diverse than other branches of medicine, and what sustains many of us in a profession that has lower prestige (and pay) than other medical specialties is a passion for a field that still values our patients' stories and the artistry of medicine.

When faced with patients who are not adhering to their prescription, I encourage them to be open about their choice. Regardless of their reasons for stopping, I keep the door open for future communication should they change their mind. This openness means I can spend weeks, and even months, simply being a companion to my patient as he or she navigates this process. Sometimes being a steadfast companion on a patient's journey toward recovery is the most valuable service a physician can provide.

THE ALLURE OF MAGIC
BULLETS

People are always looking for the single magic bullet that will totally
change everything. There is no single magic bullet.
—Temple Grandin, author

When I talk about PTSD to professional audiences, I am often asked
my opinion about an experimental treatment that someone read
about in a magazine or saw on TV. I have a healthy skepticism toward PTSD treatments that are touted as magic bullets, mostly
because they tend to get a disproportionate amount of public attention before they have been scientifically proved to be effective.
This attention raises false hopes for patients who are desperate and
often means they will be disappointed by treatments that end up
overpromising and underdelivering. Of course, if a PTSD sufferer
has exhausted all other treatment options to no avail, turning
to the experimental makes perfect sense. What I find frustrating is
when patients forgo tried and tested treatments, which they perceive
as too time-consuming or do not promise sufficient relief, for experimental products that have not been thoroughly vetted.

In 2008, reports started to emerge about how a stellate ganglion
block, an invasive manipulation of sympathetic nerve tissue, had
helped PTSD sufferers. The procedure, which consisted of injecting
a local anesthetic into sympathetic nerve tissue in the neck, had led
to immediate symptom relief in a small group of patients. The stellate
ganglion block, which took less than thirty minutes to deliver, nat-

urally caught the attention of many of my patients who heard about it on the news or read about it on the Internet. What was not made clear in much of the coverage was that a positive outcome in a few cases is not sufficient to label something a treatment. A treatment should be more effective than a placebo, so it needs to be studied under controlled conditions. It took some time for the first controlled study of the stellate ganglion block to be done, and the results, which were reported in 2016, were disappointing: the block was not superior to a sham injection in relieving PTSD. Unfortunately, these negative results did not grab headlines, yet the misleading buzz that surrounded the early reports will remain on the Internet forever.

Some other touted magic bullets that are still considered experimental, but nonetheless have generated much attention, are ketamine, MDMA, and medical marijuana.

Ketamine is a nonbarbiturate anesthetic and antagonist at the NMDA receptor. It is typically administered intravenously and has been used for years to provide pain relief to patients with severe burns. It was during this use that its dissociative properties became apparent. Ketamine may disrupt the process by which traumatic memories are laid down, as some studies show that those who received ketamine after a traumatic event were less likely to go on to develop PTSD. A 2014 paper in *The Journal of the American Medical Association* reported on a controlled study that demonstrated a rapid reduction in symptom severity following ketamine infusion in patients with chronic PTSD. It's important to note the limitations associated with ketamine: its benefits may last only a few weeks, and there is a potential for patients getting addicted to it.

The last few years have seen an interest in using MDMA (3,4-methylenedioxymethamphetamine, also known as ecstasy) to enhance the effects of psychological therapy for PTSD sufferers. The popularity of using MDMA in psychiatry has waxed and waned over the years, and some experts have welcomed its comeback. The data remain thin, however, with only a couple of small randomized controlled studies showing an improvement in traumatic stress symptoms. Such small studies cannot assure the safety of MDMA use on a long-term basis.

Once or twice a month patients will ask me whether medical marijuana would be helpful for their PTSD. Many of these patients disclose that they have used marijuana recreationally and found it very helpful, sometimes more than their prescription drugs. As the medical marijuana movement gathers more steam, I'm increasingly aware that veterans, their families, lawmakers, and politicians feel strongly that physicians should assist those who want to take medical marijuana for their PTSD symptoms, and this puts me into a bind.

Neuroscientists have put forth convincing arguments of the value in targeting the cannabinoid receptors in the brains of PTSD sufferers, but the current data to support the use of medical marijuana in the real world are scant to nonexistent. In 2016, investigators with Abraham Ribicoff Research Facilities at the Yale School of Medicine pored over thirteen studies examining the efficacy of marijuana for psychiatric symptoms. They found no controlled trials that had studied marijuana use in PTSD patients and, in essence, very little evidence to support the practice.

This lack of evidence is further complicated by my concerns about the potential of harm. Such was the case for my patient Tom, who viewed hospitals and doctors with grim suspicion. He was not shy about airing his antigovernment views and came to the VA clinic "only when I have to . . . when I have no choice." In quarterly appointments with me, I did what he would allow—a cursory check-in and a refill of his antidepressant prescription—but he needed more. He was a prickly character prone to rants and raves and bouts of depression and avoided social situations as much as possible. He needed more than a prescription, and I reminded him of that regularly.

Tom got a medical marijuana card about a year ago and told me that the drug was tremendously helpful for his nightmares and insomnia, "Way more than that pharmaceutical junk you give me!" But what started off as occasional use two to three times per week gradually creeped up to daily use. At a recent visit I asked him how much marijuana he was using. I looked him straight in the eye, waiting patiently for his answer.

Tom blushed red. "Well, I'll speak the truth, Dr. Jain. You know I have nothing to hide. I have been using it a few times a day now, not just at night. It really takes the edge off my anxiety, keeps me calm. You know I have that spot of arthritis in my right knee, so it helps with the pain, too . . . But I *never* use it when Collette is with me . . . you need to know that. I draw the line there."

Tom was divorced and shared custody of his only child, a teenage girl. On the days Collette was with him, he prepared a healthy breakfast, packed her lunch, did school drop-off and pickup, and chauffeured her to after-school cheerleading meets and study groups.

"Okay, so let me get this straight. On the days that Collette is with you, you don't use? Correct?"

Tom shook his head vigorously. "Oh, no, I use. I have to, every day, but not in front of her . . . you know, I'll take a bit before breakfast, and then a bit later, just after lunch, and then just before bed . . . depends on how hectic her schedule is . . ."

"So if I'm hearing this right, you may use medical marijuana in the morning before dropping Collette off at school? Bear with me for a second here, and consider this scenario . . . if your daughter wanted to get a ride with a kid who smoked marijuana daily or a parent who, like yourself, had a medical marijuana card, would you let her ride in their car?"

Tom's face froze. "No . . . no . . . of course not."

"But you think it is okay for her to ride with you?"

Tom shook his head gently. "I get it, Dr. Jain . . . I get it. You make a good point. I guess I thought I had it all under control . . . I am going to have to rethink what it is I'm doing here."

In their zeal to promote the beneficial effects of marijuana, proponents often downplay the downsides. Just because it is natural does not mean it is safe, and any substance that is powerful enough to alter brain chemistry can be expected to have side effects. Science is already aware that chronic exposure to marijuana can lead to addiction, and for younger adults, early and persistent marijuana use has been associated with psychosis. Marijuana also impairs an individual's attention, memory, IQ, and driving ability. For patients with PTSD, one observational study found that starting marijuana use after PTSD treatment worsened symptoms and led to more violent behavior and alcohol use. It also nullified the benefits of specialized PTSD treatment.

There are probably few people who understand the relationship between cannabis use and PTSD better than Dr. Marcel Bonn-Miller, a researcher at the University of Pennsylvania Perelman School of Medicine. I asked him if, in his cutting-edge work, he could share a perspective that might give me reason to be more optimistic about the promise of medical marijuana and share the enthusiasm my patients have about this treatment.

Bonn-Miller reminded me that the majority of studies documenting negative consequences of cannabis suffer from a major flaw: they discuss the plant as if it were homogeneous. In fact, there are many cannabinoids and other chemical compounds present within the cannabis plant, with D9-tetrahydrocannabinol (THC) and cannabidiol

(CBD) having received the most scientific attention. He told me that the first two randomized controlled trials testing THC and CBD for PTSD are currently under way but agreed that the published research on cannabinoids and PTSD remains in its infancy.

Still, I can't shake a nagging feeling that part of the enthusiasm surrounding ketamine, MDMA, and medical marijuana is based on the fact that they alleviate traumatic stress by providing patients with an altered state and not by getting to the root of the trauma symptoms. I fear the rapid relief they promise may be just too good to be true. Any medication with a potential for abuse has to be carefully considered before it is offered to someone with PTSD. We know that addiction and traumatic stress go hand in hand, and the history of using benzodiazepines for PTSD sufferers should serve as an invaluable lesson for doctors and patients.

A more realistic approach would be to accept that a significant trauma often leaves a survivor forever changed, and although there should always be hope, the notion that things will go back to "normal" is misleading. Better is to accept that the brain is complex, that every human soul is unique, and that the trauma, to varying degrees, may have become part of the survivor's DNA. The goal of treatment, then, should be to help survivors thrive in their new normal.

PART 6

Our World on Trauma

TRAUMA OF THE MASSES

A Wicked Problem

The term "wicked" in this context is used, not in the sense of evil, but rather as an issue highly resistant to resolution.
—Lynelle Briggs, former Australian public service commissioner

War permeated every year of the twentieth century, with the cumulative death toll of military personnel and civilians reaching close to 200 million. That century was also rife with civil wars linked to genocidal atrocities. Civilian survivors of war-torn countries face multiple traumas: being physically maimed, witnessing the sudden death of their loved ones, and experiencing the physical destruction of their community. Civilian rape has long been used as a weapon of war; more than twenty thousand women were raped during the Bosnian war, and in Darfur, some reports estimate that ten thousand girls and women were raped each year. This century has been marked by wars in Afghanistan and Iraq and ongoing civil conflicts worldwide, with the current civil war in Syria being a source of major concern.

Intermingled with the horrors of war are the traumas of those forced to flee conflict-ridden regions. The last seventy-five years have witnessed World War II, decolonization movements over Africa and Asia, the decline of the Soviet Union, and instability in the Middle East, incidents that collectively turned 150 million men, women, and children into refugees. Currently, Europe is experiencing a massive influx of refugees, mostly from Syria, Afghanistan, and

Iraq, who have experienced traumatizing journeys and often arrive in poor physical health.

Beyond war, human rights are being violated on a widespread scale with the global and entrenched issue of human trafficking. There are an estimated 21 million victims of forced labor worldwide. These humans are trafficked for commercial sexual exploitation, domestic servitude in private homes, the provision of body organs, bonded labor, and forced criminal activity. Children are also often trafficked and can be exploited as child soldiers, members of begging rings, or "mail-order brides" or as part of illegal adoptions. As might be expected, the people most at risk for being trafficked are those who are impoverished, have minimal education, have a prior history of abuse, or belong to a marginalized group by virtue of their gender, ethnicity, or culture. Victims are often enticed by any number of lies, including the prospect of being able to earn money that can improve their (and their family's) dire situation.

Natural disasters such as earthquakes, tsunamis, hurricanes, tornadoes, wildfires, and floods also cause mass traumatization. They wreak widespread devastation as survivors face the loss of loved ones and witness their homes and livelihoods being destroyed. In a national survey of Americans, almost 20 percent of men and 15 percent of women reported having experienced a natural disaster in their lifetime. Comparable statistics from low- and middle-income countries are not available, but reports suggest that exposure rates are higher than in the United States.

The September 11, 2001, attack on the World Trade Center was the first act of war on the US mainland since the Civil War and the worst human-made disaster in recent US history. More than 2,500 people were massacred, and tens of thousands of people were affected by the destruction of the towers and the subsequent rescue, recovery, and cleanup operations. Since those attacks, terrorism has hit France, India, Ireland, Spain, the United Kingdom, and else-where, often resulting in large-scale disasters with many civilian casualties.

Faced with the magnitude of this wicked problem of mass trau-matization, I find little value in the doomy gloom of pessimists who assume that such devastation is absolute and irreversible. Nor do I find solace in the naiveté of optimists who live in the hope of a conflict- and disaster-free world. Rather, I find myself preoccupied with more pressing questions: What is the cost of war on the human psyche? What happens when disaster and terror impact large swaths of a population in a discrete time period? What is the global impact of such mass traumatization? How do whole societies, cultures, and countries remember or forget dark periods in their history?

In the last two decades, trauma scientists, by asking crucial questions in the aftermath of war, disaster, and terror, have found answers. The science of suffering is enhancing our understanding of the psychological repercussions of such global events. Most im-portant, this hard-earned knowledge is now shedding light on how to mitigate damage and accelerate healing in the aftermath of mass traumatization.

In the pages that follow I will deconstruct this evidence, but first I will return to my own family history of trauma. In many ways, the story of the 1947 Partition is a universal narrative with echoes that can be heard in today's headlines: mass civilian casualties of conflict, countless people forced to flee, refugee camps in deplorable condi-tions, orphaned children, rape as a weapon of war, and violence in the name of religion.

I share this personal history in the hope that it will illuminate the vicissitudes of human lives and what happens when individual circumstances, decisions, and obligations collide with catastrophic global events. Alongside the inevitable history, geography, and political lessons, diving into such individual stories also yields essential truths that can pave a path toward finding new purpose for individual lives that have endured the unspeakable—a path that, ultimately, will play an essential role in resolving the wicked problem of mass traumatization.

THE 1947 PARTITION

In the first six weeks of Independence, about half as many Indians were killed as Americans died during nearly four years of the second World War. . . . It is beyond human competence to conceive, far less to endure the thought of, the massiveness of the mania of rage, the munificence of the anguish, the fecundity of hate breeding hate, perhaps for generations to come.

—"The Trial of Kali," *Time*, 1947

In 1947, my grandfather, Walaiti Shah Jain, was employed as personal assistant to the state of Punjab's commissioner. The position gave him status and a good life for his wife and six children. They lived in a roomy bungalow in Sargodha, a town in the Punjab region of British India. Like that of so many South Asians, my grandfather's last name, Jain, reveals his religious background: he was born into a family that followed the ancient dharmic religion of Jainism.

My grandfather was barely of age when both his parents died and his elder brother, Kharaiti, and Kharaiti's wife, Parmeshewari, stepped in as his guardians. Studying always came easily to him, though, especially languages, and he mastered English, a mandatory subject in the schools of British India, with ease. This talent served him well; he was able to get a job in the Indian Civil Service and was earning enough to make him eligible for an arranged marriage to a suitable bride.

But once again loss loomed. His wife died giving birth to their first child, a son named Roshan. Shortly after that, Kharaiti suddenly succumbed to an infectious illness. Still, my grandfather somehow found a way to forge on. By 1947, he was remarried to my grand-mother Vidya and together they had five children. He had continued to ascend the ranks and was now in an influential position in the Indian Civil Service.

On his day off, Walaiti would don jodhpurs to go horseback riding and later, at home with his children, would hand-make their favorite treat, *anjeer burfi*, a rich fudge of figs, pistachio nuts, and evaporated milk. In the evenings, he would read them books such as *The Arabian Nights* and other fantastical stories of witches and wizards. During the hot summer months, when the commissioner left for the cooler climate of the hill stations, Walaiti would also shift his entire family to the picturesque hillside resort of Murree. In contrast to many of his relatives, my grandfather developed a deep belief in the value of modern education and financed Roshan's medical studies. My grandfather had even loftier plans for my dad: to send him to England for his higher education.

My grandmother was born at the turn of the twentieth century in Chittagong, a large seaport city on the banks of the Karnaphuli River near the Bay of Bengal in northeastern India. She spoke English (a rarity among Indian women of that time), played the harmonium beautifully, and was an accomplished cook. Her marriage to Walaiti required her to permanently relocate thousands of miles away to the state of Punjab. It was there she would endow their five children with the richness of her Bengali heritage—an ear for music and a love of the written word.

I wonder if my grandfather had any inkling of the terror 1947 would bring. A third wave of personal tragedy was about to hit him, and, as luck would have it, that wave would be submerged under the tsunami of a world in turmoil. I wonder if he sensed that the ground beneath his feet had already started to shift; that the only India he knew, British India, was on the verge of disintegrating.

***

At its peak the British Empire ruled over almost half a billion people spanning a quarter of the earth's total surface. The extent of its reach around the globe ensured that the sun was always shining on at least one of its colonies, and thus it became known as "the empire upon which the sun never sets." The British rule of India, a time period known as the Raj, formally started in the eighteenth century. India soon became a major source of British wealth as she was rich in natural resources such as gold, diamonds, silk, cotton, and pepper, a spice so sought after by the British that they called it "black gold." India was also a source of cheap labor and an indigent population who could be inducted into the British armies in addition to being a massive market for British-made goods. It was easy to see how India became known as "the jewel in the crown"—the crown, of course, being a British one.

British-made goods were often responsible for the decline of local Indian industry. With the growing Indian population, the land-holdings of many farmers often became too small to remain viable, and it was not uncommon for monsoons to fail and ruin a small landowner. Unemployment among working-class Indians was on the rise, and more and more people felt the angst of economic insecurity. As the frequency of hardships increased, so, too, did Indian discontent with the British.

During World War I, 2 million Indians fought for the British, and tens of thousands of them were killed. For that sacrifice, Indians expected a reward in the form of "home rule." But they received what was tantamount to nothing, and, as if to add insult to injury, the British became more oppressive. British landlords lived in grand residences with manicured lawns, played cricket, and drove Rolls-Royces, while Indian farmworkers faced unjustified oppression:

arrests without a warrant, physical beatings, illegal seizures of land, demands for services without pay, and the refusal of water.

The British decided how Indians would live, what they could buy, and what they could sell. Fighting against those unjust laws would propel India toward freedom from British oppression.

By the early 1920s, Mohandas K. Gandhi, an Indian lawyer, had become a national hero. In response to Great Britain's Rowlatt Acts, which gave the British in India free rein to root out "revolutionary" elements and to detain them without trial, Gandhi organized *hartals*, or general strikes, of Indian workers. The Mahatma (great soul), as Gandhi was called by the people, started a program of peaceful noncooperation with the British that advocated the boycotting of the British goods that were responsible for the decay of local industries. He encouraged Indians to spin their own cloth to free themselves from reliance on British imported cloth and popularized the strategy by traveling with his own spinning wheel.

Gandhi went on to win the hearts of millions of his fellow Indians and called for immediate independence from the Raj. By August 1942, the Quit India Movement, a civil disobedience organization, was launched. In his "Karo ya Maro" ("Do or Die") speech, Gandhi made a call for determined, but passive, resistance to British oppression to inspire his fellow Indians to claim freedom from their colonial ruler.

Intellectually, Indians of my grandfather's generation were raised to view themselves as citizens of the empire; they grew up singing the British anthem, aspired to wear British clothes, and dreamed of educating their children in British institutions. But spiritually, millions of Indians were experiencing a new awakening as Gandhi offered them a vision of a different existence: an India solely for Indians.

***

By 1947, the British had made concrete plans to leave India. Steps for a transfer of power after two centuries of colonial rule were under way, and staggered elections had been going on since the winter of 1945, with provincial ministries already being formed. Was my grandfather worried about his future in the new India? Did he sense the intensity with which millions of Muslims wanted a separate homeland carved out for themselves, called Pakistan, which would rest on the foundation of Muslim nationalism?

The newspapers would have been full of stories about Muhammed Ali Jinnah, the leader of the All-India Muslim League, and Jawaharlal Nehru, the leader of the Indian National Congress, the two parties that were the obvious front-runners in the race to take over the reins of power after the British left. Did my grandfather think Pakistan would really come into existence? And did he have any inkling what Pakistan would be carved out of?

But personal tragedy has a way of overpowering one's life no matter the urgency of world events. For Walaiti the calamity came in the spring of 1947 in the form of a deadly virus. His youngest child, Kamala, affectionately known as Choti, or "Little One," was only three years of age when she became sick with smallpox. Within days her little body succumbed to the rapid infection.

After Choti's death, my grandmother Vidya Vati quickly lost interest in life, eventually becoming confined to her bed, where she would lie quietly with a blank expression, not eating or drinking. Walaiti decided to move the family to the city of Jhelum, where the construction of their new home was nearing completion. He also sent word for his widowed sister-in-law, Parmeshewari, to come to help with the children. She arrived with her beloved son, her only source of financial security in her old age.

By now India was descending into chaos. Street violence and rioting were carried out in the name of freedom, and intense fearfulness became part of life in Punjab. Communal violence escalated, and prominent areas of major cities were destroyed in arson attacks. Despite joint appeals for peace by Gandhi and Jinnah, by the end of May 1947, fighting and destruction spread to the cities of Lahore and Gurgaon. Tired of the quarrels and fearful that the whole economic future of the subcontinent would be undermined if they continued to postpone freedom, Indian politicians agreed to partition the country, and on June 3, 1947, a plan was made public.

A boundary commission led by Cyril Radcliffe, a British judge, was hurriedly formed and charged with the mammoth task of carving out borders. Radcliffe had never set foot in India prior to his assignment to the commission. His border lines cut through homes, jute fields, and rice paddies, spreading chaos and mayhem on the ground. The Partition, as it came to be known, proved to be a disaster. It resulted in millions of Muslims moving to Pakistan and millions of non-Muslims (Hindus, Sikhs, Jains, and Christians) moving from Pakistan to India at a moment's notice. The new nations were grossly unprepared for what would become the largest population movement in recorded history.

Vidya's condition did not improve, and by early August she died. I can only imagine that my grandfather's world was now in turmoil: his daughter and wife dead in the space of a few months and his remaining children too young to fully process what had happened. Two weeks after Vidya's death, in mid-August, the boundary lines were revealed to the public and placed Walaiti and his family a mere 100 miles from the border. *But, as Jains, they were on the wrong side of the border.* Their home now came under the territory of Pakistan.

Things seemed to settle down for a while, and many people believed they could live as a religious minority in the new democracy of Pakistan, and their Muslim counterparts, with settled lives in India, hoped for the same on their side of the border. So Parmeshewari's son set off back to his hometown to resume his job, leaving his mother to stay behind to help his grieving uncle manage his young family.

But it was a deceptive calm. News came that Parmeshewari's son had been murdered in the violence that was reerupting all over Punjab. Gangs of rioters deliberately derailed trains and massacred passengers; women and children did not escape the brutality, with rape and kidnapping occurring at alarming rates. Fearing violence and discrimination, millions of people were forced to leave their homes in India and Pakistan, traveling by rail, foot, trucks, and cars in search of safety on the other side of the border.

Parmeshewari was devastated that her beloved son had been murdered, but the danger of staying in Pakistan was getting harder to ignore. The family hurriedly prepared to leave, packing essential belongings and planning to get on the next bus to India. But then Parmeshewari took my grandfather aside: she wanted him to go to her home in Gujranwala and retrieve a cache of family jewelry hidden there. With her son murdered, she faced financial destitution. She was the widow of his elder brother, and he owed her that favor.

Within days my grandfather put his children onto a bus that took them on a journey from Jhelum via Lahore over the Atari border to Amritsar, India. He placed Roshan, now in his early twenties, in charge of the other children. He and Parmeshewari would stay, retrieve her jewels, and follow shortly.

Every day, the siblings ran to greet the buses arriving from Pakistan, scrutinizing the faces of disembarking passengers in search of their beloved father. Weeks passed, and despondency fell over Walaiti's children as they realized that their father was not coming. Finally, a family friend wrote with the news that Walaiti had been stabbed to death in the Partition violence.

In a few short months, Walaiti's children's lives went from being filled with opportunity and promise to becoming totally unprotected. The home in Jhelum that their father had lovingly built for his family, with a private water well, five spacious bedrooms, and a mezzanine, would go to a Pakistani family in the surreal series of exchanges that came to define the post-Partition months.

My grandfather's decision to delay his departure for India cost him his life and threw the destiny of his children to the winds.

***

The 1947 Partition was a tragedy of epic proportions. In the words of Stanford University's South Asian and Islamic Studies librarian Dr. C. Ryan Perkins:

> Up to two million people lost their lives in the most horrific of manners. The darkened landscape bore silent witness to trains laden with the dead, decapitated bodies, limbs strewn along the sides of roads, and wanton rape and pillaging. There was nothing that could have prepared the approximately 14 million refugees for this nightmare.

Somehow that monumental atrocity has passed largely unacknowledged by the world. There are likely many reasons why the story of the Partition is publicly undertold, a big one being that India and Pakistan, as fledgling nations, may not have had the luxury of memorializing the dead and the demands of the living had to take precedence. There is, however, an additional explanation that trauma scientists would offer: the powerful human drive to deny the unspeakable. Repression, dissociation, and denial can operate on a societal level. But the science of suffering tells us that there is a big price to pay for such collective denial. Atrocities don't remain buried forever. As powerful as the desire is to deny, in the long run it does not work.

Science may not have had an agreed-upon definition of PTSD in 1947, but that does not mean it did not exist. What happened to the millions upon millions of traumatized survivors? A hint about the answer to this question was offered by the Partition historian Yasmin Khan:

> People were not well equipped with the language of psychiatry... it was too much to hope for any systematic understanding of the collective trauma which a generation had experienced. Partition had a widespread psychological impact which may never be fully recognized or traced.

More recently, the concerned voices of South Asian activists have been growing louder. They are highlighting the problems of the "silence" surrounding the Partition and the long-lasting psychological impact not only on survivors but also on their children. Indian scholars have also commented on the "spiral of silence" surrounding Partition-linked violence. They argue that the unacknowledged collective trauma has engendered spirals of violence between Hindus and Muslims that continue to be vigorously reenacted across the Indian subcontinent. Such ongoing reenactments do not bode well for the future relationship of these two nuclear-armed neighbors.

In 2011, Guneeta Singh Bhalla, a Berkeley physicist and the granddaughter of a Partition survivor, left the world of science to found the 1947 Partition Archive, a nonprofit organization dedicated to institutionalizing the people's history of Partition. Today, the archive holds four thousand survivor stories that have been preserved from three hundred cities and twelve countries and in twenty-two languages by more than five hundred dedicated citizen historian volunteers. Their mission transcends religion and nationality, aiming to honor all Partition survivors through a process of assisted narration.

Guneeta Singh Bhalla once told me that every time she visits South Asia on archive business she is met with the question "Why are you raking up the past like this?" Perhaps the most effective answer is that every week, the archive is contacted by scores of aging survivors across the South Asian diaspora who want to tell their Partition stories, drawn by an intuition about the healing power of giving their testimony. These oral histories showcase what trauma scientists have known for some time: that remembering and narrating individual stories about terrible events are necessary, not only for the healing of the survivor but in forming a foundation for the restoration of the overarching social order.

WAR, DISASTER, AND TERROR

Hard-Earned Knowledge and Lessons for the Future

We learn from history that we learn nothing from history.
—George Bernard Shaw

In the late 1990s, researchers embarked on an epidemiological study that took a close look at civilian survivors of four post-conflict, low-income countries: Algeria (after the Islamic Salvation Front's series of population massacres), Cambodia (after the Khmer Rouge's genocide), Ethiopia (after the 1991 war that separated Eritrea from Ethiopia), and Gaza (after the first intifada). Their results, which were published in *The Journal of the American Medical Association*, showed rates of PTSD that lay in the 16 to 40 percent range, considerably higher than what is found in trauma survivors who reside in high- and middle-income countries. A 2003 national survey found the rate of PTSD to be over 40 percent in Afghanistan, a country that has seen almost four decades of war and conflict, destruction of its infrastructure, and depletion of vital human resources. Such studies were among the first to define the magnitude of the psychological toll that war in low-income countries takes on civilian survivors.

More recently, European scientists have been documenting rates of PTSD among refugees arriving from Syria, Afghanistan, and Iraq at epidemic proportions. General research on refugees' mental health has now yielded clear lessons. First, it is safe to assume that refugees who have come from countries with a history of political violence have been exposed to multiple traumatic experiences in their home countries. Many have a history of being tortured after being imprisoned on political charges, and these individuals are at an even higher risk for PTSD.

Second, there are serious implications of not treating refugees who have PTSD. A 2017 study of over 300 Congolese refugees found that trauma survivors suffer not only from the core PTSD symptoms but also from impaired cognitive functioning. Such impairments hamper their abilities to hold a job, be an effective parent, and manage the tasks of day-to-day living, not to mention integrate successfully into their new host country.

Finally, it is vital not to forget that a massive portion of the refugee population comprises children who have been exposed to extreme violence. Their prognosis worsens if they do not have access to healthy nutrition, clean water, education, and the social stimulation that their growing brains and bodies need. Stable settlement and social support in the host country are vital in restoring the children's psychological well-being, yet refugee children, especially unaccompanied minors, often remain vulnerable to ongoing exploitation, poverty, abuse, and neglect even when they have resettled in a more stable country.

Important scientific findings about the long-term psychological consequences of atrocities have emerged from studies of aging Jewish survivors of the genocide committed by Nazi Germany. Even though Holocaust survivors, as a group, proved resilient in terms of their overall physical and mental health and life expectancy, among those who had faced other traumas over the subsequent years, PTSD was rampant at rates of over 50 percent. Holocaust survivors with PTSD often also had clinical depression that appeared rooted in survivor's guilt. This guilt-ridden melancholia was characterized by intense feelings of inferiority, self-blame, and criticism and by a sense that one must struggle to compensate for having failed to live up to expectations. In a thoughtful analysis of more than 200,000 Holocaust survivors, researchers at the University of Haifa found that those who had fled from countries with higher levels of genocide, and subsequently became refugees, were more likely to die by suicide later in life. Feelings of guilt are a deadly dimension for those who have not only narrowly escaped death but were forced to leave loved ones behind in the process.

In recent years, trauma scientists have also quantified rates of trauma exposure and PTSD in survivors of human trafficking. In one study, researchers interviewed more than a thousand men, women, and children from Cambodia, Thailand, and Vietnam who survived trafficking and asked them about the specific nature of their experiences while also assessing if they had clinically significant mental health problems. The results, which were published in *The Lancet*, showed that almost 50 percent of the group experienced physical and sexual violence during the period they were trafficked and almost 40 percent had current symptoms of post-traumatic stress. As might be expected, the more hazardous their living and working conditions, the more likely their odds of subsequently developing symptoms of depression, anxiety, and PTSD. In a small study of female survivors of sexual trafficking in Nepal, researchers found extremely high levels of anxiety and depression (almost 90 percent), and almost 30 percent of the survivors had PTSD. Similar results were found in another study done with women survivors of sex trafficking who had returned to their homes in Moldova.

As has been seen in survivors of prolonged trauma, the psychological distress experienced by survivors of trafficking persists well beyond the time spent under their traffickers' control. Survivors live lives plagued by unhealthy coping strategies, low self-esteem, and an inability to build healthy and trusting relationships. Such downstream consequences need to be factored in when considering the design of rescue, recovery, and reintegration efforts for the survivors of human trafficking. If not given due consideration, survivors will remain susceptible to future revictimization.

***

Reassuringly, rates of PTSD after natural disasters, or "acts of God," are generally lower than those found after human-made disasters such as war. Still, among the wide range of psychological consequences of surviving a natural disaster, PTSD remains sufficiently frequent and debilitating.

It is important to be aware of the variability in the experiences of disaster survivors. Some survivors may have witnessed the disaster directly and narrowly escaped death; others may have survived less dangerous, but nonetheless harrowing, aftershocks, such as their home being destroyed. This variability explains why Dr. Sandro Galea, dean of the Boston University School of Public Health, and his colleagues found such a broad range of PTSD prevalence rates following natural disasters: "approximately 5 percent to 60 percent in the first 1–2 years after a disaster."

Intensity of exposure to a disaster also explains the higher rates of PTSD found in first responders who are tasked to fight disasters on the front lines. One study found a 50 percent rate of PTSD among firefighters who fought bushfires in southeastern Australia. Other research, done after the Chi-Chi earthquake in Taiwan, found similar rates of PTSD in Taiwanese firefighters.

The young and old are also more vulnerable after natural disasters. After Hurricane Katrina, studies of children who came from schools in the hardest-hit parishes showed that 45 percent of them reported significant symptoms of PTSD in the immediate aftermath, with that number dropping to 30 percent a year later. Four years after the hurricane, the percentage of traumatized children remained higher than expected. Not surprisingly, vulnerable older adults (those who were already sick, homebound, or dependent on others for day-to-day living) were most vulnerable to developing PTSD in the aftermath of Katrina.

A similar trajectory of suffering in the elderly occurred after the 2011 Great East Japan earthquake, which caused a tsunami and a nuclear power plant accident. The tsunami warning urged residents to evacuate, but the elderly were unable to act quickly enough and made up a big percentage of the casualties. Elderly survivors who escaped continued to suffer because they were now isolated and had lost contact with their communities after being forced to relocate. Mental health professionals reported high levels of stigma among the elderly survivors toward seeking mental health attention. One year after the disaster, research findings hinted at levels of PTSD among displaced elderly survivors to be almost 60 percent.

The predisaster condition of disaster-hit communities matters a great deal. The reality of pre-Katrina poverty and social adversity meant that many families were already struggling before Katrina hit. Furthermore, poverty and social adversity determined who bore the brunt of the devastation. African American residents of New Orleans made up almost 85 percent of those living below the poverty line and were more likely to live in the lower-lying, flood-prone sections of the city worst hit by the hurricane.

The gigantic Asian tsunami of December 26, 2004, killed more than 220,000 people in twelve countries and displaced more than

1.6 million people. In Sri Lanka, more than a million people were affected; the tsunami displaced more than 800,000 people, destroyed homes, and killed 36,000. Ninety percent of those killed were from fishing communities and belonged to the lower socioeconomic classes. Psychiatrists in Sri Lanka found significant challenges in caring for survivors in a country where mental health resources were scarce to nonexistent. In the months that followed, depression, PTSD, and alcohol abuse were often observed. Attempts to alleviate the psychological suffering of survivors was further hindered in a country that was resource poor and even before the tsunami had been struggling with the economic and political fallout of civil war.

Researchers who studied the aftermath of the 2001 terrorist attacks in New York found that most survivors did *not* develop PTSD, and their distress diminished and resolved naturally over time. These findings have been replicated in other countries where terrorist attacks were associated with mass casualties and massive destruction of property. Though this is encouraging, it's important not to forget that low percentages can still translate into large numbers of sufferers. For instance, one study estimated that one year after the terrorist attacks of September 11, 2001, there were 200,000 cases of related PTSD.

Terror also seeps beyond the direct victims. For instance, psychological repercussions of terrorism have been found among *indirect* victims, including relatives and close friends of the dead and injured and the general community living in the targeted area. Studies have shown that 17 to 29 percent of these relatives and friends and up to 4 percent of the general community can develop PTSD after an act of terror.

Again, terrorism research echoes the previous findings of the unique risks that first responders face in such situations. Following the 2001 terrorist attacks on the World Trade Center, tens of thousands of both trained and untrained disaster responders were involved in the rescue, recovery, and cleanup. In one study of over 3,000 responders, nearly one-fifth developed PTSD; half of them still had active PTSD more than ten years after the attacks. World Trade Center exposure, especially to death and human remains, was strongly associated with having PTSD years later.

Actions to Accelerate Healing

In addition to the essentials of food, shelter, and water, social support through family, friends, or community has proved vital for recovery in the aftermath of disasters. Such findings spurred the 2006 development of Psychological First Aid by experts at the National Child Traumatic Stress Network and the National Center for PTSD. The manual was designed for disaster response workers to use during their first contact with trauma survivors experiencing acute psychological distress. It focuses on the fundamentals: protecting survivors from further harm; reassuring them that the trauma is over; connecting them with family and friends and other essential resources; and giving them the opportunity to talk to a compassionate listener who is trained to respect their dignity, culture, and capacity.

A version of Psychological First Aid has been successfully piloted by the World Health Organization (WHO) in Haiti, Guinea, Liberia, and Sierra Leone and has been offered widely in war-torn Syria and to thousands of displaced people in Greece and Nigeria. Psychological First Aid is a first step in formalizing a procedure that offers protection to *all* disaster survivors. It holds the promise of curbing the development of adverse mental health consequences because disaster survivors do better if they feel, or are helped to feel, safe and connected to others.

With its focus on pragmatic design, narrative exposure therapy (NET) is a short-term treatment tailored to meet the needs of a diverse cultural population of PTSD sufferers who have survived war, organized violence, or natural disasters or who have been forced to flee their homelands. For the better part of the last two decades, NET researchers have tested the treatment extensively. It has been offered with good success to unaccompanied refugee minors living in Europe, Syrian refugees living in Canada, Iraqi refugees living in the United States, former Ugandan child soldiers, Sri Lankan child survivors of the 2004 Indian Ocean tsunami, and Chinese survivors of the Sichuan earthquake.

Another outreach program designed to target and assist individuals who have been traumatized is trauma risk management (TRiM), a peer support system originally developed by the British armed forces that aims to ensure that trauma-exposed personnel are properly supported and encouraged to seek timely help should they develop mental health problems that fail to resolve spontaneously. Research on TRiM shows that it does no harm, and it is an accepted, sustainable program that may have a positive effect in the form of reduced absenteeism from work. TRiM may hold value for first responders, police, and emergency room personnel, who are also at routine risk of occupation-related traumatic exposure.

In response to the July 7, 2005, suicide bombs that were detonated on the London transport system, killing 56 people and injuring 784, Dr. Chris Brewin and his colleagues launched a two-year Trauma Response Programme. By doing active outreach, they connected with almost 1,000 survivors of the bombings (an estimated 4,000 people were impacted). The team invited those survivors to be screened for traumatic stress and other mental health conditions attributable to the terror attacks. Those who screened positive were offered a more in-depth clinical evaluation and, if warranted, treatment. They were followed for a year, and their level of psychological distress was tracked by the research team. The results were promising; 217 entered treatment, with PTSD being the most common diagnosis. Treatment was effective, with patients scoring low on measures of mental health symptoms several months later.

What Brewin and his colleagues found was that the assumption that survivors who needed psychological assistance would show up for care did not hold true. Rather, the researchers were proactive in their outreach. They obtained lists from hospitals that treated survivors, charities involved in disaster relief efforts, government agencies, and the police. In addition, they set up a dedicated telephone support line, sent letters to local family doctors, and advertised via mass media campaigns.

Why the need for such active outreach? Perhaps the invisible wounds caused by psychological injury don't send one's alarm bells ringing to get help the way a broken leg or a skin wound does. Or the "normal" symptoms experienced in the immediate aftermath of a terror attack are similar to the symptoms of PTSD, so it can be hard to know when a "normal" reaction becomes a problem. Many people probably feel very lucky to have survived a terrorist attack and may feel guilt or shame about experiencing an emotional reaction other than gratitude. Or it may simply be a matter of not knowing where to go for help or which type of mental health professional could assist them.

Other programs deployed to assist survivors of terrorism have yielded a similar lesson: when mental health services are offered and survivors are connected to them, they will use them with good benefit. Though research is showing the clear advantages of proactive outreach after terrorism, these findings raise many pivotal questions for communities that experience terrorism but do not have the resources for such initiatives. Proactive outreach efforts cost money; who should pay for them? If survivors need services over a long period of time, who is responsible for ensuring that the health care system can meet that demand?

Lessons for the Future

The scientific findings are clear: societal interventions that aim to help survivors of mass traumatization recover must *explicitly* address traumatic stress. Mass traumatization demands a systematic, coordinated response that provides active outreach, identifies vulnerable subgroups, and, if necessary, offers psychological treatment. For such responses to succeed requires resources, funds, and unequivocal societal support.

Unfortunately, the PTSD epidemic among refugees and civilian survivors of war remains inadequately acknowledged by the wider health community and politicians. There remains a dangerous lag between what they need, in terms of mental health resources, and what they actually receive. This lag is most obvious for survivors who reside in low-resource countries. The state of affairs is especially tragic considering that the mental health community has developed effective psychological therapies specifically tailored to meet the complex needs of civilian survivors of war and refugees.

At minimum, systematic screening for trauma and related psychiatric disorders should be offered to all civilian survivors of war. Beyond screening, the mental health community needs to be prepared to do culturally sensitive outreach to subgroups reluctant to seek help for a variety of reasons, including language barriers, reluctance to talk freely with a stranger, stigma about disclosing mental distress, and cultural or religious inhibitions.

Indeed, identifying atrocity survivors who have PTSD may be a necessary first step in promoting societal healing. In a 2002 study of more than 2,000 Rwandans who had survived the 1994 genocide, Rwandans with PTSD were significantly less likely than their trauma-exposed peers who did not have PTSD to have faith that the criminal prosecution of the perpetrators of the genocide would yield justice and were less open to reconciliation efforts. In a 2005 study of almost 3,000 survivors of the civil war in Uganda, researchers found that survivors with PTSD were more likely to identify violence as the means of resolving the war than were their trauma-exposed counterparts who did not have PTSD.

The mental health burden of war that is placed upon civilian survivors is seldom granted the priority and resources it needs. Beyond the usual lip service, trite words of sympathy and rhetoric, there is a dire need for systematic action. Along with postwar efforts to rebuild schools, hospitals, and homes, there must also be well-defined pathways that ensure the psychological rehabilitation of the severely traumatized.

As citizens of a twenty-first-century global village, we all have too much to lose if such pathways fail to materialize.

AN AMERICANIZATION OF
HUMAN SUFFERING?

I love the majesty of human suffering.

—Alfred de Vigny

A few years ago, I was a visiting professor in a department of psychiatry at a prestigious medical school in India and was giving a faculty lecture on PTSD. I had just delivered the lecture and was fielding questions from the audience when one of the distinguished older professors interrupted, "Very interesting and all . . . but we don't have much of a PTSD problem in India."

The room fell silent for a few seconds, and then mutterings broke out throughout the audience. I shifted awkwardly at the lectern, stunned at the timing of that sweeping statement. I had just finished citing the work of Indian scholars documenting India's vulnerability to natural disasters, on account of its unique geoclimatic conditions, and the need for a disaster mental health strategy. I had cited statistics from the country's own National Crime Records Bureau, which had reported that rape and domestic violence were up by 7 percent since 2010. I had even referenced studies from the medical school's own emergency department that described how India accounts for nearly 10 percent of the world's road traffic accidents and the imperative need for a coordinated psychological response to assist road traffic accident survivors. Natural disasters, domestic violence, rape, and an epidemic of road traffic accidents—Indians were no strangers to trauma.

The professor's dismissive statement spoke to a raging argument in the global mental health community. At the heart of the controversy was this idea: *PTSD is essentially a European and American problem.* I was saved by a comment from the back row. A young female doctor cautiously raised her hand. "With all due respect, sir, I don't think I can agree with the statement that we don't have a PTSD problem in India. I offer three reasons for this. First, our people, especially the poor, are so used to trauma being a fact of their daily life that they are resigned to accept it. They have a fatalistic attitude so don't even acknowledge trauma as trauma, even though they may be traumatized. Second, as doctors I don't think we are well trained to even ask the right questions to elicit PTSD symptoms. Third, we live in a country where most people remain very reluctant to even acknowledge that they are experiencing any emotional or psychological discomfort."

In response to her reasoning, academic jostling broke out, and the meeting moderator, eager to push on, diverted my attention to other questions from audience members.

***

In the late 1990s, WHO's World Mental Health Surveys were sent out to twenty-eight countries, garnering a combined sample size of over 200,000 respondents. The promise of those surveys was their statistical ability to yield PTSD rates that would override data from smaller local studies that were limited in scope. When WHO compared the prevalence of trauma exposure and resulting PTSD in high-, middle-, and low-income countries, they found that although the risk of exposure to traumatic events was essentially similar across countries, the risk of developing PTSD was uniformly lower than the rates found in the United States. For example, Colombia reported a lifetime prevalence of PTSD of close to 1.8 percent, Nigeria 0 percent, and China 0 percent. All rates significantly lower than the 6.8 percent reported in American studies.

Those surprising results sparked controversy in the global mental health community. What is the value of a diagnosis that does not have worldwide applicability? The conclusion that some mental health professionals were now drawing from the results was this: *PTSD is an Americanization of human suffering.*

The controversy surrounding the World Mental Health Survey data continues to this day. There are those who do not *deny* trauma exposure in low- and middle-income countries but view it more as a trigger for mental health issues such as clinical depression, anxiety disorders, and substance abuse. Locals are simply more accepting of trauma, the analysis suggests, and are therefore not rendered so horrified, fearful, or helpless as their American counterparts when they do experience it. This reaction has been touted as a form of paradoxical resiliency.

In this argument, I sense a naive romanticism for the way more traditional societies and cultures function. This misplaced nostalgia overlooks the fact that women, children, the poor, and the marginalized are often hardest hit by trauma yet, depending on their country of origin, may not have an adequate voice to express their true reactions. The danger of embracing the notion of paradoxical resiliency too readily is that it overlooks the suffering of the most vulnerable and disadvantaged.

While this debate continues, one factor might help explain the discrepancies in the worldwide rates of PTSD: culture. History, language, customs, traditions, and religion play a huge role not only in conceptualizing traumatic stress but in shaping the mental health of a whole community and how the community recovers from trauma, too.

Examples of how various cultures define trauma-related distress, as collated by the psychiatrists Devon E. Hinton and Roberto Lewis-Fernández, are *susto* (fright), *nervios* (nerves), and *ataque de nervios* (attack of nerves) in the Latino population; *khyal* (wind) *attacks* and *weak heart* among Cambodian refugees; *possession* in Guinea and Bissau and among Mozambican, Ugandan, and Bhutanese refugees; *haypatensi* (hypertension) among civil war victims in Sierra Leone; *ihahamuka* (lungs without breath), a syndrome characterized by the sudden onset of shortness of breath, among Rwandan genocide survivors; *iiaki* (sorrow/sadness) among Quechua speakers of the Peruvian highlands; and *masilango* (extreme fear) among the Mandinka.

The discrepancies in global PTSD data may also be a consequence of what happens when human suffering is overmedicalized by focusing too narrowly on the biological consequences of trauma exposure on the human brain and body at the expense of other, equally relevant, dimensions such as the political, economic, social, and moral.

Dr. Rupinder K. Legha, a fellow in the Department of Global Health and Social Medicine at Harvard Medical School, spent more than two years developing community-based mental health services throughout rural Haiti and offered this perspective:

> The meaningfulness of diagnosing PTSD [is challenged] in settings of continued insecurity, such as Haiti, where trauma is anything but "post" and constitutes the fabric of daily life. . . . PTSD as a diagnostic category, along with its symptom clusters, provided a starting point for making sense of these scenarios but could not capture this breadth of human suffering, and neither could it speak to the perva-

siveness of trauma, poverty, and suffering across generations and throughout the country.

Still, viewing PTSD as a solely American problem is an over-simplification. Rather, the current PTSD diagnosis needs further expansion and refinement so it has more cross-cultural relevance. The range of what qualifies as a symptom of traumatic stress needs to capture the suffering of those who express emotional and psychological discomfort in different ways, and culture-specific syndromes will need further exploration to see how well they map onto PTSD symptoms or if they are something distinct.

Controversy, criticism, and debates aside, the danger of rushing to dismiss the global relevance of PTSD is that doctors will stop looking for it and patients with symptoms of post-traumatic stress will be misdiagnosed. Funding for clinical programs and research monies will be redirected to other priorities. The PTSD diagnosis, as it stands, offers us a starting point (albeit an imperfect one) from which to make sense of global human suffering. To completely discard its worldwide relevance would be like throwing the baby out with the bathwater.

PART 7

A New Era

An Ounce of Prevention

PREVENTION WITH
PRECISION

Truth is ever to be found in simplicity, and not in the multiplicity
and confusion of things.
—Isaac Newton

There is a little-known fact about the history of psychiatry: for
centuries, prevention was actually deemed an essential part of
mental health care. By the mid-1950s, preventive psychiatry was
striving to combat the social or environmental causes of mental
illness by focusing on strengthening families, encouraging healthy
lifestyles, and having psychiatrists advocate in relevant legal and
policy matters. But in the ensuing decades, with a lack of political
will and public funding and the surge in popularity of psychiatric
medication, preventive psychiatry became a forgotten chapter in the
history of the field.

The historical failure of preventive psychiatry means that conversations about PTSD typically focus on treatment: prescribing better
pills, developing more powerful therapies, encouraging sufferers to
get treatment, or targeting the knock-on effects of PTSD, such as
addiction and suicide. Understanding the causes of PTSD leads to
discussions about biology, gene deletions, misfiring brain structures,
and neurotransmitters gone awry. We often neglect the option of
prevention. But in recent years, preventive psychiatry has started
to make a comeback as clinicians working on the front lines feel
the limitations of a sole focus on treatment.

Another development that bodes well for the success of preventive psychiatry is that the broader field of medicine is now embracing the idea of biological adversity, or how factors such as our behaviors, zip code, and environment are often bigger players in determining our health than biology and genetics. The wider health care community is now starting to take more seriously the devastating toll inequality in income and food supply, housing insecurity, and low socioeconomic status take on human health.

Today, preventive efforts involve the talent of teams from all types of professional backgrounds who are harnessing the power of big data, electronic medical records, genomic sequences, and sophisticated research methodologies and merging them with the social and environmental factors known to cause disease. Through this strategy scientists can start to untangle the relationships among all these factors with a level of precision that was missing in previous preventive efforts.

Some developments worthy of specific mention are recent efforts to prevent mass shootings, family violence, and sexual violence.

Preventing Mass Shootings

Mass shootings traumatize survivors, witnesses, families, first responders, and whole communities. Researchers pooled case study data from dozens of incidents spanning more than four decades including the 1999 Columbine High School shootings in Littleton, Colorado, and the 2007 Virginia Tech shooting. PTSD was found in 10 to 36 percent of the survivors. The impact of such shootings was found to extend beyond the primary survivors to encompass whole communities often subjected to the subsequent media intrusion. Indeed, even having a distant connection to a mass shooting can cause significant psychological distress—a finding that suggests this type of gun violence is particularly malignant.

After the June 12, 2016, mass shooting at a gay nightclub in Orlando, Florida, the American Medical Association announced gun violence to be a public health crisis. Effective solutions for the prevention of such violence need to incorporate the relevant political dimensions and require physicians to enter the realm of law, policy making, and advocacy.

Dr. Renee Binder, a psychiatrist at the University of California, San Francisco, and past president of the American Psychiatric Association, did just that when she advocated for the passage of the 2014 Gun Violence Restraining Order bill in California. This law, the first of its kind in the United States, enables family members to ask police to temporarily remove guns from the possession of individuals who are at risk of becoming violent. I spoke to Binder about how she approached this complicated issue. She told me:

> The whole issue of guns needs to be framed in terms of public safety, that is, why is there a concern about gun ownership? When people have guns at home, there is a greater risk of completed suicide, certainly there is concern about accidents to family members and then there is concern about homicide. Some people can handle guns safely and know how to work with guns but there are certain times in people's lives where they should not have access to guns . . . and this is not necessarily related to mental illness. It could be you getting fired from your job, you are very upset, or you feel mistreated, in cases of intimate partner violence or where people are abusing alcohol and drugs and becoming very agitated. Even persons who have some kind of dementia and are not as careful as they used to be.

Preventing Family Violence

The Nurse-Family Partnership, founded by Dr. David Olds, a pediatrician at the University of Colorado, involves families who are vulnerable to trauma receiving intensive home visits by professionals *before* a child is born. Studies have shown that families who receive this intervention have lower levels of child abuse and neglect (including injuries and accidents) and their children do better in school and in overall markers of emotional well-being. These findings also have considerable economic value, considering that child abuse and neglect cost the United States up to $124 billion annually. Globally, a variety of preventive interventions for reducing harsh or abusive parenting in low- and middle-income countries have also been moderately successful, but there remains an urgent need for interventions that are sustainable in low-resource settings.

To address the serious problem of intimate partner violence (IPV), researchers at the National Center for PTSD designed a ten-week trauma-informed couples therapy called Strength at Home. Acknowledging that soldiers exposed to the trauma of war are at increased risk of perpetrating IPV, researchers identified at-risk couples who had been experiencing relationship difficulties *before* IPV became a problem. Researchers compared a control group who were assigned a therapist offering a supportive therapy to a group of couples who received the Strength at Home training. The latter group did better, reported less physical violence and psychological abuse, and was more likely to complete their therapy when compared to the control group.

Preventing Sexual Violence

In a joint venture among Stanford University researchers, the nonprofit No Means No, and the African Institute for Health and Development, girl students in Nairobi, Kenya, are being taught how to ward off sexual assault using a six-week empowerment and self-defense program. The program seeks to quash the cultural notion that girls should be obedient even when faced by an attacker. The location of the study is particularly important considering that almost half of Kenyan women report that they were sexually assaulted when they were children.

The preliminary findings have been encouraging, with more than half of the almost two thousand high school girls who completed the course then using the skills to fend off sexual harassment or rape. Michael Baiocchi and Clea Sarnquist, the Stanford researchers involved in the study, are using sophisticated statistics to illuminate the precise causal pathways that make the intervention work, in the hope that it can be replicated in other settings.

For every dollar we spend on treatment, a dollar should be spent on prevention, and every time we highlight the value of treatment, the importance of prevention should be reiterated. The twenty-first century has given birth to a new and more precise version of preventive psychiatry that is proving to be impactful in different ways and, if it gains enough momentum, could make a significant dent in the PTSD problem. The primary preventions described thus far are prevention in its purest form. By preventing mass shootings, family violence, and sexual assault, we remove the trauma, and without these common traumatic events, PTSD related to such violence will simply cease to exist.

THE GOLDEN HOURS

Better three hours too soon than a minute too late.

—William Shakespeare, *The Merry Wives of Windsor*

Primary prevention is not always possible, and PTSD researchers have ventured into the realm of secondary prevention as a result. Secondary prevention intervenes in the window of time after trauma exposure but before the onset of PTSD, an opportunity to strike before it's too late. This window of time has come to be referred to as the *golden hours*, a time during which medical intervention could set a pathway toward recovery.

The PTSD literature is flush with enticing leads about the way medications and psychological therapies can be harnessed to prevent the onset of PTSD in those who have survived trauma. Dr. Gustav Schelling, a German physician caring for very sick patients in an intensive care unit (ICU), was used to reports of patients developing PTSD related to their near-death experiences. He observed that patients who were given hydrocortisone as part of the care for their critical illness experienced fewer signs and symptoms of PTSD after they recovered.

Cortisol is known to impair the retrieval of long-term memory, and scientists have hypothesized that hydrocortisone, delivered as a pill or an intravenous treatment, might prevent the onset of PTSD after trauma. Schelling tested his observation in randomized controlled studies and found that hydrocortisone administered during ICU treatment was associated with not only a significant reduction of PTSD symptoms in survivors but also improvements in their overall health. Another cutting-edge approach uses the drug mifepristone, which also impacts cortisol levels, but instead of providing an artificial and temporary boost in levels, it resets the way the body produces cortisol in the first place.

Emergency room physicians commonly give morphine, an opioid medication, to people who have survived life-threatening physical injuries such as severe motor vehicle accidents, bomb explosions, or gunshot wounds. Scientists have known for some time that being in extreme pain at the time of a traumatic event increases the odds of developing PTSD. Opioids also act to reduce the release of noradrenaline from the brain, a release that is known to go into overdrive in the PTSD brain, and recent molecular studies hint that the genes for the brain's opioid receptors may play a role in how the expression of fear is regulated in the amygdala.

Early work suggests that using opioids on a short-term basis to aggressively reduce pain after physical trauma may also help prevent the onset of PTSD related to the same trauma. One such study, published in *The New England Journal of Medicine*, followed almost 700 combat-injured military personnel serving in Iraq who were given morphine very soon after surviving a severe injury and found they were significantly less likely to develop PTSD. This study yielded encouraging findings, but there is an important caveat: it is doubtful that morphine would be valuable for the prevention of PTSD following severe psychological trauma when the survivor did not sustain painful physical injuries.

Less progress has been made in investigating which psychological therapies might work in the golden hours to prevent PTSD, due in part to the disappointing results that came from the routine use of critical incident stress debriefing (CISD) after traumatic incidents in the 1980s. CISD was designed to take place within hours or days of a traumatic event and typically included all emergency personnel responding to a disaster scene. It consists of a single four-hour session that encourages the group to share their emotional reactions to and experiences of the trauma.

Unfortunately, subsequent studies found that CISD was not only ineffective in preventing PTSD but actually appeared to do more harm than good. Exactly why is unknown, but some explanations point to the timing of CISD being too soon after the trauma and the overly zealous one-size-fits-all approach of including everyone involved. A more tailored "watchful waiting" approach is favored now, in which trauma survivors are identified and educated about how to get help but not required to talk about the incident unless and until they feel a need to do so.

The finding that CISD might harm trauma survivors meant that researchers shied away from testing psychological interventions in the golden hours—that is, until a team led by Dr. Barbara Olasov Rothbaum, a psychologist at Emory University, piloted a modified prolonged exposure (PE) intervention for delivery within hours after a trauma. Distinctly different from debriefing, its aim was to intervene early enough to prevent the consolidation of trauma memories in survivors.

In Rothbaum's study, 130 patients who presented to the emergency room of a hospital in Georgia were followed over several months. The patients had experienced a variety of traumas from rape to nonsexual assault and motor vehicle accidents. The study participants were either assigned to receive a modified PE intervention, usually within twelve hours of their trauma exposure, or assigned to a control group. The intervention consisted of three brief sessions that focused on breathing relaxation, exposure exercises, attention to cognitions, and self-care. Those assigned to the modified PE arm of the study reported fewer symptoms of PTSD and depression in the three months following the trauma.

More recently, researchers from the University of Oxford attempted to disrupt memory consolidation in the golden hours by using the computer game Tetris. Engaging in a visually absorbing task soon after surviving trauma could, they hypothesized, distract the brain and prevent it from over-consolidating those early visual memories of trauma.

The team recruited seventy-one individuals who survived motor vehicle crashes while they were still in the emergency department. Half of them were asked to think about the worst moments of the accident and then were asked to play Tetris for twenty minutes. The other half were asked to write down a log of what they had done since coming to the hospital.

The results, which were published in the journal *Molecular Psychiatry*, are promising. When compared to the log completers, participants who played Tetris were less likely to report post-trauma intrusive memories and related psychological distress in the week that followed their car accident.

While important concerns will need to be addressed before such "golden hour" interventions can be implemented into routine practice, the promise of interventions that could prevent the future suffering of so many is hard to ignore.

REACHING THE
HARD TO REACH

Making PTSD Treatment More Accessible

"Location, location, location."
—Real estate maxim

Until interventions in the golden hours become reality, frontline mental health professionals have little choice but to focus their attention on how to treat survivors with PTSD. The effect of not getting PTSD treatment in a timely fashion is clear: if one is untreated and still has PTSD after one to two years, the chance of remission is drastically reduced. From an economic standpoint, PTSD sufferers miss an average of four days of work per month, resulting in a loss of almost $3 billion per year in productivity in the United States alone. Unfortunately, only a minority of PTSD sufferers get treatment.

All these facts combined make a compelling case for early intervention, in which we accept that PTSD has taken hold but seek to soften its blow on our patients' quality of life. Perhaps the swiftest way to better reach PTSD sufferers as early as possible is for psychiatrists to start paying less attention to *what* treatments they are offering and more attention to *where* patients are offered treatment.

Since the 1990s, there has been an accumulation of research showing that the majority of patients with mental illness actually present to their primary care doctor, not a psychiatrist's office; when they do, their mental illness often goes undiagnosed, or, if they get care, it may not be of the highest quality. These findings prompted a few health care organizations to push toward the integration of mental health and primary care.

Integrated care started with simply adding a social worker, psychiatric nurse, or psychologist to the staff of a primary care clinic and then progressed to implementing sophisticated tools for screening patients for mental illness. There has also been a push to get psychiatrists to move their location and work alongside their colleagues in primary care, providing ongoing consultation and lending their specialty expertise. Though such initiatives remain few and far between, they have been shown to improve the identification and treatment of psychiatric conditions.

For the last several years, I have provided integrated care, and my experience has been transformative. I've found that many of the barriers to seeking help dissolve when a psychiatrist shifts location to a primary care clinic. Rather than receiving an anonymous referral to a mental health clinic on a different campus, patients see a psychiatrist right there in their primary care clinic, someone who works closely with their regular, trusted doctor, which helps the stigma and ambivalence melt away. It feels as though I am seeing the patients I have always seen except that I am reaching them twenty years earlier, at a point in time when their PTSD symptoms are less entrenched and more amenable to treatment. Beyond my hunches, research results show that PTSD sufferers who receive care in such integrated clinics fare better than those treated in traditional settings.

Emergency rooms are another place in which PTSD interventions are being integrated into the care of trauma survivors. In such programs, mental health professionals connect with trauma survivors in the emergency room, offering them tailored interventions, dependent upon their level of psychological distress, over the posttrauma weeks and months. Such programs are yielding promising results for survivors of IPV, physical assaults, motor vehicle accidents, and workplace injuries and appear, at the very least, to provide early identification and assistance and, at best, to prevent the onset of PTSD.

Similar success has been seen in studies of mothers of premature infants hospitalized in neonatal intensive care units (NICUs). Mothers who developed early signs of traumatic stress related to witnessing their infant's preterm birth and NICU hospitalization were offered a skills-based intervention that was developed to reduce symptoms of PTSD, anxiety, and depression. This brief intervention, which included elements of trauma-focused cognitive behavioral therapy (CBT), was effective in reducing future PTSD.

Beyond primary care clinics, emergency rooms, and ICUs, mental health professionals are now playing an active role in schools. Educators who work in school districts located in violent inner cities have long observed how psychological trauma plays a key role in the academic failure and behavioral problems they witness in their students. The combination of scientific advances in understanding PTSD and collective educator wisdom has been responsible for a recent movement toward "trauma-informed schooling." Rather than punishing traumatized children with behavioral problems, this movement aims to train teachers and staff to seek alternative solutions that will not retraumatize a child. Students are now being taught to recognize when they are triggered and to cope with and manage in healthier ways.

Peer Support and the Promise of Technology

Though efforts to expand access to care are encouraging, they do not address the overarching issue that when treatment is made available to PTSD sufferers, many still won't accept it. In recent years, there has been much innovation that aims to better meet PTSD sufferers where they are. My own research has focused on piloting peer support programs for veterans with PTSD. In these programs, certified veteran peer specialists, in remission from PTSD, are hired as part of the mental health treatment team to offer support to veterans with PTSD who are still struggling. As might be expected, it's much easier for sufferers to open up and connect with a peer who has passed through similar strife.

Veterans who have gone through peer support programs report being more socially engaged, hopeful, and empowered about their futures and more engaged in their mental health care. Peer support is just one example of how PTSD treatment is being reengineered to reach more people. Another exciting trend to make treatments more acceptable is harnessing the power of technology to make the delivery of treatment more widely available.

The shortage of mental health professionals in the United States translates into a problem in availability of care for PTSD sufferers. Technology has provided a partial solution. Mental health professionals based at better-staffed hospitals can supplement services at underserved clinics by using videoconferencing technology. Videoconferencing allows for real-time, interactive, face-to-face communication between doctor and patient through a television, computer, tablet, or smartphone screen.

For skeptics who fear that such visits may be impersonal or dilute the rapport between doctors and PTSD sufferers or that technical hitches will hamper the quality of treatment, it appears that there is little cause for concern. Many studies have shown that PTSD treatment delivered in this way is as good as in-person treatment. There has also been a move to offer this service to patients directly in their homes, and research is again showing that little is lost in terms of effectiveness or quality. Moreover, offering patients treatment in the comfort of their home can save them travel time and costs and may be particularly beneficial to PTSD sufferers who have high levels of avoidance symptoms.

In attempts to save therapists time without compromising the success of treatment, researchers have also developed online versions of CBT for PTSD. Patients work through online programs with remote guidance from a therapist. Not only is Internet-delivered CBT acceptable to patients, but therapists noted a 25 percent reduction in the time involved in using this version over the time involved in providing face-to-face CBT. Most important, participants reported a positive relationship with their web therapist.

PTSD Coach is a smartphone application (app) that was created by the National Center for PTSD in partnership with the Department of Defense's National Center for Telehealth and Technology. The app is available to anyone who has a smartphone and is designed to be a self-help tool that does not require the involvement of a mental health professional. Since its launch it has been downloaded more than 150,000 times by people in more than eighty countries and has received high ratings from both iPhone and Android smartphone users.

Preliminary studies have found that app users report high levels of satisfaction and find the app helpful. In a recent trial, almost fifty adult sufferers who were not in PTSD treatment were randomized either to use PTSD Coach as a self-help option or to go on a wait list (i.e., receive no treatment). After one month, reduction in PTSD symptoms was found to be larger in the app group than in the wait list group. The implications of such findings are considerable given that smartphones have found their way into the palms of nearly two-thirds of Americans and PTSD Coach does not require the involvement of a mental health professional.

Dr. Eric Kuhn, a psychologist and researcher at the National Center for PTSD, was part of the original team that created PTSD Coach.

Since its launch, he has devoted his time to figuring out how to use this technology to help PTSD sufferers. I asked him his thoughts about the future of technological innovation in PTSD treatment, and he said:

> I'm excited about the potential of machine learning and artificial intelligence. A big nut I'd like to help crack is how we can bring our effective cognitive behavioral therapy (CBT) interventions more fully into technological interventions. Successfully identifying and challenging unhelpful PTSD cognitions requires highly skilled CBT therapists but as the technology improves, I think some of the typical cognitions could be modified with technology. Help for some harder ones, particularly around guilt and self-blame that are more idiosyncratic, are further off on the horizon.

Dr. Josef Ruzek is a psychologist at Stanford University who specializes in developing technological interventions to treat PTSD in trauma survivors. Ruzek views technology as being integral to how mental health professionals can best reach the hard to reach. He told me:

> In ten years almost everyone will have a smartphone and I'd like to see us bundle mental health technology into these gadgets. What I envisage is a suite of fifteen or so Web- and phone-based interventions for PTSD and related problems such as insomnia or problem drinking. People could either use this suite by themselves or they could get help from peer support counselors. These technologies don't have to be perfect, but as a first-tier option, they would probably have great impact.

THE POWER OF SOCIAL NETWORKS

They burned the flag and they demonstrated against us; it's on the cover of the paper today. They have no respect. They have no idea what's going on over there, Mom—the men that are sacrificing their lives. People are dying every day over there, and nobody back here even seems to care. It's a bunch of goddamn shit if you ask me!
—Ron Kovic, *Born on the Fourth of July*

Regardless of the type of trauma, receiving social support after traumatic events can prevent the onset of PTSD. Even if an individual develops PTSD, a positive social network can help the symptoms heal. In fact, optimizing social support in the early period after a traumatic event has become a standard part of what would be considered excellent treatment. In this way, PTSD goes far beyond the biology of an individual human and extends to our society.

The power of positive social networks to heal also explains the damage that negative social experiences can have. The National Vietnam Veterans' Readjustment Study found that the most important protective factor against developing postwar PTSD was how the veterans *perceived* the social support they received in their posttrauma life. This finding provides an invaluable lesson: attempts to support survivors of trauma, no matter how well intentioned, may have little impact if they are not tailored to the specific needs of those we are trying to aid.

Dr. Marylene Cloitre, a psychologist at New York University and the National Center for PTSD, explained the nuances of social support that she observed in her work with survivors of 9/11:

> The community around survivors feels awkward and doesn't know what to do, so they start moving away. Combine this with the fact that survivors, who are sad or irritable, are not the most attractive people to engage with to begin with. I say to patients sometimes, it's unfair, that in a way, not only are you suffering but you're also responsible for making people around you comfortable with you.

The power of social networks to heal the traumatized is perhaps best illustrated in the aftermath of disaster, and in the twenty-first century, social media technology has utterly disrupted the way humans connect after disaster strikes.

In 2012, Facebook's CEO, Mark Zuckerberg, took a trip to Japan and told Japan's prime minister that the terrible tsunami that had struck the country in 2011 had inspired him to find ways to help people after natural disasters through social media. Indeed, social media (e.g., blogs, chat rooms, discussion forums, YouTube, LinkedIn, Facebook, and Twitter) have played an increasing role in disaster management. Social media have been used to disseminate crucial information, including relaying victims' requests for assistance and monitoring users' activities to establish their location.

Can social media technology be leveraged to bolster the social networks of postdisaster survivors and, in turn, prevent PTSD?

After the 2010 Haitian earthquake, survivors used social media to tell their stories, and their narratives, in turn, drove the mainstream media's response to the tragedy. During Hurricane Katrina, online spaces became virtual instantiations of the damaged and broken physical environments from which survivors were now barred. These virtual instantiations of physical communities were then used as points of connection and sites on which to exchange social support. After the shootings at Virginia Tech and Northern Illinois University, students participated in numerous online activities related to the shootings and found them beneficial to their recovery.

Social media technology holds promise for disaster survivors because of the very nature of digital networking, which is unlike anything humankind has seen before. Social media rely on peer-to-peer networks that are often collaborative, decentralized, and community driven, so survivors can seek support from beyond their immediate, conventional social network.

Of course, there are downsides, too, with fake news, blind authorship, presentations of opinion as fact, and privacy and security concerns being just a few. And then, of course, there is the digital divide: access to social media is predicated on the assumption that the disaster survivors have the necessary tools. Those with a low socioeconomic status are typically in most need after a disaster and, of course, least likely to have the means to purchase the technology needed to access social media.

Science has yet to discover whether social media can really bolster the social networks of postdisaster survivors enough to prevent PTSD. Still, increasing support for *all* survivors in postdisaster settings remains crucial, and in this regard the promise of integrating social media technology into future efforts is tremendous.

THE SCIENCE OF
RESILIENCE

That which does not kill us makes us stronger.
—Friedrich Nietzsche

When I was a child, I gravitated to movies about survivors who, despite being dealt many a tough blow, from being orphaned to poverty stricken, mauled, or maimed, beat all odds to build inspiring lives. I remember the feel-good factor that accompanied those tales, a sense that the human spirit was limitless.

As a physician and PTSD specialist, I have found that the appeal of the favorite movies of my youth has faded with every day spent on the front lines caring for real people who have survived trauma. The movie portrayals offered a sanitized version of what it means to survive under unspeakable circumstances. The hardness of survival, the scars it leaves, and the toll it can take on the inner workings of a life are what I now bear witness to.

An Iraq War veteran seeks treatment for his PTSD because he acknowledges that it is impacting his ability to be a good father. A woman who survived childhood incest realizes that she must learn to trust people if she wants to move forward in her life. A traumatized immigrant who has spent a thirty-year marriage taking his anger out on his wife now realizes that his family's problems stem from his own behavior. These sufferers carry flaws that sabotage their day-to-day existence, deflecting them off their life's course. But they do move forward.

I also meet those whose lives are ravaged by trauma. They are submerged so deeply in the resultant chaos and the whirlwind of emotions and pain that they are unable to come up for air. This variability in how humans deal with trauma raises a question: In the aftermath of experiencing the unspeakable, why do some seek oblivion or revenge, while others are able to transcend the horrors of the past?

In recent decades, PTSD researchers, most notably Dr. Steven Southwick and his team at Yale University School of Medicine, have found an inspired way to answer this question. They shifted their focus away from those with PTSD to the much larger percentage of those who, after experiencing trauma, do not develop PTSD. What are the unique strengths of these individuals? How do they approach adversity? How do they bounce back after facing trauma and tragedy? In essence, what are the secrets of their resilience after facing the unspeakable?

From a scientific perspective, resilience is hard to define. For starters, it appears to be multidimensional, so, for example, a survivor of a horrific car accident could prove to be resilient when it comes to taking care of his psychological well-being and physical health but show less resilience in his work productivity or maintaining his interpersonal relationships. Resilience is also dynamic, in that it changes over a lifetime, so, for example, a survivor of childhood sexual abuse may be resilient in her twenties but in her thirties, while raising her own children and facing the stressor of a divorce, may become less so.

Resilience also plays out on many levels, from the genetic to the neurobiological, the developmental, and the psychological. Our brains have a stress response apparatus that includes the hypothalamic-pituitary-adrenal axis, sympathetic nervous system, and serotonergic system. These highly intricate and interwoven systems rely on genes to express their activity levels, with some brains being able to mount a better response to stress than others. Indeed, genetic factors may account for one-third of the overall risk of developing PTSD following exposure to traumatic events. Scientists have also identified brain circuits that operate more efficiently in certain individuals who have been exposed to trauma. The brains of these people are primed to send strong signals to the amygdala, keeping it in check and allowing the prefrontal cortex to plan and execute actions under stressful circumstances.

An overprotected childhood, free of adversity, does little to foster resilience. Indeed, childhood exposures to moderate levels of stress, even repeated exposures, can lay the foundation for future resilience as the child gets a head start on developing the grit needed to master inevitable future life trauma. It is imperative to note that *moderate* stress is the sweet spot in terms of a correlation with future resiliency. Childhoods filled with repeated exposure to severe stress damage natural resiliency and children's ability to respond effectively to future trauma exposure.

What is often overlooked when considering any individual's resilience in the face of a particular trauma is what the person has already experienced *before* dealing with the current situation. For instance, a terrorist bomb detonates on a busy city street, killing, maiming, and causing widespread destruction and chaos. A survivor with a history of moderate lifetime stress speaks up about the attack, comforts and aids other survivors, and before long returns to his or her normal routine. Another survivor who has been resilient in the face of a personal history of severe childhood abuse and neglect may, after surviving this terror attack, be unable to bounce back naturally, the bombing being a last straw of sorts.

Researchers have also identified a set of psychological traits and habits of those who show resilience in the aftermath of trauma. These individuals tend to respond with an active coping style; they face their fears head-on and work through their problems, accepting and dealing with the emotions they are experiencing. This contrasts to a more passive, and hence less resilient, coping style, which relies on denial, avoidance, or simply resigning oneself to the situation.

Individuals who are resilient maintain a positive outlook on life; they view the trauma as being temporary and can visualize a positive ending. Having a strong moral compass or life mission or engaging in spiritual and religious practices can also help survivors cope after tragedy. Using mental agility or cognitive flexibility to come up with creative solutions and find meaning in the aftermath of tragedy are additional attributes of the naturally resilient. Tapping into the benefits of physical exercise is also important. Regular physical exercise leads to a release of the brain's natural chemicals and neuro-transmitters. These, in turn, alleviate stress and anxiety, lift mood, and improve memory and learning.

Individuals who are resilient are also able to regulate their emotions more effectively. Consider a person who experiences a near-miss car accident on a busy highway. An emotionally reactive person may respond with road rage, a reflexive response that hampers the ability to think straight and can lead to an irrational decision such as chasing after the alleged perpetrator. Resilient individuals are able to reframe the situation: "He probably did not cut in on purpose . . . maybe he did not see me . . . thank goodness there was no accident."

Superhumans or the Beneficiaries of Endowed Gifts?

The survivor movies I watched as a child often tapped into a myth that is still propagated in popular culture: some humans are super-human; they are born with nerves of steel, an impeccable attitude, hardy determination, and mounds of natural talent. They are impervious to their surroundings and will flourish wherever you put them, whatever tragedy they face.

Though I don't doubt the existence of superhumans, I would argue that more often than not their traits are not inherent but rather endowed, as gifts, by their early caregivers, environment, and community.

Take, for instance, the resilient trait of having a positive outlook. A recent study examined data from World War II and Korean War veterans and took a close look at the relationship between the odds of their having PTSD and a variety of life experiences. The researchers asked about the veterans' prewar life (Did you have a history of childhood trauma? Did you come from a cohesive family?), their war zone experience (What level of combat were you exposed to? Did your military unit have good cohesion?), and also their postwar life (What was your homecoming experience? Have you faced other stressful life events?). Among their many findings was this: "A supportive childhood family environment can have *lifelong* protective effects, whereas a conflict-ridden family environment can set one up for lifelong patterns of pessimistic appraisals." Findings like these pose the question, How much of an individual's positive outlook in the aftermath of trauma is attributable to the early examples set by his or her parents, family, teachers, and friends?

Resilience also plays out on a societal level in that the resilience of the wider community to which you belong has a knock-on effect on your own capacity, as an individual, to be resilient. The zip code where you live is a prime determinant of your capacity to be resilient in the face of trauma. For example, a refugee who moves her family from a war-torn, middle-income country to a politically stable, high-income country endows an extra dose of resilience upon the future lives of her children. Parents who scrimp and save to move their kids from a violent inner city to a more affluent suburb have gifted future resilience to their children. Can the children, then, take sole credit for their future resilience? Of course they can take credit for making the most of the opportunities that living in a more resilient community has afforded them, but they cannot claim credit for the gift of being transplanted into a certain zip code by their parents.

The myth of the resilient superhuman is probably best exemplified when we look at the relationship between social support and resilience. Studies suggest that social support fosters resilience by dampening down the fight-or-flight response and releasing oxytocin, a brain chemical that reduces fear, increases self-confidence, and encourages the individual to respond to stress in an active rather than passive manner.

Consider this scenario: A young college student is raped by another student; she is traumatized and distressed but seeks help from her parents and the relevant authorities, who respond in a supportive way. She receives immediate medical care, and the perpetrator is placed on suspension while her allegation is investigated. Her parents arrange for her to come home and take a short leave from her classes. She becomes fearful and has nightmares and intrusive memories of the rape, so her parents insist that she see a mental health professional. They seek a referral for a good therapist from a close family friend who is a local family doctor. The personal connection means her request for help is fast-tracked; she is seen within days and offered psychological reassurance, and within weeks she is on the road to recovery. Though the subsequent legal case, media attention, and interruption of her studies is harrowing, she traverses it with unwavering support from her family and advocates from within the college and legal and activist organizations. Her attacker is eventually jailed, and she returns to campus to complete her studies.

Compare it to this scenario: A young college student is raped by another student; she is traumatized and distressed but seeks help from her parents and the relevant authorities. Her father chides her for being "stupid" and accuses her of "letting this happen." He questions her account, insinuates that she is exaggerating, and withholds emotional support when she cannot offer much physical "proof" that the rape happened. Her mother is more sympathetic but is unable to assert her opinion over her dominating husband's stance. She falls silent and turns away when her daughter looks to her for sympathy. The student becomes perplexed and distressed and fails to follow through with the paperwork the college needs to lodge her allegation and investigate it. Because she is a recipient of financial aid, her father instructs her to "not make a fuss" with the college because she will "mess up her future." She follows his advice but experiences overwhelming fear, nightmares, and intrusive memories of the rape. Her distress is exacerbated by the fact that she frequently sees the perpetrator on campus. A friend suggests that she seek help at the local student health center, even offers to make an appointment, but her demanding class schedule and the part-time job she needs for supplemental income to pay for her housing mean she cannot follow through with her appointment. Unfortunately her condition only deteriorates, she turns to alcohol for relief of her symptoms, and within weeks she is skipping classes and her grades start to drop. Eventually she drops out of college.

The oft-quoted dictum "What does not kill you makes you stronger" implies that if you can just survive through a period of adversity, it will leave you better off in the long run, wiser and stronger, better able to deal with whatever your future life may throw at you. This dictum warrants some analysis in light of these two scenarios. Did the first college student go on to thrive in the face of adversity because of sheer willpower, endurance, or an inherent character? Or was it the support of her loved ones and the wider validation by her community that provided the protective shield necessary for her healing? Was this a support system that she was born into, and, if so, can she take full credit for it? No doubt she can take credit for her choice to make the most of the help that was offered to her, but where would she have been without that protective surrounding? Would her situation have been that different from that of the other rape survivor?

What about the reverse? What if the second college student had somehow been able to tap into a supportive social network, similar to the one that was available to the first college student? Would she have fared better?

Perhaps, then, a more apt saying might be "There but for the grace of God go I," a favorite among seasoned mental health professionals.

Resilience in Action

In the aftermath of trauma exposure, who is most likely to develop PTSD? Big-data studies have identified the following risk factors: being socially disadvantaged, being younger, being a woman, having a prior history of trauma exposure or a history of childhood trauma, having a family history of psychiatric illness, dissociating at the time of the trauma, and having limited posttrauma social support. When one considers this risk profile, it becomes clear that the same way resilience is often endowed in the form of gifts to an individual, the reverse holds true, too. Much of what makes a human vulnerable to developing PTSD, or worse, in the aftermath of trauma appears to be beyond the individual's control.

There is an exciting shift under way that addresses this gap by empowering individuals with the knowledge, skills, and training to make them more resilient *before* they are exposed to trauma or shortly thereafter. Hardiness training, Skills for Psychological Recovery, and cue-centered treatment are just some examples of programs that have been developed and are in the early phases of being tested.

As might be expected, many of the advances in resiliency training have arisen from studies done with military and first responders for whom trauma exposure is an occupational hazard. At a basic level, trainings typically involve briefings, informational leaflets, and videos that aim to educate participants about the way one's brain and body normally respond to trauma and the signs of PTSD. More intense efforts involve the teaching of specific coping skills, anxiety-reducing techniques, and the importance of maintaining social supports so that the emotional impact of trauma can be curtailed. This skills training can be done through cognitive exercises, role playing, and live demonstrations.

Stress inoculation training (SIT) is worthy of mention because it is widely acknowledged as one of the more effective approaches. The philosophy behind SIT aims to "inoculate" participants by actually exposing them to low-level stressors by using virtual reality technology or actual simulations and teaching them how to respond and how to control their bodies' physiological reactions to stress with relaxation training and stress management techniques.

Dr. Carl C. Bell, a psychiatrist at the University of Illinois at Chicago, led a program geared toward youth homicide prevention that aims to target risk factors and also accentuate protective factors. The Aban Aya Youth Project took place in twelve public schools in Chicago. It focused on rebuilding the social fabric surrounding kids in a given community, improving self-esteem through improved academic performance, and providing them with opportunities to increase their social and emotional skills by learning anger management, peer mediation, and conflict resolution techniques. The program reported many encouraging outcomes, including reducing violent behavior, school delinquency, and illicit drug use among boys.

Though it remains to be seen whether such programs can be replicated on a large scale, their promise is enticing: by leveraging what is known about the science of resilience, there is an opportunity to level the playing field so that more people are given the opportunity to thrive and survive in the aftermath of trauma.

AFTERWORD:
A PRECIOUS INHERITANCE

My father would often walk me home from elementary school, holding my hand with a firm grip that made me feel secure and warm inside. Our thirty-minute walk would be filled with his voice taking me on a nonstop journey all over the countries of the intellectual kingdom from philosophy, geography, and history to politics, ethics, and science.

His lesson would start as he greeted me at the blue railings of the school entrance and continue as we crossed the tiny wooden bridge that ran over a trickling reservoir and onto the sidewalk, where I skipped alongside him, avoiding all the cracks. He would continue as we passed rows of emerald green privet bushes encircling tiny squares of English gardens that sat under grey clouds, holding the perpetual promise of rain. He would pause briefly to ensure our safe crossing of the intersection at the busy main road but then take up again with his ideas of how a hospital should best provide health care to the rich and the poor, the importance of aerobic exercise to human health, what a crime it is to waste the earth's precious resources, and how ancient Indian thought held the answers to much of mankind's misery, if only we would take the time to study and understand it.

As a girl barely aged ten, I assumed that was the way all fathers spoke to their children. It was only with the passage of time and exposure to the ways of the world that I would come to appreciate his uniqueness: an insatiable curiosity, perceptual clarity, encyclopedic memory, and brain chock-full of creative ideas. What I had no idea of at that time was that it was precisely those intrinsic attributes, his cognitive flexibility, that would be vital to his survival after 1947.

He had a powerhouse intellect that allowed him to do the mental somersaults that ensured his resiliency in the face of adversity.

Decades after our walks home from school I shared with Dad a piece I had published about nightmares, traumatic stress, and imagery rehearsal therapy (IRT). After reading it, with his usual care and attention to detail, he was prompted to disclose something he rarely spoke about. He told me how, in 1947, as a ten-year-old boy, when his father had put him on the bus from Jhelum to Amritsar, he had had no idea that he was leaving his home forever. When, a short time later, he had been told that his father had been murdered before crossing the border, he had felt his whole world collapse. For years after 1947, he still dreamed of being reunited with his father. In his dreams, he would experience a feeling of suffocation and the sensation that someone, or something, was trying to kill him. As a teenager, he figured out a way to overcome those nightmares, and the method he described to me was a rudimentary form of IRT. I remember marveling how, as a teenager, he had had the cognitive ability to hack out a solution to solve his problem.

Another example of his cognitive flexibility is his uncanny ability to access his inner child, almost at will. I can recall so many childhood incidents where one moment Dad would be raging and ranting about the tiniest of matters, and the next minute, sitting on the sofa, watching a TV sitcom, he would laugh out loud till his eyes filled with tears. Years later, he told me how, as a child laborer, when life had felt especially oppressive, he would find some way to go to the cinema. It was during those times, sitting in the dark, absorbed in the music, drama, and comedy of the latest Raj Kapoor or Dilip Kumar Bollywood epic that he could forget all the harshness of life and once again become a child. He told me how he would intentionally laugh hard, as if he did not have a care in the world, and that there was something about that forced expression that was healing for him.

I think it is safe to say that many of Dad's intrinsic abilities might have been squandered if it had not been for his brother Roshan. In the fledgling India, with no child welfare protection laws, Dad was put to work in a factory, packaging yarn, for nine hours a day, six days of the week. The money he earned covered household expenses not only for himself but for his younger siblings. School was not mandatory and, moreover, was expensive, and the benefits of employment were more tangible to Dad: he made money, earned his keep, and could have some semblance of independence. He was soon convinced that school was a waste of time and a factory job was all he needed to get by. Plus he had little respect for authority, and as he entered puberty, his fierce intellect was misguidedly citing all sorts of reasons for why he did not need an education.

But then, just as a child's life can become marred by tragedy, it can also have a remarkable resiliency to heal. For my father, the seeds of hope were planted by Roshan. In 1947, Roshan was in his early twenties, a medical student who was engaged to be married. After my grandfather's death, Roshan was in charge of his four younger siblings, so he quit medical school and tried to find employment. His job search took him all over north India, and, whenever possible, he would send money back home for his brothers and sisters. During those chaotic times, Roshan became sick with rheumatic fever, which damaged the valves of his heart. He could work only sporadically, and under the pressure of his failing health and declining fortunes, his engagement was also broken off.

Still, despite that bleakness, Roshan would periodically return from his out-of-state work to doggedly try to convince Dad to return to school. But Dad was consumed by rage at Roshan. The extended family with which Dad was living never told him that Roshan was sending money home, and the pain of his perceived abandonment was so intense in Dad's young mind that he used it to power his anger toward Roshan and do the opposite of what he was telling him to do.

In 1949, Roshan secured local employment and returned home. When he arrived, Dad, who was all set to ignore him, could not help but be taken aback at his gaunt appearance. The vitality appeared to have been sucked out of him, and even the mildest exertion left him gasping for breath. Still, despite his failing health, he did not shy away from arguing with Dad about the importance of a formal education.

During one of their arguments, Roshan became very short of breath, and, as he was overcome with waves of uncontrollable cough-ing, his face turned almost blue. Dad watched as Roshan fumbled in his pocket searching for his digitalis medication, then collapsed onto a chair, looking beat and exhausted. Dad, momentarily stunned by what he had witnessed, said nothing but over the coming days ac-quiesced to Roshan's request that he reenroll in school.

Roshan paid for Dad's school fees, supplies, and books and hired a private tutor so that Dad could make up for his two-year hiatus from school. In November 1950, Roshan died from complications of rheumatic heart disease, but the legacy of education he left gave Dad a new lease of life. He graduated from high school and college and went on to get a master's degree in English literature.

The obstacles were many, and he would often work two jobs, in addition to attending school, to make ends meet. But with an educa-tion, Dad's destructive attitudes started to be replaced by a passion for knowledge, intellectual curiosity, and a yearning for independent thought. Over time, his formal education would grant him passage to England, where he would work and raise a family. In an ironic twist, the land of India's former colonial ruler would prove a gentler place for him to live in.

Whenever he would hit troubled times in life, he would return to great books to find answers that would restore meaning. I do not know anyone who treasures the carefully written word more than my father. So, more than fifty years ago, when Indian society dictated that he mute his elation at the birth of a daughter, he found educated reasons to fiercely defy such ignorance. To top that, he started to make big plans to ensure that all his children would receive the finest education. In this way, my uncle Roshan created a family legacy that I would continue to reap the rewards of. The name Roshan, translated from Hindi, means "Shining Light."

In my mind, the biggest boon a formal education granted my father was that it made him eligible to marry my mother. My parents' marriage was arranged, and only that ancient method of forging unions could explain their pairing, for I am convinced that if left to his own devices, Dad would have been unable to attract someone like Mom into his life. Her upbringing could not have been more different from his. She was born and raised in a village where her family had lived for generations, and her childhood was surrounded by a plethora of doting relatives in a place where every kid in the village belonged to all the adults. The opportunities for laughter were endless, and she had little pressure on her to do much of anything. School was serious, but there was no college in the village, and because it was unthinkable to send girls away for schooling, Mom's level of education was predetermined to end at high school.

Her different start in life blessed her with a grounded nature and endless capacity for love, in contrast to Dad's more wavering affections and propensity to be mistrustful, even of those who wish him well. She has endless patience and is by nature cheerful, optimistic, and accommodating in her dealings with others, a perfect antidote to Dad's more mercurial mood, general impatience, and more entitled posturing in his interpersonal dealings. In my eyes, the protective effect of her love for him has been immeasurable.

I cherish those memories of my childhood walks with Dad because it was during those times that he was his best self. He had a childlike fascination about the world, was deeply compassionate, and was connected to humankind. I feel the cumulative boons of those walks to this day. His boldness was infectious and left me with the confidence to be aspirational in my own life. In contrast to those walks, there was much I witnessed about Dad while growing up that was painful to be around. He could be unreasonably tough on me and frequently outspoken, to the point of its being uncomfortable. He refused to accept injustices small or large, real or misperceived, and often insisted on standing in his own truth even if it meant sucking up all the oxygen in the room.

Today, I have a deeper understanding of what I was witnessing: my father's ongoing internal battle, a fight not only for survival but for making meaning out of tragedy. The events of 1947 were a physical force that derailed his life. At some point early on, it seems he decided that he was not going to let that force take him down, but surviving presented him with a dilemma. He could not simply forget or bury his past, because to do so would mean losing a piece of himself in the process. He would live, but the trauma would have to live alongside him; he could give that traumatic force a different shape and direction, but he could not deny its existence.

He chose to use the traumatic force of 1947 to give his life mission and purpose, resolving to honor his parents' memory by restoring his family name to what it had once been. In that way, he preserved the traumatic legacy of 1947 as a sort of precious inheritance that, despite all its darkness, also held universal truths. I believe that process of making meaning ultimately anchored my father, enabling him to survive and thrive despite the heavy odds stacked against him. In doing so, he veered away from the paths of hatred, revenge, or oblivion that can consume the lives of so many of those who have survived trauma.

HOW THIS BOOK WAS WRITTEN

Never in the history of medicine has patients' confidentiality and medical professionalism been so scrutinized and regulated. This climate rightfully raises ethical dilemmas for any physician who writes about his or her profession for a lay audience. The physician writers Rita Charon, Jack Coulehan, and Danielle Ofri have published careful arguments that articulate some fundamental considerations: writing about patients should never cause them harm (emotional, spiritual, financial, or psychological), and physician writers should always engage in an honest appraisal of who will benefit most by their publication. The patient? The physician? The larger society?

The ethical issues for physician writers are ever evolving in a dynamic landscape, and although there remains no right answer on how to resolve such conflicts, in this book I implemented the following safeguards. The reader should consider *The Unspeakable Mind* a work of nonfiction but understand that to protect individual patients' privacy the stories depicted are composites of real encounters brought together to illustrate various situations. I decided that the specifics of a case were less critical in this type of work and could be re-created into a composite without compromising the truth. All patient composites were deidentified by excluding information that is very specific to each patient. To further protect patients' privacy, I chose not to write about rare cases.

Additional safeguards include always writing in a way that intends to honor my patients, is respectful, and enriches the public discourse about PTSD. I deliberately did not write graphic trauma accounts as I did not want to cause unnecessary distress to readers who have a trauma history. In addition to keeping the faith of my patients, I have followed the wise advice of the physician writer Jack Coulehan to also "keep faith with the reader" by being transparent about how I have chosen to write about patients.

Though the conversations with family members and colleagues described in this book depict true events, real names have been withheld to protect the privacy of the individuals concerned. The book's dialogue is either based on notes taken during the time or reconstructed from memory. In some places time has been compressed or the order of events has been changed for the sake of narrative cohesion. Other sections of the book relay memories of incidents I personally experienced as a child and later as a medical student, resident, research fellow, psychiatrist, and PTSD specialist. This period spans more than three decades, so if my memory has failed me, the fault is mine.

I have written in some detail about my own family history of trauma and the lives of my ancestors. All this information came from several detailed conversations I had with my parents, who were subsequently given the opportunity to read these sections and to correct matters of fact. My father's story of his life before, during, and after 1947 comes from his memories of the events as they transpired in addition to details he gleaned from subsequent conversations with various family elders, all of whom are now deceased. Both of my parents have their stories, as told through assisted narration, documented in the 1947 Partition Archive. Since 2016, I have served in an advisory role to the archive.

Over the decade it has taken to write this book, I have been the fortunate beneficiary of the wisdom of global leaders in the field of PTSD practice and science. Many of them are formally acknowledged at the end of this book, and although it is not practical for me to name every single individual here, the fact remains that they have all been influential in my personal development as a PTSD specialist and researcher.

A significant portion of this book also involves describing and deconstructing a massive body of scientific data. It is important to note the existence of a bias in funding sources for PTSD research. High-income-country institutions fund the bulk of PTSD research, so the data we have often come from populations who reside in such countries. Furthermore, the PTSD research that is conducted in middle- and low-income countries is often funded by institutions or agencies that receive funding from high-income countries or governments. It could be argued that this funding leads to a cultural bias in research design and agenda. Still, the reality is that some of the most devastating and deadliest traumas take place in low- and middle-income countries. For these reasons, I felt an urgency to present whatever science has discovered about PTSD in such countries but, for the sake of completion, have acknowledged the inherent bias.

Another issue is one of generalizability. Advancing the science and understanding of PTSD is integral to the mission of the Veterans Administration. Thus, much of the highest-quality PTSD data comes from studies done with research subjects who are veterans. In *The Unspeakable Mind*, I often generalize the findings from these studies to civilian populations. I am mindful of the scientific limits of such generalizability but make this jump only when, from a clinician viewpoint, it did not feel it was misleading to do so. The treatment of children with PTSD is beyond the scope of this book and not specifically addressed in Part 5. The reader is referred to the Resources section for further details.

I have endeavored to credit all referenced science in an extensive notes section. If I have failed to correctly acknowledge a person or source, I would like to be given the opportunity to correct this. With regard to my choice of research studies to present to the reader, I have given preference to the most up-to-date studies that have used controlled statistical designs and revealed findings worthy of note. These selection criteria mean that many naturalistic data, case studies, or observational data from the fields of criminology, anthropology, and sociology have been omitted. There are some areas of the field in which the quality of science is subpar; in such cases I have summarized the best available evidence. I have avoided the excessive use of off-putting scientific and medical jargon and have endeavored to do so without compromising the precise language that my profession demands.

Prior to publication, I sent this manuscript to several colleagues for their expert review and input. I asked them to point out any glaring omissions or errors or where the writing was scientifically subpar. Their detailed commentary and careful feedback were subsequently incorporated into the final manuscript. These generous souls have been formally acknowledged at the end of this book.

Parts of this book, in different forms, have appeared on *PLOS Blogs* and KevinMD.com and in *Psychology Today STAT,* and *Canadian Medical Association Journal.* Many of the expert quotes that appear in the book were excerpted from earlier extensive interviews which have been published elsewhere. The references for these original interviews can be found in the notes section. The excerpts that appear in this book have, on occasion, been edited for clarity and brevity.

ACKNOWLEDGMENTS

I am profoundly grateful for the following:

My patients who have provided, over and over, the inspiration for a book like this to have a soul.

The support of close colleagues at the VA Palo Alto Healthcare System, National Center for PTSD, and Stanford University. It is a blessing to work in an ecosystem of dedicated clinicians, researchers, and educators. I am especially inspired by the courage of the clinical teams who are required to wade into the messy parts of people's psyches. Their work is challenging, often unsung, and invariably carried out under tough circumstances. Yet they show up, every day, ready to engage in this extreme support of experiential empathy.

Steve Lindley and Craig Rosen who took a chance on me and have graciously mentored my career since I first arrived at Stanford in 2009. Marylene Cloitre and Joe Ruzek, from the National Center for PTSD, who welcomed me into an intellectual home quite unlike any I have ever known. Samina Iqbal, a truly gifted VA physician leader, who has long understood the importance of integrated care and who, almost a decade ago, paved the way for me to be able to provide this important service for women veterans. Andy Pomerantz who, as National Mental Health Director for Integrated Care, led the charge to have high quality, patient-centered integrated care available to all American veterans. The bold leadership of Tina Lee, Laura Roberts, and Jerry Yesavage, whose actions ensure the stability of the environments required for academic psychiatry to thrive.

The Michael Alan Rosen Foundation for generously supporting my PTSD research since 2011.

The monthly journal club, which has been an unexpected boon. Being in the company of such passionate and naturally skeptical physicians has made me a better doctor. Special thanks to Kathy Sanborn for introducing me to this group and to Anna Lembke and Harriet Roeder for leading this special program. My students, who are truly the brightest and the best and make me hopeful about the future of our profession.

Many early teachers and colleagues who, at pivotal moments of my career, encouraged me to write: Pete Carlson, Carl Chan, Joe Layde, Laura Roberts, and Carol Tsao deserve specific mention. Robert Higgo, Tony Meyer, Dinshah Gagrat, Vani Ray, and Krishna Mylavarapu all superb psychiatrists who have shaped my identity by emphasizing the importance of artistry and service in the practice of psychiatry.

Jon Lehrmann who has remained a constant mentor in my life for the better part of the last twenty years. He was the first person ever to tell me that I could write, and actively encouraged me to get my work published. Jon is a tireless champion for those who live with mental illness, an extraordinary role model for psychiatrists, and one of the most generous and compassionate people I have ever had the pleasure to know.

The physician writer Audrey Shafer, who is a pioneer in the field of medical humanities and has been a beloved mentor and true advocate for my career and writing ambitions. Her huge heart and passion for educating future generations of physicians in the arts and humanities is a continual source of inspiration to me.

Hans Steiner who, via the Pegasus Physician Writers' groups, has provided so many Stanford doctors endless opportunities for rejuvenation and creative collaboration. As a world leader in treating trauma-related conditions, he has been a true believer, not only in this book, but in me, too. His clarity of vision and passion for preserving all that is good and true in the art of caring for patients has meant so much.

Irv Yalom, whose teaching novels and textbooks I have cherished since my days as a psychiatry resident. I consider myself very lucky to have had the opportunity to spend time, share words, and break bread with a psychiatrist who has had such a profound, positive, and lasting influence on our field.

Daniel Mason and Sandeep Jauhar, both wildly accomplished physician writers who have my deepest admiration. They have helped me navigate the various intricacies of the publishing world and supported me over many a hurdle. I am blessed to have been able to rely on their comradery through such uncertain times.

Over the years, the essays, books, and journalism of these additional doctor authors have, in a variety of ways, influenced my own approaches to writing about medicine: Atul Gawande; Siddhartha Mukherjee; Andrew Solomon; Abraham Verghese; Kay Redfield Jamieson; Nancy Andreason; Louise Aronson; Paul Kalanithi; Danielle Ofri; and Jerome Groopman.

The following landmark textbooks which proved to be invaluable resources as I wrote this book: *The Handbook of PTSD: Science and Practice*; *Trauma and Recovery: The Aftermath of Violence-From Domestic Abuse to Political Terror*; *Achilles in Vietnam: Combat Trauma and the Undoing of Character*; and *Traumatic Stress: The Effects of Overwhelming Experience on Mind, Body, and Society.*

Charles Marmar, Matthew Friedman, Erik Kandel, Rachel Yehuda, Anna Lembke, Victor Carrion, Joan Cook, Rebecca Moore, Craig Rosen, Marcel Bonn Miller, Renee Binder, Eric Kuhn, Joe Ruzek, and Marylene Cloitre gave their valuable time to answer my questions about their specific areas of expertise. Their generosity allowed me to infuse the book with their deep perspectives and cutting-edge approaches.

My parents, who shared their memories of our family history and of growing up in India in the years and decades that followed Partition. They also read this book and provided invaluable feedback and my father made extensive notes to help me write the sections of the book that relay our family history. To them, I have dedicated this book.

Laurel Braitman, Jackie Genovese, and the Pegasus Physician Writers who read parts of this manuscript when it was in its initial stages. A special thanks to Richard Shaw who has been a thoughtful and optimistic presence through this journey.

Anna Lembke, Bill Boddie, and Ellie Beam who carefully read and provided constructive feedback on select chapters from the final manuscript. I am especially grateful for the expert commentary of Priya Satia, a Stanford professor of British history, as I wrote the chapter about the 1947 Partition.

Christine Silk, Shelley Preston, Kathryn Azevedo, Pria Anand, Craig Rosen, Jon Lehrmann, Hans Steiner, Raziya Wang, and Alka Mathur are all cherished friends and colleagues who went above and beyond and read the entire manuscript. Your collective wisdom and considered input gave me that much needed boost to get this project over the finish line.

Ann Tennier, who provided her signature care and attention to copy-editing this manuscript as it passed through many incarnations. Becky Hall also helped with copy-editing the proposal and early chapters, and Hannah Holt ensured the appropriate organization and cataloguing of research articles.

Hem, Gogi, Kim, Danielle, Sarah, Surag, Maddy, Trevor, Alpesh, Nagappan, Ty, Brian, and Jason—all amazing family and friends who were quick to chime in with much-needed feedback on the title and other related woes.

My agent, Trena Keating, whose faith in my abilities has been a godsend. A true advocate for new voices, her compassionate intelligence and stellar editorial talent were pivotal to my realization that *this* was the book I was meant to write. I feel deeply fortunate for her reassuring and wise counsel throughout all phases of this unfamiliar journey.

My editor at Harper, Gail Winston, who is the type of editor that writers dream of having. Over the three years it has taken me to write this book I have been blessed with regular and quick access to her impeccable judgment and editorial magic. Her deep passion for the material was palpable and her dazzling expertise means this book ended up better and bolder in ways that I could not have imagined possible.

Gail's entire team and colleagues at Harper who have provided ongoing expertise and assistance at key stages of this process. Sofia Groopman was immensely helpful in providing guidance in the initial stages of manuscript preparation. Emily Taylor deserves special mention as her prompt assistance, professionalism, and obsessive attention to detail has proved invaluable during the final stages of bringing this book to life.

For S and K, who are both my unintentional muses and the source of such deep delight. I hope that life will always bring you love, the real kind that challenges you to be the best human you can possibly be. And I hope that you always choose to do meaningful work, work that is bigger than yourself.

Finally, while it is true that it has taken a village to bring this book to life the fact remains that this book would not exist were it not for R. Thank you for infusing my life with the peace, joy, and harmony necessary for creativity to thrive. If my talent has taken a shape in this world it is because of your love, friendship, and unflinching support.

NOTES

Prologue

xiv diagnostic checklist: American Psychiatric Association, *Diagnostic and Statistical Manual of Mental Disorders*, 5th ed. (Arlington, VA: American Psychiatric Association, 2013), 271–80.

Introduction

xvii experiencing many such traumas: Fran H. Norris and Laurie B. Slone, "Epidemiology of Trauma and PTSD," in *Handbook of PTSD: Science and Practice*, 2nd ed., ed. Matthew J. Friedman, Terence Martin Keane, and Patricia A. Resick (New York: Guilford Press, 2014), 100–21.

xviii suffer and also need help: Paula P. Schnurr, "A Guide to the Literature on Partial PTSD," *PTSD Research Quarterly* 25, no. 1 (2014): 1–3, https://www.ptsd.va.gov/professional/newsletters/research-quarterly/v25n1.pdf.

xix alcoholism: Duncan G. Campbell, Bradford L. Felker, Chuan-Fen Liu, Elizabeth M. Yano, JoAnn E. Kirchner, Domin Chan, Lisa V. Rubenstein, and Edmund F. Chaney, "Prevalence of Depression-PTSD Comorbidity: Implications for Clinical Practice Guidelines and Primary Care-Based Interventions" *Journal of General Internal Medicine* 22, no. 6 (2007): 711–18, https://doi.org/10.1007/s11606-006-0101-4.

xix anxiety: Leslie K. Jacobsen, Steven M. Southwick, and Thomas R. Kosten, "Substance Use Disorders in Patients with Posttraumatic Stress Disorder: A Review of the Literature," *The American Journal of Psychiatry* 158, no. 8 (2001): 1184–90, https://doi.org/10.1176/appi.ajp.158.8.1184.

xix higher risk of death by suicide: Jitender Sareen, Tanya Houlahan, Brian J. Cox, and Gordon J. G. Asmundson, "Anxiety Disorders Associated with Suicidal Ideation and Suicide Attempts in the National Comorbidity Survey," *The Journal of Nervous and Mental Disease* 193, no. 7 (2005): 450–54.

xix heart disease to obesity: Paula P. Schnurr, *Trauma and Health: Physical Health Consequences of Exposure to Extreme Stress* (Washington, DC: American Psychological Association, 2005).

xix sufferers are often hard to reach: Philip S. Wang, Michael Lane, Mark Olfson, Harold A. Pincus, Kenneth B. Wells, and Ronald C. Kessler,

"Twelve-Month Use of Mental Health Services in the United States: Results from the National Comorbidity Survey Replication," *Archives of General Psychiatry* 62, no. 6 (2005): 629–40, https://doi.org/10.1001/archpsyc.62.6.629.

xix developing depression, anxiety, and PTSD themselves: Eve B. Carlson and Joseph Ruzek, "PTSD and the Family," U.S. Department of Veterans Affairs, last modified February 23, 2016, accessed January 7, 2018, https://www.ptsd.va.gov/professional/treatment/family/ptsd-and-the-family.asp.

xix can last for generations: Yael Danieli, *International Handbook of Multigenerational Legacies of Trauma* (New York: Plenum Press, 2010).

xx indexed in the medical literature: Derek Summerfield, "The Invention of Post-traumatic Stress Disorder and the Social Usefulness of a Psychiatric Category," *The British Medical Journal* 322, no. 7278 (2001): 95–98, http://www.ncbi.nlm.nih.gov/pmc/articles/PMC1119389/.

The Road Trip with My Father

4 chaos and violence: Urvashi Butalia, *The Other Side of Silence: Voices from the Partition of India* (Durham, NC: Duke University Press, 2003).

4 forced to flee: C. Ryan Perkins, "1947 Partition of India & Pakistan," https://exhibits.stanford.edu/1947-partition/about/1947-partition-of-india-pakistan.

5 a horrible happening: Judith L. Herman, *Trauma and Recovery: The Aftermath of Violence—From Domestic Abuse to Political Terror* (New York: Basic Books, 2015), 1.

A Pressing Public Health Concern

10 "The ordinary human response": Judith L. Herman, *Trauma and Recovery: The Aftermath of Violence—From Domestic Abuse to Political Terror* (New York: Basic Books, 2015), 34.

11 rates of exposure: For a detailed breakdown of the epidemiology of PTSD, I refer the reader to Fran H. Norris and Laurie B. Slone, "Epidemiology of Trauma and PTSD," in *Handbook of PTSD: Science and Practice*, 2nd ed., ed. Matthew J. Friedman, Terence Martin Keane, and Patricia A. Resick (New York: Guilford Press, 2014), 100–21.

11 The most frequently reported: Arieh Shalev, Israel Liberzon, and Charles Marmar, "Post-traumatic Stress Disorder," *The New England Journal of Medicine* 376, no. 25 (2017): 2459–69.

11 more than 70 percent: C. Benjet, E. Bromet, E. G. Karam, et al., "The Epidemiology of Traumatic Event Exposure Worldwide: Results from the World Mental Health Survey Consortium," *Psychological Medicine* 46, no. 2 (2016): 327–43.

11 Clinician-Administered PTSD Scale: F. W. Weathers, D. D. Blake, P. P. Schnurr, et al., *The Clinician-Administered PTSD Scale for DSM-5 (CAPS-5)*, 2013, interview schema available from the National Center for PTSD at www.ptsd.va.gov.

13 public health concern: Kathryn M. Magruder, Katie A. McLaughlin, and Diane L. Elmore Borbon, "Trauma Is a Public Health Issue," *European Journal of Psychotraumatology* 8, no. 1 (2017): 1375338.

13 the higher this rate climbs: Anna Kline, Maria Falca-Dodson, Bradley Sussner, et al., "Effects of Repeated Deployment to Iraq and Afghanistan on the Health of New Jersey Army National Guard Troops: Implications for Military Readiness," *American Journal of Public Health* 100, no. 2 (2010): 276–83.

13 Similar statistics are seen: Mark I. Singer, Trina Menden Anglin, Li-Yu Song, and Lisa Lunghofer, "Adolescents' Exposure to Violence and Associated Symptoms of Psychological Trauma," *The Journal of the American Medical Association* 273, no. 6 (1995): 477–82. Tanya N. Alim, Dennis S. Charney, and Thomas A. Mellman, "An Overview of Posttraumatic Stress Disorder in African Americans," *Journal of Clinical Psychology* 62, no. 7 (2006): 801–13.

13 the odds of developing: Thomas M. Stein, "Mass Shootings," in *Disaster Medicine*, ed. David E. Hogan and Jonathan L. Burstein (Philadelphia: Lippincott Williams & Wilkins, 2011), 451.

13 Rape is the trauma: Ronald C. Kessler, Amanda Sonnega, Evelyn Bromet, et al., "Posttraumatic Stress Disorder in the National Comorbidity Survey," *Archives of General Psychiatry* 52, no. 12 (1995): 1048–60.

13 particularly in the first year: Isaac R. Galatzer-Levy, Yael Ankri, Sara Freedman, et al., "Early PTSD Symptom Trajectories: Persistence, Recovery, and Response to Treatment: Results from the Jerusalem Trauma Outreach and Prevention Study (J-TOPS)," *PloS One* 8, no. 8 (2013): e70084, https://doi.org/10.1371/journal.pone.0070084.

14 only a third: Philip S. Wang, Michael Lane, Mark Olfson, et al., "Twelve-Month Use of Mental Health Services in the United States: Results from the National Comorbidity Survey Replication," *Archives of General Psychiatry* 62, no. 6 (2005): 629–40, https://doi.org/10.1001/archpsyc.62.6.629.

14 average of twelve years: Philip S. Wang, Patricia Berglund, Mark Olfson, et al., "Failure and Delay in Initial Treatment Contact After First Onset of Mental Disorders in the National Comorbidity Survey Replication," *Archives of General Psychiatry* 62, no. 6 (2005): 603–13, https://doi.org/10.1001/archpsyc.62.6.603.

14   "Such unhealed PTSD": Jonathan Shay, *Achilles in Vietnam: Combat Trauma and the Undoing of Character* (New York: Scribner, 2005), xx.

14   2015 research findings: Charles R. Marmar, William Schlenger, Clare Henn-Haase, et al., "Course of Posttraumatic Stress Disorder 40 Years After the Vietnam War: Findings from the National Vietnam Veterans Longitudinal Study," *JAMA Psychiatry* 72, no. 9 (2015): 875–81, http://dx.doi.org/10.1001/jamapsychiatry.2015.0803.

14   "The effect on quality of life": Shaili Jain, "The National Vietnam Veterans Longitudinal Study (NVVLS) and the Implications for the Science and Practice of PTSD: An Interview with Dr. Charles Marmar," *PLOS Blogs*, September 16, 2015, http://blogs.plos.org/mindthebrain/2015/09/16/the-national-vietnam-veterans-longitudinal-study-nvvls-and-the-implications-for-the-science-and-practice-of-ptsd-an-interview-with-dr-charles-marmar/.

A Brief History of Trauma

16   "Stat consult": Reprinted from Shaili Jain, "The Psych Consult," *Canadian Medical Association Journal* 182, no. 17 (2010): 1888–89. © Canadian Medical Association 2010. This work is protected by copyright and the making of this copy was with the permission of the *Canadian Medical Association Journal* (www.cmaj.ca) and Access Copyright. Any alteration of its content or further copying in any form whatsoever is strictly prohibited unless otherwise permitted by law.

19   As far back: Source material for this chapter taken from Lars Weisaeth, "The History of Psychic Trauma," in *Handbook of PTSD: Science and Practice*, 2nd ed., ed. Matthew J. Friedman, Terence Martin Keane, and Patricia A. Resick (New York: Guilford Press, 2014), 38–59.

Old Wine in a New Bottle? From Shell Shock to Battered Women to PTSD

21   Traumatic stress has accrued: Lars Weisaeth, "The History of Psychic Trauma," in *Handbook of PTSD: Science and Practice*, 2nd ed., ed. Matthew J. Friedman, Terence Martin Keane, and Patricia A. Resick (New York: Guilford Press, 2014), 38–59, at 39.

22   psychological injury of World War I: Marc-Antoine Crocq and Louis Crocq, "From Shell Shock and War Neurosis to Posttraumatic Stress Disorder: A History of Psychotraumatology," *Dialogues in Clinical Neuroscience* 2, no. 1 (2000): 47–55, http://www.ncbi.nlm.nih.gov/pmc/articles/PMC3181586/.

22   "Psychiatry as a profession": Bessel A. van der Kolk, Lars Weisaeth, and Onno van der Hart, "History of Trauma in Psychiatry," in *Traumatic*

Stress: The Effects of Overwhelming Experience on Mind, Body, and Society, ed. Bessel A. van der Kolk, Alexander C. McFarlane, and Lars Weisaeth (New York: Guilford Press, 2007), 47.

23   the need to protect them: Lars Weisaeth, "The History of Psychic Trauma," in *Handbook of PTSD: Science and Practice*, 2nd ed. by Matthew J. Friedman, Terence Martin Keane, and Patricia A. Resick (New York: Guilford Press, 2014), 53.

23   compensatory research to test its legitimacy: Mardi Horowitz, Nancy Wilner, and William Alvarez, "Impact of Event Scale: A Measure of Subjective Stress," *Psychosomatic Medicine* 41, no. 3 (1979): 209–18. A key step to this substantial progress was the development, in 1979, of an Impact of Event Scale by the psychiatrist Mardi Horowitz. It offered a way to measure the psychological distress caused by various traumas. Now scientists could begin to cross the sea of myths that this elusive condition had been submerged in over the centuries.

23   "invent" the condition: Derek Summerfield, "The Invention of Post-Traumatic Stress Disorder and the Social Usefulness of a Psychiatric Category," *BMJ : British Medical Journal* 322, no. 7278 (2001): 95–98, http://www.ncbi.nlm.nih.gov/pmc/articles/PMC1119389/.

24   Epidemiological, clinical, and biological markers: Eric Vermetten, Dewleen Baker, Rakesh Jetly, and Alexander Mcfarlane, "Concerns over Divergent Approaches in the Diagnostics of Posttraumatic Stress Disorder," *Psychiatric Annals* 46 (2016): 498–509, https://doi.org/10.3928/00485713-20160728-02.

24   In the latest *DSM*: American Psychiatric Association, *The Diagnostic and Statistical Manual of Mental Disorders*, 5th ed. (Arlington, VA: American Psychiatric Association, 2013), 271–80.

Rocky Roads: Overdiagnosis and Underrecognition

25   PTSD remains steeped in controversy: A. Barbano, W. Van der Mei, R. Bryant, D. Delahanty, T. DeRoon-Cassini, Y. Matsuoka, A. Shalev, (2018), "Clinical Implications of the Proposed ICD-11 PTSD Diagnostic Criteria," *Psychological Medicine*, (2008): 1–8, DOI: 10.1017/S0033291718001101, https://www.ncbi.nlm.nih.gov/pubmed/29754591.

26   Many trauma survivors report: Peretz Lavie, "Sleep Disturbances in the Wake of Traumatic Events," *The New England Journal of Medicine* 345, no. 25 (2001): 1825–32, https://doi.org/10.1056/NEJMra012893.

26   *post-traumatic growth*: Richard G. Tedeschi and Lawrence G. Calhoun,

"The Posttraumatic Growth Inventory: Measuring the Positive Legacy of Trauma," *Journal of Traumatic Stress* 9, no. 3 (1996): 455–71, https://www.ncbi.nlm.nih.gov/pubmed/8827649.

26 "Approximately 3/4 of Vietnam veterans": Shaili Jain, "The National Vietnam Veterans Longitudinal Study (NVVLS) and the Implications for the Science and Practice of PTSD: An Interview with Dr. Charles Marmar," *PLOS Blogs*, September 16, 2015, http://blogs.plos.org /mindthebrain/2015/09/16/the-national-vietnam-veterans-longitudinal -study-nvvls-and-the-implications-for-the-science-and-practice-of-ptsd -an-interview-with-dr-charles-marmar/.

27 Genetic factors probably account: Karestan C. Koenen, Ananda B. Amstadter, and Nicole R. Nugent, "Gene-Environment Interaction in Posttraumatic Stress Disorder: An Update," *Journal of Traumatic Stress* 22, no. 5 (2009): 416–26, https://doi.org/10.1002/jts.20435.

27 Though these markers hint: Sehrish Sayed, Brian M. Iacoviello, and Dennis S. Charney, "Risk Factors for the Development of Psychopathology Following Trauma," *Current Psychiatry Reports* 17, no. 8 (2015): 70, https://doi.org/10.1007/s11920-015-0612-y.

27 traumatic events can serve as triggers: Dean G. Kilpatrick, Kenneth J. Ruggiero, Ron Acierno, et al., "Violence and Risk of PTSD, Major Depression, Substance Abuse/Dependence, and Comorbidity: Results from the National Survey of Adolescents," *Journal of Consulting and Clinical Psychology* 71, no. 4 (2003): 692–700.

27 "What many people do not understand": Shaili Jain, "PTSD and the DSM-5: A Conversation with Dr. Matt Friedman," *PLOS Blogs*, November 10, 2015, http://blogs.plos.org/blog/2015/11/10/ptsd-and-the-dsm-5-a-conversation -with-dr-matt-friedman/.

28 partial PTSD: Jacques Mylle and Michael Maes, "Partial Posttraumatic Stress Disorder Revisited," *Journal of Affective Disorders* 78, no. 1 (2017): 37–48, https://doi.org/10.1016/S0165-0327(02)00218-5.

A Disorder of Memory

38 *physiological reactions to cues*: American Psychiatric Association, *The Diagnostic and Statistical Manual of Mental Disorders*, 5th ed. (Washington, DC: American Psychiatric Association, 2013), 271.

39 *amnesia is common*: Jonathan Shay, *Achilles in Vietnam: Combat Trauma and the Undoing of Character* (New York: Scribner, 2005), 172.

41 lag period: Richard J. McNally, "Progress and Controversy in the Study

of Posttraumatic Stress Disorder," *Annual Review of Psychology* 54, no. 1 (2003): 229–52, https://doi.org/10.1146/annurev.psych.54.101601.145112.

42 PTSD is often described: Chris R. Brewin, "Remembering and Forgetting," in *Handbook of PTSD: Science and Practice*, 2nd ed., ed. Matthew J. Friedman, Terence Martin Keane, and Patricia A. Resick (New York: Guilford Press, 2014), 200–18.

42 indelible images: Robert Jay Lifton, *Death in Life: Survivors of Hiroshima* (University of North Carolina Press, 1991), 482.

43 Neuropsychology categorizes normal memories: Larry R. Squire and Stuart M. Zola, "Structure and Function of Declarative and Nondeclarative Memory Systems," *Proceedings of the National Academy of Sciences of the United States of America* 93, no. 24 (1996): 13515–22, http://www.ncbi .nlm.nih.gov/pmc/articles/PMC33639/.

43 Traumatic memories are also stored: Martin A. Conway and Christopher W. Pleydell-Pearce, "The Construction of Autobiographical Memories in the Self-Memory System," *Psychological Review* 107, no. 2 (2000): 261–88.

44 *fear structures*: Peter J. Lang, "A Bio-Informational Theory of Emotional Imagery," *Psychophysiology* 16, no. 6 (1979): 495–512, https://doi.org /10.1111/j.1469-8986.1979.tb01511.x.

44 applying it to the neuropsychology: Edna B. Foa and Michael J. Kozak, "Emotional Processing of Fear: Exposure to Corrective Information," *Psychological Bulletin* 99, no. 1 (1986): 20–35.

44 unwittingly act as triggers: David A. Ross, Melissa R. Arbuckle, Michael J. Travis, et al., "An Integrated Neuroscience Perspective on Formulation and Treatment Planning for Posttraumatic Stress Disorder: An Educational Review," *JAMA Psychiatry* 74, no. 4 (2017): 407–15, https://doi.org/10.1001 /jamapsychiatry.2016.3325.

44 The hippocampus: Ann M. Rasmussen and Chadi G. Abdallah, "Biomarkers for Treatment and Diagnosis," *PTSD Research Quarterly* 26, no. 1 (2015): 1–4, http://www.ptsd.va.gov/professional/newsletters/research-quarterly/ V26N1.pdf.

44 long-term memories: Jonathan E. Sherin and Charles B. Nemeroff, "Posttraumatic Stress Disorder: The Neurobiological Impact of Psychological Trauma," *Dialogues in Clinical Neuroscience* 13, no. 3 (2011): 263–78, http://www.ncbi .nlm.nih.gov/pmc/articles/PMC3182008/.

45 are memories made: Eric R. Kandel, *The Disordered Mind: What Unusual Brains Tell Us About Ourselves* (Farrar, Straus and Groux, 2018), 186–89.

45 synaptic connections between nerve cells: Eric R. Kandel, "The Molecular

Biology of Memory Storage: A Dialog Between Genes and Synapses (Nobel Lecture)," *Bioscience Reports* 21, no. 5 (2001): 565 LP-611, doi: 10.1023/A:1014775008533.

45 this attribute proved fundamental: Michael Robertson and Garry Walter, "Eric Kandel and *Aplysia californica*: Their Role in the Elucidation of Mechanisms of Memory and the Study of Psychotherapy," *Acta Neuropsychiatrica* 22, no. 4 (2010): 195–96, https://doi.org/10.1111/j.1601 -5215.2010.00476.x.

46 "PTSD very likely has prion mechanisms": Shaili Jain, "Prions, Memory and PTSD: A Conversation with Nobel Prize Winning Neuroscientist Dr. Eric R. Kandel," *PLOS Blogs: Mind the Brain* (blog), August 12, 2015, http:// blogs.plos.org/mindthebrain/2015/08/12/prions-memory-and-ptsd-a -conversation-with-nobel-prize-winning-neuroscientist-dr-eric-r-kandel/.

Nightmares

49 The classic PTSD nightmare: E. Hartmann, "Nightmare After Trauma as Paradigm for All Dreams: A New Approach to the Nature and Functions of Dreaming," *Psychiatry* 61, no. 3 (1998): 223–38.
Bessel A. van der Kolk, R. Blitz, W. Burr, et al., "Nightmares and Trauma: A Comparison of Nightmares After Combat with Lifelong Nightmares in Veterans," *The American Journal of Psychiatry* 141, no. 2 (1984): 187–90, https://doi.org/10.1176/ajp.141.2.187.

49 Some people with PTSD: Milton Kramer, "The Biology of Dream Formation: A Review and Critique," *The Journal of the American Academy of Psychoanalysis* 30, no. 4 (2002): 657–71. Pallavi Nishith, Patricia A. Resick, and Kim T. Mueser, "Sleep Difficulties and Alcohol Use Motives in Female Rape Victims with Posttraumatic Stress Disorder," *Journal of Traumatic Stress* 14, no. 3 (2001): 469–79, https://doi.org/10.1023/A:1011152405048.

53 insomnia is a distinct problem: Maurice M. Ohayon and Colin M. Shapiro, "Sleep Disturbances and Psychiatric Disorders Associated with Posttraumatic Stress Disorder in the General Population," *Comprehensive Psychiatry* 41, no. 6 (2000): 469–78, https://doi.org/10.1053/comp.2000.16568. Barry Krakow, Patricia L. Haynes, Teddy D. Warner, et al., "Nightmares, Insomnia, and Sleep-Disordered Breathing in Fire Evacuees Seeking Treatment for Posttraumatic Sleep Disturbance," *Journal of Traumatic Stress* 17, no. 3 (2004): 257–68, https://doi.org/10.1023/B:JOTS.0000029269.29098.67. T. C. Neylan, C. R. Marmar, T. J. Metzler, et al., "Sleep Disturbances in the Vietnam Generation: Findings from a Nationally Representative Sample of Male Vietnam Veterans," *The American Journal of Psychiatry* 155, no. 7

(1998): 929–33, https://doi.org/10.1176/ajp.155.7.929. T. M. Brown and P. A. Boudewyns, "Periodic Limb Movements of Sleep in Combat Veterans with Posttraumatic Stress Disorder," *Journal of Traumatic Stress* 9, no. 1 (1996): 129–36.

53   PTSD sufferers do not sleep: Anne Germain and Tore A. Nielsen, "Sleep Pathophysiology in Posttraumatic Stress Disorder and Idiopathic Nightmare Sufferers," *Biological Psychiatry* 54, no. 10 (2017): 1092–98, https://doi .org/10.1016/S0006-3223(03)00071-4.

53   Two decades of research: Victor I. Spoormaker and Paul Montgomery, "Disturbed Sleep in Post-traumatic Stress Disorder: Secondary Symptom or Core Feature?," *Sleep Medicine Reviews* 12, no. 3 (2017): 169–84, https:// doi.org/10.1016/j.smrv.2007.08.008.

53   imagery rehearsal therapy: For more information about imagery rehearsal therapy (IRT), as well as other therapies, see Standards of Practice Committee, R. Nisha Aurora, Rochelle S. Zak, Sanford H. Auerbach, et al., "Best Practice Guide for the Treatment of Nightmare Disorder in Adults," *Journal of Clinical Sleep Medicine* 6, no. 4 (2010): 389–401, http://www.ncbi.nlm .nih.gov/pmc/articles/PMC2919672/.

Flashbacks

56   functional magnetic resonance imaging: Matthew G. Whalley, Marijn C. W. Kroes, Zoe Huntley, et al., "An fMRI Investigation of Posttraumatic Flashbacks," *Brain and Cognition* 81, no. 1 (2013): 151–59, https://doi .org/10.1016/j.bandc.2012.10.002.

An Unlived Life: The Hidden Cost of Avoidance

60   avoidance: David A. Ross, Melissa R. Arbuckle, Michael J. Travis, et al., "An Integrated Neuroscience Perspective on Formulation and Treatment Planning for Posttraumatic Stress Disorder: An Educational Review," *JAMA Psychiatry* 74, no. 4 (2017): 407–15, https://doi.org/10.1001/jama psychiatry.2016.3325.

61   Avoidance occurs on two levels: American Psychiatric Association, *The Diagnostic and Statistical Manual of Mental Disorders*, 5th ed. (Arlington, VA: American Psychiatric Association, 2013), 271.

62   autobiographical memories: Jasmeet P. Hayes, Michael B. VanElzakker, and Lisa M. Shin, "Emotion and Cognition Interactions in PTSD: A Review of Neurocognitive and Neuroimaging Studies," *Frontiers in Integrative Neuroscience* 6 (October 2012): 89, https://doi.org/10.3389 /fnint.2012.00089.

64 *Staring at the Sun*: Irvin D. Yalom, *Staring at the Sun: Overcoming the Terror of Death* (San Francisco: Jossey-Bass, 2009).

Denial Land: When Trauma Memories Are Deeply Buried

66 extreme denial stays fixed: American Psychological Association, "Memories of Childhood Abuse," http://www.apa.org/topics/trauma/memories.aspx.

Carrying Sorrows in the Blood: Cortisol, Epigenetics, and Generational Trauma

70 Carrying Sorrows in the Blood: This phrase comes from the unpublished poem "A Life" by Audrey Shafer.

72 one's vulnerability to developing PTSD: L. E. Duncan, A. Ratanatharathorn, A. E. Aiello, et al., "Largest GWAS of PTSD (N=20 070) Yields Genetic Overlap with Schizophrenia and Sex Differences in Heritability," *Molecular Psychiatry* 23 (2017): 666–73, http://dx.doi.org/10.1038/mp.2017.77. Janine Naß and Thomas Efferth, "Pharmacogenetics and Pharmacotherapy of Military Personnel Suffering from Post-Traumatic Stress Disorder," *Current Neuropharmacology* 15.6 (2017): 831–860, PMC, Web, doi: 10.2174 /1570159X15666161111113514, https://www.ncbi.nlm.nij.gov/pmc/articles /PMC5652029/.

72 Epigenetics: Rachel Yehuda and Linda M. Bierer, "The Relevance of Epigenetics to PTSD: Implications for the DSM-V," *Journal of Traumatic Stress* 22, no. 5 (2009): 427–34, https://doi.org/10.1002/jts.20448.

73 hypothalamic-pituitary-adrenal (HPA) axis: David A. Ross, Melissa R. Arbuckle, Michael J. Travis, et al., "An Integrated Neuroscience Perspective on Formulation and Treatment Planning for Posttraumatic Stress Disorder: An Educational Review," *JAMA Psychiatry* 74, no. 4 (2017): 407–15, https://doi.org/10.1001/jamapsychiatry.2016.3325.

73 cortisol: Nikolaos P. Daskalakis, Amy Lehrner, and Rachel Yehuda, "Endocrine Aspects of Post-traumatic Stress Disorder and Implications for Diagnosis and Treatment," *Endocrinology and Metabolism Clinics of North America* 42, no. 3 (2013): 503–13, https://doi.org/https://doi .org/10.1016/j.ecl.2013.05.004. Farha Motiwala, "Do Glucocorticoids Hold Promise as a Treatment for PTSD?," *Current Psychiatry* 12, no. 9 (2013): 59–60.

73 the salivary cortisol of pregnant women: Rachel Yehuda, Stephanie Mulherin Engel, Sarah R. Brand, et al., "Transgenerational Effects of Posttraumatic Stress Disorder in Babies of Mothers Exposed to the World Trade Center

Attacks During Pregnancy," *The Journal of Clinical Endocrinology & Metabolism* 90, no. 7 (2005): 4115–18, http://dx.doi.org/10.1210/jc.2005-0550.

74   "The message is simple": Shaili Jain, "Cortisol, the Intergenerational Transmission of Stress, and PTSD: An Interview with Dr. Rachel Yehuda," *PLOS Blogs Network*, June 8, 2016, http://blogs.plos.org/blog/2016/06/08 /cortisol-the-intergenerational-transmission-of-stress-and-ptsd-an-interview -with-dr-rachel-yehuda/.

74   Other studies: Jonathan G. Shaw, Steven M. Asch, Rachel Kimerling, et al., "Posttraumatic Stress Disorder and Risk of Spontaneous Preterm Birth," *Obstetrics and Gynecology* 124, no. 6 (2014): 1111–19, https://doi .org/10.1097/AOG.0000000000000542.

74   rooted in historical events: There are many communities throughout the world that have suffered group trauma. For a wider perspective, I refer the reader to *International Handbook of Multigenerational Legacies of Trauma*, ed. Yael Danieli (Boston: Springer, 1998).

75   Are these collective sorrows: In recent years, a fringe cadre of mental health professionals has been advocating for recognition of the impact of historical *group* trauma on the present-day lives of the descendants of African slaves. The concept of post-traumatic slave syndrome was first proposed in the social sciences world well over a decade ago by the social worker Dr. Joy DeGruy, who argued that centuries of slavery in the United States, followed by structural racism and oppression, have led to a widespread multigenerational trauma in black America. DeGruy argues that the ubiquitous nature of structural racism means that the collective trauma of slavery has never been allowed sufficient time to be expressed, understood, and alleviated, a problem compounded by the resistance of American society to fully acknowledge the horrors of slavery. As a result, the traumatic oppression of centuries of slavery on the collective African spirit remains so overwhelming that the behaviors of enslaved Africans, which may have at one time provided a survival advantage, remain entrenched generations later but have now taken on a self-defeating form. Post-traumatic slave syndrome remains an unofficial description that has not been embraced by the medical establishment. See Joy DeGruy Leary, *Post Traumatic Slave Syndrome: America's Legacy of Enduring Injury and Healing* (Milwaukie, OR: Uptone Press, 2005). See also Omar G. Reid, Sekou Mims, and Larry Higginbottom, *Traumatic Slavery Disorder: Definition, Diagnosis, and Treatment* (Charlotte, NC: Conquering Books, 2005). W. E. Cross, "Black Psychological Functioning and the Legacy of Slavery: Myths and Realities,"

in Yael Danieli, ed. *International Handbook of Multigenerational Legacies of Trauma* (Boston: Springer, 1998), 387–402. Related to this, Paul Farmer discusses structural violence in rural Haiti, the importance of understanding the historical, social, and economic factors in which afflictions are embedded; see Paul Farmer, "An Anthropology of Structural Violence," *Current Anthropology* 45, no. 3 (2004): 305–25, doi:10.1086/382250.

A Wildness in the Bones: Acute Awareness and Shady Moods

78 "fight-or-flight" reaction: David A. Ross, Melissa R. Arbuckle, Michael J. Travis, et al., "An Integrated Neuroscience Perspective on Formulation and Treatment Planning for Posttraumatic Stress Disorder: An Educational Review," *JAMA Psychiatry* 74, no. 4 (2017): 407–15, https://doi.org/10.1001/jamapsychiatry.2016.3325.

78 The amygdala: Jonathan E. Sherin and Charles B. Nemeroff, "Post-traumatic Stress Disorder: The Neurobiological Impact of Psychological Trauma," *Dialogues in Clinical Neuroscience* 13, no. 3 (2011): 263–78, http://www.ncbi.nlm.nih.gov/pmc/articles/PMC3182008/.

78 In this study: Scott L. Rauch, Paul J. Whalen, Lisa M. Shin, et al., "Exaggerated Amygdala Response to Masked Facial Stimuli in Posttraumatic Stress Disorder: A Functional MRI Study," *Biological Psychiatry* 47, no. 9 (2000): 769–76, https://doi.org/https://doi.org/10.1016/S0006-3223(00)00828-3.

79 In a 2004 study: Lisa M. Shin, Scott P. Orr, Margaret A. Carson, et al., "Regional Cerebral Blood Flow in the Amygdala and Medial Prefrontal Cortex During Traumatic Imagery in Male and Female Vietnam Veterans with PTSD," *Archives of General Psychiatry* 61, no. 2 (2004): 168–76, https://doi.org/10.1001/archpsyc.61.2.168.

81 the circuits of her brain: Jonathan E. Sherin and Charles B. Nemeroff, "Post-traumatic Stress Disorder: The Neurobiological Impact of Psychological Trauma," *Dialogues in Clinical Neuroscience* 13, no. 3 (2011): 263–78, http://www.ncbi.nlm.nih.gov/pmc/articles/PMC3182008/.

81 A 2016 study: Benjamin T. Dunkley, Elizabeth W. Pang, Paul A. Sedge, Rakesh Jetly, Sam M. Doesburg, and Margot J. Taylor, "Threatening Faces Induce Fear Circuitry Hypersynchrony in Soldiers with Post-Traumatic Stress Disorder," *Heliyon* 2, no. 1 (2016): e00063, https://doi.org/10.1016/j.heliyon.2015.e00063.

82 host of other plausible possibilities: Daniel R. Weinberger and Eugenia Radulescu, "Finding the Elusive Psychiatric 'Lesion' with 21st-Century Neuroanatomy: A Note of Caution," *The American Journal of Psychiatry*

173, no. 1 (2016): 27–33, https://doi.org/10.1176/appi.ajp.2015.15060753. Benjamin T. Dunkley, Elizabeth W. Pang, Paul A. Sedge, et al., "Threatening Faces Induce Fear Circuitry Hypersynchrony in Soldiers with Post-traumatic Stress Disorder," *Heliyon* 2, no. 1 (2016): e00063, https://doi.org/10.1016/j.heliyon.2015.e00063.

Dissociation: The Two-Thousand-Yard Stare

84   These experiences are occasionally felt: Benjamin J. Sadock and Virginia A. Sadock, eds., *Kaplan & Sadock's Comprehensive Textbook of Psychiatry*, 7th ed. (Baltimore: Lippincott Williams & Wilkins, 2000), vol. I, 805.

84   dissociative subtype of PTSD: Ruth A. Lanius, Erika J. Wolf, Mark W. Miller, et al., "The Dissociative Subtype of PTSD," in *Handbook of PTSD: Science and Practice*, 2nd ed., ed. Matthew J. Friedman, Terence Martin Keane, and Patricia A. Resick (New York: Guilford Press, 2014), 235–50.

85   "Functional brain imaging studies show": Shaili Jain, "PTSD and the DSM-5: A Conversation with Dr. Matt Friedman," *PLOS Blogs*, November 10, 2015, http://blogs.plos.org/mindthebrain/2015/11/10/ptsd-and-the-dsm-5-a-conversation-with-dr-matt-friedman/.

85   *emotional overmodulation*: Ruth A. Lanius, Eric Vermetten, Richard J. Loewenstein, et al., "Emotion Modulation in PTSD: Clinical and Neuro-biological Evidence for a Dissociative Subtype," *The American Journal of Psychiatry* 167, no. 6 (2010): 640–47, https://doi.org/10.1176/appi.ajp.2009.09081168.

85   betrayal trauma theory: Richard J. McNally, "Betrayal Trauma Theory: A Critical Appraisal," *Memory* 15, no. 3 (2007): 280–311, https://doi.org/10.1080/09658210701256506.

86   found this dissociative form: Dan J. Stein, Karestan C. Koenen, Matthew J. Friedman, et al., "Dissociation in Posttraumatic Stress Disorder: Evidence from the World Mental Health Surveys," *Biological Psychiatry* 73, no. 4 (2013): 302–12, https://doi.org/10.1016/j.biopsych.2012.08.022.

Bodily Wounds

92   link between PTSD and poor physical health: Paula P. Schnurr, Jennifer S. Wachen, Bonnie L. Green, and Stacey Kaltman, "Trauma Exposure, PTSD, and Physical Health," in *Handbook of PTSD: Science and Practice*, 2nd ed., ed. Matthew J. Friedman, Terence Martin Keane, and Patricia A. Resick (New York: Guilford Press, 2014), 502–22, at 502.

93   having PTSD is associated: Martin D. Marciniak, Maureen J. Lage,

Eduardo Dunayevich, et al., "The Cost of Treating Anxiety: The Medical and Demographic Correlates That Impact Total Medical Costs," *Depression and Anxiety* 21, no. 4 (2005): 178–84, https://doi.org/10.1002/da.20074.

93   They described three ways: Paula P. Schnurr and Bonnie L. Green, "Understanding Relationships Among Trauma, PTSD, and Health Outcomes," in *Trauma and Health: Physical Consequences of Exposure to Extreme Stress*, ed. Paula P. Schnurr and Bonnie L. Green (Washington, DC: American Psychological Association, 2004), 247–75.

93   PTSD patients have shorter telomeres: Zahava Solomon, Noga Tsur, Yafit Levin, et al., "The Implications of War Captivity and Long-Term Psychopathology Trajectories for Telomere Length," *Psychoneuroendocrinology* 81, suppl. C (July 2017): 122–28, https://doi.org/10.1016/j.psyneuen.2017.04.004.

93   link between PTSD and accelerated aging: James B. Lohr, Barton W. Palmer, Carolyn A. Eidt, et al., "Is Post-traumatic Stress Disorder Associated with Premature Senescence? A Review of the Literature," *The American Journal of Geriatric Psychiatry* 23, no. 7 (2015): 709–25, https://doi.org/10.1016/j.jagp.2015.04.001.

93   host of neurological, gastrointestinal, autoimmune, and joint conditions: Huan Song, Fang Fang, and Grunnar Tomasson, "Association of Stress-Related Disorders with Subsequent Autoimmune Disease," *JAMA* 319, no. 23 (2018): 2388–2400. doi:10.1001/jama.2018.7028, https://jamanetwork.com/journals/jama/fullarticle/2685155.

93   having PTSD increases the odds: Jitender Sareen, Brian J. Cox, Ian Clara, and Gordon J. G. Asmundson, "The Relationship Between Anxiety Disorders and Physical Disorders in the U.S. National Comorbidity Survey," *Depression and Anxiety* 21, no. 4 (2005): 193–202, https://doi.org/10.1002/da.20072. Aoife O'Donovan, Beth E. Cohen, Karen Seal, et al., "Elevated Risk for Autoimmune Disorders in Iraq and Afghanistan Veterans with Posttraumatic Stress Disorder," *Biological Psychiatry* 77, no. 4 (2015): 365–74, https://doi.org/10.1016/j.biopsych.2014.06.015.

93   the combined toll: D. Ford, "Depression, Trauma, and Cardiovascular Health," in Schnurr and Green, eds., *Trauma and Health*, 73–97.

93   the behavioral pathways: A. A. Rheingold, R. Acierno, and H. S. Resnick, "Trauma, Posttraumatic Stress Disorder, and Health Risk Behaviors," in Schnurr and Green, eds., *Trauma and Health*, 217–43.

94   Having PTSD means: Angelica L. Zen, Shoujun Zhao, Mary A. Whooley, and Beth E. Cohen, "Post-traumatic Stress Disorder Is Associated with Poor Health Behaviors: Findings from the Heart and Soul Study," *Health Psychology* 31, no. 2 (2012): 194–201, https://doi.org/10.1037/a0025989.

Ian M. Kronish, Jenny J. Lin, Beth E. Cohen, et al., "PTSD and Medications Adherence in Patients with Uncontrolled Hypertension," *JAMA Internal Medicine* 174, no. 3 (2014): 468–70, doi: 10.1001/jamainternmed.2013.12881.

94   relationship between PTSD and death: William E. Schlenger, Nida H. Corry, Christianna S. Williams, et al., "A Prospective Study of Mortality and Trauma-Related Risk Factors Among a Nationally Representative Sample of Vietnam Veterans," *American Journal of Epidemiology* 182, no. 12 (2015): 980–90, http://dx.doi.org/10.1093/aje/kwv217.

A Soldier's Heart: PTSD and Cardiac Disease

98   untreated PTSD may have flipped: Dimpi Patel, Nathaniel D. Mc-Conkey, Ryann Sohaney, et al., "A Systematic Review of Depression and Anxiety in Patients with Atrial Fibrillation: The Mind-Heart Link," *Cardiovascular Psychiatry and Neurology* (April 2013): 159850, https://doi.org/10.1155/2013/159850.

98   The nuanced relationship: Steven S. Coughlin, "Post-traumatic Stress Disorder and Cardiovascular Disease," *The Open Cardiovascular Medicine Journal* 5 (July 2011): 164–70, https://doi.org/10.2174/1874192401105010164.

99   A research team: Beth E. Cohen, Charles Marmar, Li Ren, et al., "Association of Cardiovascular Risk Factors with Mental Health Diagnoses in Iraq and Afghanistan War Veterans Using VA Health Care," *The Journal of the American Medical Association* 302, no. 5 (2009): 489–92, https://doi.org/10.1001/jama.2009.1084.

99   A 2014 joint study: Laura D. Kubzansky, Paula Bordelois, Hee Jin Jun, et al., "The Weight of Traumatic Stress: A Prospective Study of Posttraumatic Stress Disorder Symptoms and Weight Status in Women," *JAMA Psychiatry* 71, no. 1 (2014): 44–51, https://doi.org/10.1001/jamapsychiatry.2013.2798.

100 Follow-up studies: Andrea L. Roberts, Jessica C. Agnew-Blais, Donna Spiegelman, et al., "Posttraumatic Stress Disorder and Incidence of Type 2 Diabetes Mellitus in a Sample of Women: A 22-Year Longitudinal Study," *JAMA Psychiatry* 72, no. 3 (2015): 203–10, https://doi.org/10.1001/jamapsychiatry.2014.2632.

100 more likely to have: Jennifer A. Sumner, Laura D. Kubzansky, Mitchell S. V. Elkind, et al., "Trauma Exposure and Posttraumatic Stress Disorder Symptoms Predict Onset of Cardiovascular Events in Women," *Circulation* 132, no. 4 (July 29, 2015): 251–59, https://doi.org/10.1161/CIRCULATIONAHA.114.014492.

100 prospective twin study: Viola Vaccarino, Jack Goldberg, Cherie Rooks, et al., "Post-traumatic Stress Disorder and Incidence of Coronary Heart Disease: A Twin Study," *Journal of the American College of Cardiology* 62, no. 11 (2013): 970–78, https://doi.org/https://doi.org/10.1016/j .jacc.2013.04.085.

100 PTSD appears to be: Donald Edmondson and Roland von Känel, "Post-traumatic Stress Disorder and Cardiovascular Disease," *The Lancet Psychiatry* 4, no. 4 (2017): 320–29, https://doi.org/10.1016/S2215 -0366(16)30377-7. More recent research concludes that post-traumatic stress disorder is a risk factor for incident cardiovascular disease as well as a common psychiatric consequence of cardiovascular disease events that might worsen the outcome of the cardiovascular disease. Recent findings from the World Trade Center–Heart study offer additional evidence. World Trade Center attack–related post-traumatic stress disorder in first responders was found to be a risk factor for myocardial infarction and stroke, in men and women, and independent of recognized cardiovascular risk factors and depression. Molly Rench, Zoey Laskaris, Janine Flory, et al., "Post-Traumatic Stress Disorder and Cardiovascular Disease," *Circulation II*, no. 7 (2018), https://www.ahajournals.org/doi/10.1161/CIRCOUTCOMES .117.004572.

100 a condition that impacts: James B. Lohr, Barton W. Palmer, Carolyn A. Eidt, et al., "Is Post-traumatic Stress Disorder Associated with Premature Senescence? A Review of the Literature," *The American Journal of Geriatric Psychiatry* 23, no. 7 (2015): 709–25, https://doi.org/10.1016/j .jagp.2015.04.001.

Russian Roulette: The Perilous Bond Between Traumatic Stress and Addiction

105 when Purdue Pharma introduced: Art Van Zee, "The Promotion and Marketing of OxyContin: Commercial Triumph, Public Health Tragedy," *American Journal of Public Health* 99, no. 2 (2009): 221–27, https://doi .org/10.2105/AJPH.2007.131714.

105 She told me that: Shaili Jain, "The Prescription Pain Pill Epidemic: A Conversation with Dr. Anna Lembke," *PLOS Blogs*, March 1, 2017, http:// blogs.plos.org/mindthebrain/2017/03/01/the-prescription-pain-pill -epidemic-a-conversation-with-dr-anna-lembke/.

106 chronic pain: Eeman Akhtar, et al., "The Prevalence of Post-Traumatic Stress Disorder Symptoms in Chronic Pain Patients in a Tertiary Care Setting:

A Cross-Sectional Study," *Pyschosomatics* 3182, no. 18 (2018), https://doi.org/10.1016/j.psym.2018.07.102.

106 the significant overlap: see J. Siqveland, T. Ruud, and E. Hauff, "Post-traumatic Stress Disorder Moderates the Relationship Between Trauma Exposure and Chronic Pain," *European Journal of Psychotraumatology* 8, no. 1 (2017): 1375337, https://doi.org/10.1080/20008198.2017.1375337.

106 one study reporting: Hagit Cohen, Lily Neumann, Yehoshua Haiman, et al., "Prevalence of Post-traumatic Stress Disorder in Fibromyalgia Patients: Overlapping Syndromes or Post-traumatic Fibromyalgia Syndrome?," *Seminars in Arthritis and Rheumatism* 32, no. 1 (2002): 38–50, https://www.sciencedirect.com/science/article/pii/S0049017202000136.

106 a 2012 study: Karen H. Seal, Ying Shi, Gregory Cohen, et al., "Association of Mental Health Disorders with Prescription Opioids and High-Risk Opioid Use in US Veterans of Iraq and Afghanistan," *The Journal of the American Medical Association* 307, no. 9 (2012): 940–47, https://doi.org/10.1001/jama.2012.234.

107 over 60 percent of addicted persons: Jenna L. McCauley, Therese Killen, Daniel F. Gros, et al. "Posttraumatice Stress Disorder and Co-Occuring Substance Use Disorders: Advances in Assessment and Treatment," *Clinical Pyschology: A Publication of the Division of Clinical Psychology of the American Psychological Association* 19, no. 3 (2012): 10.1111/cpsp.12006. PMC. Web. Sept. 12, 2018. https://www.ncbi.nlm.nih.gov/pmc/articles/PMC3811127/.

107 I am constantly on the lookout: David M. Ledgerwood and Aleks Milosevic, "Clinical and Personality Characteristics Associated with Post Traumatic Stress Disorder in Problem and Pathological Gamblers Recruited from the Community," *Journal of Gambling Studies* 31, no. 2 (2015): 501–12, https://doi.org/10.1007/s10899-013-9426-1.

108 "self-medicate": Denise A. Hien, Huiping Jiang, Aimee N. C. Campbell, et al., "Do Treatment Improvements in PTSD Severity Affect Substance Use Outcomes? A Secondary Analysis from a Randomized Clinical Trial in NIDA's Clinical Trials Network," *The American Journal of Psychiatry* 167, no. 1 (2010): 95–101, https://doi.org/10.1176/appi.ajp.2009.09091261.

108 rarely ends well: Samuel T. Wilkinson, Elina Stefanovics, and Robert A. Rosenheck, "Marijuana Use Is Associated with Worse Outcomes in Symptom Severity and Violent Behavior in Patients with Posttraumatic Stress Disorder," *The Journal of Clinical Psychiatry* 76, no. 9 (2015): 1174–80, https://doi.org/10.4088/JCP.14m09475.

109 it ties my hands: There are some programs that address both simulta-

neously, but they are not readily available. See, e.g., Mehmet Sofuoglu, Robert Rosenheck, and Ismene Petrakis, "Pharmacological Treatment of Comorbid PTSD and Substance Use Disorder: Recent Progress," *Addictive Behaviors* 39, no. 2 (February 2014): 428–33, https://doi.org/10.1016/j .addbeh.2013.08.014.

Broken Smiles: The Toxicity of Childhood Adversity

113 Her relationship with Evie: M. Denise Dowd, "Early Adversity, Toxic Stress, and Resilience: Pediatrics for Today," *Pediatric Annals* 46, no. 7 (2017): e246–49, https://doi.org/10.3928/19382359-20170615-01.

114 more than double: Christina W. Hoven, Cristiane S. Duarte, Christopher P. Lucas, et al., "Psychopathology Among New York City Public School Children 6 Months After September 11," *Archives of General Psychiatry* 62, no. 5 (2005): 545–52, https://doi.org/10.1001/archpsyc.62.5.545.

114 Parents and caregivers: John A. Fairbank, Frank W. Putnam, and William W. Harris, "Child Traumatic Stress: Prevalence, Trends, Risk, and Impact," in *Handbook of PTSD: Science and Practice*, 2nd ed., ed. Matthew J. Friedman, Terence Martin Keane, and Patricia A. Resick (New York: Guilford Press, 2014), 121–45.

115 This feeling of guilt is a strong predictor: Ann-Christin Haag, Daniel Zehnder, and Markus A. Landolt, "Guilt Is Associated with Acute Stress Symptoms in Children After Road Traffic Accidents," *European Journal of Psychotraumatology* 6 (October 2015), https://doi.org/10.3402/ejpt .v6.29074.

115 "Kids may find themselves thinking or talking about the trauma": Shaili Jain, "Dealing with Psychological Trauma in Children: Answers from Neuroscience, Community Initiatives, and Clinical Trials for Treating Childhood PTSD," *PLOS Blogs*, April 1, 2013, http://blogs.plos.org /mindthebrain/2013/04/01/dealing-with-psychological-trauma-in -children-answers-from-neuroscience-community-initiatives-and-clinical -trials-for-treating-childhood-ptsd/.

116 children with PTSD have altered neurobiology: Xueling Suo, Du Lei, Fuqin Chen, et al., "Anatomic Insights into Disrupted Small-World Networks in Pediatric Posttraumatic Stress Disorder," *Radiology* 282, no. 3 (2016): 826–34, https://doi.org/10.1148/radiol.2016160907.

116 The children with PTSD made more errors: Victor G. Carrion, Brian W. Haas, Amy Garrett, et al., "Reduced Hippocampal Activity in Youth with Posttraumatic Stress Symptoms: An fMRI Study," *Journal of Pediatric Psychology* 35, no. 5 (2010): 559–69, https://doi.org/10.1093/jpepsy/jsp112.

116 children with PTSD also had abnormalities: Victor G. Carrion, Carl F. Weems, Christa Watson, et al., "Converging Evidence for Abnormalities of the Prefrontal Cortex and Evaluation of Midsagittal Structures in Pediatric PTSD: An MRI Study," *Psychiatry Research* 172, no. 3 (2009): 226–34, https://doi.org/10.1016/j.pscychresns.2008.07.008.

116 In 2016, Carrion's team: Megan Klabunde, Carl F. Weems, Mira Raman, and Victor G. Carrion, "The Moderating Effects of Sex on Insula Subdivision Structure in Youth with Posttraumatic Stress Symptoms," *Depression and Anxiety* 34, no. 1 (2017): 51–58, https://doi.org/10.1002/da.22577.

117 started investigating the relationship: Centers for Disease Control and Prevention, "Adverse Childhood Experiences (ACEs)," April 1, 2016, http://www.cdc.gov/violenceprevention/acestudy/index.html. Jack P. Shonkoff, "Capitalizing on Advances in Science to Reduce the Health Consequences of Early Childhood Adversity," *JAMA Pediatrics* 170, no. 10 (2016): 1003–07, https://doi.org/10.1001/jamapediatrics.2016.1559.

118 take on risky behaviors: Hannah Carliner, Katherine M. Keyes, Katie A. McLaughlin, et al., "Childhood Trauma and Illicit Drug Use in Adolescence: A Population-Based National Comorbidity Survey Replication—Adolescent Supplement Study," *Journal of the American Academy of Child & Adolescent Psychiatry* 55, no. 8 (2017): 701–08, https://doi.org/10.1016/j.jaac.2016.05.010.

118 The study also found: These findings have been replicated in other studies. See, e.g., Edith Chen, Nicholas A. Turiano, Daniel K. Mroczek, and Gregory E. Miller, "Association of Reports of Childhood Abuse and All-Cause Mortality Rates in Women," *JAMA Psychiatry* 73, no. 9 (2016): 920–27, https://doi.org/10.1001/jamapsychiatry.2016.1786.

118 "Adverse childhood experiences": Vincent J. Felitti, "The Origins of Addiction: Evidence from the Adverse Childhood Experiences Study," February 16, 2004, http://www.nijc.org/pdfs/Subject%20Matter%20Articles/Drugs%20and%20Alc/ACE%20Study%20-%20OriginsofAddiction.pdf, 4. These findings have been replicated in other settings and countries, too. See Kristine A. Campbell, Tonya Myrup, and Lina Svedin, "Parsing Language and Measures Around Child Maltreatment," *Pediatrics* 139, no. 1 (January 2017), https://doi.org/10.1542/peds.2016-3475.

118 family violence increasingly recognized: Pia R. Britto, Stephen J. Lye, Kerrie Proulx, et al., "Nurturing Care: Promoting Early Childhood Development," *The Lancet* 389, no. 10064 (2017): 91–102, https://doi.org/10.1016/S0140-6736(16)31390-3.

118 at risk of falling short: Margaret Chan, Anthony Lake, and Keith Hansen,

"The Early Years: Silent Emergency or Unique Opportunity?," *The Lancet* 389, no. 10064 (2017): 11–13, https://doi.org/10.1016/S0140 -6736(16)31701-9.

119 potentially devastating: Bruce D. Perry, Gene Griffin, George Davis, et al., "The Impact of Neglect, Trauma, and Maltreatment on Neurodevelopment," in *The Wiley Blackwell Handbook of Forensic, Neuroscience,* ed. Anthony R. Beech, Adam J. Carter, Ruth E. Mann, and Pia Rotshtein (Hoboken, NJ: John Wiley and Sons, 2018). Adam Schickedanz, Neal Halfon, Narayan Sasrry, et al., "Parents' Adverse Childhood Experiences and Their Children's Behavioral Health Problems," *Pediatrics* 142, no. 2 (2018), doi: 10.1007/s00406-005-0624-4.

119 long term impact: R.F. Anda, V.J. Felitti, J.D. Bremner, et al., "The Enduring Effects of Abuse and Related Adverse Experiences in Childhood: A Convergence of Evidence from Neurobiology and Epidemiology," *Eur Arch Psychiatry*, Clin Neurosci 256 no. 3 (2006), https://www.ncbi.nlm.nih.gov /pubmed/16311898.

Senescence: Traumatic Stress in Late Life

123 traumatic memories can emerge or reemerge: Joan M. Cook, Avron Spiro III, and Danny G. Kaloupek, "Trauma in Older Adults," in *Handbook of PTSD: Science and Practice*, 2nd ed., ed. Matthew J. Friedman, Terence Martin Keane, and Patricia A. Resick (New York: Guilford Press, 2014), 351–67.

123 "I think events such as": Shaili Jain, "The Golden Years: Traumatic Stress and Aging—An Interview with Joan Cook," *PLOS Blogs*, October 6, 2016, http://blogs.plos.org/mindthebrain/2016/10/06/the-golden-years -traumatic-stress-and-aging-an-interview-with-joan-cook/.

124 She studied Holocaust survivors: Y. Danieli, "As Survivors Age—Part I," *National Center for Post Traumatic Stress Disorder Clinical Quarterly* 4, no. 1 (1994): 1–7. Y. Danieli, "As Survivors Age—Part II," *National Center for Post Traumatic Stress Disorder Clinical Quarterly* 4, no. 2 (1994): 20–24.

124 PTSD sufferers are almost twice as likely: Kristine Yaffe, Eric Vittinghoff, Karla Lindquist, et al., "Post-traumatic Stress Disorder and Risk of Dementia Among U.S. Veterans," *Archives of General Psychiatry* 67, no. 6 (2010): 608–13, https://doi.org/10.1001/archgenpsychiatry.2010.61. Omar Meziab, Katharine A. Kirby, Brie Williams, et al., "Prisoner of War Status, Posttraumatic Stress Disorder, and Dementia in Older Veterans," *Alzheimer's & Dementia* 10, no. 3 (suppl.) (2014): S236–41, https://doi.org /https://doi.org/10.1016/j.jalz.2014.04.004. One study of almost five

hundred veterans compared those who had PTSD with those who had PTSD and had also been prisoners of war (POWs) and hence subjected to intense physical harm, psychological stress, isolation, and nutritional deprivation during the time of their captivity. The risk of developing dementia in old age was even higher for the POW group than for those who had PTSD alone.

125 older adults with PTSD: Recent research echoes these findings. Posttraumatic stress disorder symptoms were negatively related to measures of psychomotor speed/attention and learning/working memory in middle-aged women; see Jennifer A. Sumner, Kaitlin Hagan, Fran Grodstein, et al., "Posttraumatic Stress Disorder Symptoms and Cognitive Function in a Large Cohort of Middle-Aged Women," *Depression and Anxiety* 34, no. 4 (2017): 356–66, https://doi.org/10.1002/da.22600. This study adds to a growing body of literature that suggests that mental disorders are associated with worse cognitive function over the life course. The sample comprised 14,029 middle-aged women in the Nurses' Health Study II. Researchers measured lifetime trauma exposure, lifetime PTSD symptoms, and past-week depressive symptoms in 2008; cognitive function was measured in 2014–2016.

125 Late-onset stress symptomatology: Lynda A. King, Daniel W. King, Kristin Vickers, et al., "Assessing Late-Onset Stress Symptomatology Among Aging Male Combat Veterans," *Aging & Mental Health* 11, no. 2 (2007): 175–91, https://doi.org/10.1080/13607860600844424.

125 LOSS may be a psychological mechanism: Eve H. Davison, Anica Pless Kaiser, Avron Spiro III, et al., "From Late-Onset Stress Symptomatology to Later-Adulthood Trauma Reengagement in Aging Combat Veterans: Taking a Broader View," *The Gerontologist* 56, no. 1 (2016): 14–21, https://doi.org/10.1093/geront/gnv097.

Complex Trauma

132 Sharon was also HIV positive: D. J. Brief, A. R. Bollinger, M. J. Vielhauer, et al., "Understanding the Interface of HIV, Trauma, Post-traumatic Stress Disorder, and Substance Use and Its Implications for Health Outcomes," *AIDS Care* 16, suppl. 1 (2004): S97–120, https://doi.org/10.1080/095401 20412301315259.

135 *complex PTSD*: Judith Herman, *Trauma and Recovery: The Aftermath of Violence—From Domestic Abuse to Political Terror* (New York: Basic Books, 2015), 119.

137 phenomenon of reenactment: Judith Herman, *Trauma and Recovery: The Aftermath of Violence—From Domestic Abuse to Political Terror* (New York: Basic Books, 2015), 53.

137 perhaps the most compelling: Kevin Lalor and Rosaleen McElvaney, "Child Sexual Abuse, Links to Later Sexual Exploitation/High-Risk Sexual Behavior, and Prevention/Treatment Programs," *Trauma, Violence & Abuse* 11, no. 4 (2010): 159–77, https://doi.org/10.1177/1524838010378299. Bessel A. van der Kolk, "The Compulsion to Repeat the Trauma: Re-enactment, Revictimization, and Masochism," *Psychiatric Clinics of North America* 12, no. 2 (June 1989): 389–411, http://www.traumacenter.org/products/pdf_files/Compulsion_to_Repeat.pdf.

Intimate Violence: A Secret Pandemic

139 If a woman cannot be safe: Aysha Taryam, "It's Time for a Law Against Domestic Violence in the UAE," *The Gulf Today*, October 18, 2015, http://gulftoday.ae/portal/111e4a1c-3cfa-4cd6-a2c3-52eb7a21ad6d.aspx.

143 nearly one in four women: Centers for Disease Control and Prevention, "Intimate Partner Violence: Consequences," August 22, 2017, http://www.cdc.gov/violenceprevention/intimatepartnerviolence/consequences.html. Almost 14 percent of women in the United States have been injured as a result of IPV, and in 2010, more than one thousand females were murdered by an intimate partner. Annually, IPV costs our society more than $8.3 billion with the increased health care costs for victims of IPV persisting as much as fifteen years after the cessation of abuse. Globally, IPV features among the top ten causes of years of life lost due to premature mortality and disability. See Mark L. Rosenberg, Alexander Butchart, James Mercy, et al., "Interpersonal Violence," in *Disease Control Priorities in Developing Countries*, 2nd ed., ed. Dean T. Jamison, Joel G. Breman, Anthony R. Measham, et al. (Washington, DC: International Bank for Reconstruction and Development/World Bank; New York: Oxford University Press, 2006), https://www.ncbi.nlm.nih.gov/books/NBK11721/.

143 "Over the course of human history": Elaine J. Alpert, "Domestic Violence and Clinical Medicine: Learning from Our Patients and from Our Fears," *Journal of General Internal Medicine* 17, no. 2 (2002): 162–63, https://doi.org/10.1046/j.1525-1497.2002.11229.x.

143 a common consequence of IPV: Jacqueline M. Golding, "Intimate Partner Violence as a Risk Factor for Mental Disorders: A Meta-Analysis," *Journal of Family Violence* 14, no. 2 (1999), 99–132, https://doi.org/10.1023/A:1022079418229.

143 IPV is a classic example: Rachel Kimerling, Julie C. Weitlauf, Katherine M. Iverson, et al., "Gender Issues in PTSD," in *Handbook of PTSD: Science and Practice*, 2nd ed., ed. Matthew J. Friedman, Terence Martin Keane, and Patricia A. Resick (New York: Guilford Press, 2014), 317–19.

A Danger to Others: Hurt People Hurt Other People

153 "Trauma breeds further trauma": Bessel A. van der Kolk, *The Body Keeps the Score: Brain, Mind, and Body in the Healing of Trauma* (New York: Penguin Books, 2015), 350.

154 effects of sexual violence: Nancy Wolff, Jessica Huening, Jing Shi, and B. Christopher Frueh, "Trauma Exposure and Posttraumatic Stress Disorder Among Incarcerated Men," *Journal of Urban Health* 91, no. 4 (2014): 707–19, https://doi.org/10.1007/s11524-014-9871-x.

Angry Loving: The Stubborn Imprint of Inner-City Poverty

157 Themes emerged from the stories I heard: U.S. Department of Justice, Office of Justice Programs, "Bureau of Justice Statistics Special Report: Black Victims of Violent Crime," August 2007, https://www.bjs.gov/content /pub/pdf/bvvc.pdf.

157 perpetuated more frequently: James J. Mazza and William M. Reynolds, "Exposure to Violence in Young Inner-City Adolescents: Relationships with Suicidal Ideation, Depression, and PTSD Symptomatology," *Journal of Abnormal Child Psychology* 27, no. 3 (1999): 203–13, https://link.springer. com/article/10.1023%2FA%3A1021900423004.

157 combat veterans: Chalsa M. Loo, "PTSD Among Ethnic Minority Veterans," February 23, 2016, http://www.ptsd.va.gov/professional/treatment/cultural /ptsd-minority-vets.asp.

157 teenagers living in: Margaret Dempsey, Stacy Overstreet, and Barbara Moely, "'Approach' and 'Avoidance' Coping and PTSD Symptoms in Inner-City Youth," *Current Psychology* 19, no. 1 (March 2000): 28–45, https://link .springer.com/article/10.1007/s12144-000-1002-z. Bradley D. Stein, Lisa H. Jaycox, Sheryl Kataoka, et al., "Prevalence of Child and Adolescent Exposure to Community Violence," *Clinical Child and Family Psychology Review* 6, no. 4 (December 2003): 247–64, https://link.springer.com/article /10.1023/B:CCFP.0000006292.61072.d2. Mark I. Singer, Trina Menden Anglin, Li yu Song, and Lisa Lunghofer, "Adolescents' Exposure to Violence and Associated Symptoms of Psychological Trauma," *The Journal of the American Medical Association* 273, no. 6 (February 8, 1995): 477–82, https://jamanetwork.com/journals/jama/article-abstract/386889. Tanya N.

Alim, Dennis S. Charney, and Thomas A. Mellman, "An Overview of Posttraumatic Stress Disorder in African Americans," *Journal of Clinical Psychology* 62 no. 7 (2006): 801–13, https://doi.org/10.1002/jclp.20280. PTSD is rampant in the United States' most violent neighborhoods, and researchers, documenting the levels of violence experienced by thousands of inner-city residents (many of whom are African American), have found that roughly 30 percent have PTSD.

157 PTSD in African Americans: Regina G. Davis, Kerry J. Ressler, Ann C. Schwartz, et al., "Treatment Barriers for Low-Income, Urban African Americans with Undiagnosed Posttraumatic Stress Disorder," *Journal of Traumatic Stress* 21, no. 2 (2008): 218–22, https://doi.org/10.1002/jts.20313.

157 they are less likely: Michele Spoont, David Nelson, Michelle Van Ryn, and Margarita Alegria, "Racial and Ethnic Variation in Perceptions of VA Mental Health Providers Are Associated with Treatment Retention Among Veterans with PTSD," *Medical Care* 55, suppl. 9 (September 2017): S33–42, https://doi.org/10.1097/MLR.0000000000000755. Early discontinuation of mental health treatment is more common among veterans with PTSD who are of minority race or ethnicity.

157 general mistrust of medical institutions: Ethnic-minority veterans may be more likely to disclose problems or engage in treatment when paired with a clinician of the same race. See, e.g., Loo, "PTSD Among Ethnic Minority Veterans." It is important to recognize the historical antecedents of this mistrust. See Centers for Disease Control and Prevention, "U.S. Public Health Service Syphilis Study at Tuskegee," August 30, 2017, https://www.cdc.gov/tuskegee/timeline.htm.

157 family disapproval of their decision: Michele R. Spoont, Nina A. Sayer, Shannon M. Kehle-Forbes, et al., "A Prospective Study of Racial and Ethnic Variation in VA Psychotherapy Services for PTSD," *Psychiatric Services* 68 no. 3 (2017): 231–37, https://doi.org/10.1176/appi.ps.201600086.

158 one is more likely: Tanya N. Alim, Dennis S. Charney, and Thomas A. Mellman, "An Overview of Posttraumatic Stress Disorder in African Americans," *Journal of Clinical Psychology* 62, no. 7 (2006): 801–13, https://doi.org/10.1002/jclp.20280.

160 marriages of individuals with PTSD: B. K. Jordan, C. R. Marmar, J. A. Fairbank, et al., "Problems in Families of Male Vietnam Veterans with Posttraumatic Stress Disorder," *Journal of Consulting and Clinical Psychology* 60, no. 6 (1992): 916–26. Jennifer L. Price and Susan P. Stevens, "Partners of Veterans with PTSD: Research Findings," March 30, 2017, https://

www.ptsd.va.gov/professional/treatment/family/partners_of_vets
_research_findings.asp.

161 problems in their sex life: Daniel J. Cosgrove, Zachary Gordon, Jonathan
E. Bernie, et al., "Sexual Dysfunction in Combat Veterans with Post-
traumatic Stress Disorder," *Urology* 60, no. 5 (2017): 881–84, https://doi
.org/10.1016/S0090-4295(02)01899-X. D. S. Riggs, C. A. Byrne, F. W.
Weathers, and B. T. Litz, "The Quality of the Intimate Relationships of
Male Vietnam Veterans: Problems Associated with Posttraumatic Stress
Disorder," *Journal of Traumatic Stress* 11, no. 1 (1998): 87–101, https://doi
.org/10.1023/A:1024409200155.

161 There is more violence: C. A. Byrne and D. S. Riggs, "The Cycle of
Trauma: Relationship Aggression in Male Vietnam Veterans with Symptoms of Posttraumatic Stress Disorder," *Violence and Victims* 11, no. 3
(1996): 213–25.

161 They are also overburdened: Zahava Solomon, Mark Waysman, Ehud
Avitzur, and Dan Enoch, "Psychiatric Symptomatology Among Wives of
Soldiers Following Combat Stress Reaction: The Role of the Social Network and Marital Relations," *Anxiety Research* 4, no. 3 (1991): 213–23,
https:/doi.org/10.1080/08917779108248775. Briana S. Nelson and David
W. Wright, "Understanding and Treating Post-traumatic Stress Disorder
Symptoms in Female Partners of Veterans with PTSD," *Journal
of Marital and Family Therapy* 22, no. 4 (1996): 455–67, https://doi
.org/10.1111/j.1752-0606.1996.tb00220.x.

161 A 2012 study: Candice M. Monson, Steffany J. Fredman, Alexandra
Macdonald, et al., "Effect of Cognitive-Behavioral Couple Therapy for
PTSD: A Randomized Controlled Trial," *The Journal of the American
Medical Association* 308, no. 7 (2012): 700–09, https://doi.org/10.1001
/jama.2012.9307.

162 "PTSD patients don't do as well": Matt McMillen, "PTSD Treatment and
Couples Therapy Go Hand in Hand," WebMD, August 14, 2012, http://
www.webmd.com/sex-relationships/news/20120814/ptsd-treatment
-couple-therapy-go-hand-in-hand?page=2.

The Fairer Sex? Rape, Secondary Injuries, and Postpartum PTSD

166 study after study shows: David F. Tolin and Edna B. Foa, "Sex Differences
in Trauma and Posttraumatic Stress Disorder: A Quantitative Review of
25 Years of Research," *Psychological Bulletin* 132, no. 6 (2006): 959–92,
https://doi.org/10.1037/0033-2909.132.6.959.

166 Though emerging evidence suggests: Sophie H. Li and Bronwyn M.

Graham, "Why Are Women so Vulnerable to Anxiety, Trauma-Related and Stress-Related Disorders? The Potential Role of Sex Hormones," *The Lancet Psychiatry* 4, no. 1 (2017): 73–82, https://doi.org/https://doi.org/10.1016 /S2215-0366(16)30358-3.

166 nearly one in five women has been raped: Lizabeth A. Goldstein, Julie Dinh, Rosemary Donalson, et al., "Impact of Military Trauma Exposures on Posttraumatic Stress and Depression in Female Veterans," *Psychiatry Research* 249 (March 2017): 281–85, https://doi.org/10.1016/j.psychres .2017.01.009.

166 "Young women attending university": Charlene Y. Senn, Misha Eliasziw, Paula C. Barata, et al., "Efficacy of a Sexual Assault Resistance Program for University Women," *The New England Journal of Medicine* 372, no. 24 (2015): 2326–35, at https://doi.org/10.1056/NEJMsa1411131.

166 rape is the type of trauma: Kaitlin A. Chivers-Wilson, "Sexual Assault and Posttraumatic Stress Disorder: A Review of the Biological, Psychological and Sociological Factors and Treatments," *McGill Journal of Medicine* 9, no. 2 (2006): 111–18, http://www.ncbi.nlm.nih.gov/pmc/articles /PMC2323517/.

169 Around 1 to 6 percent of women who experience birth trauma: Shaili Jain, "Perinatal Psychiatry, Birth Trauma and Perinatal PTSD: An Interview with Dr. Rebecca Moore," *PLOS Blogs*, August 24, 2016, http://blogs.plos .org/blog/2016/08/24/perinatal-psychiatry-birth-trauma-and-perinatal -ptsd-an-interview-with-dr-rebecca-moore/.

169 Statistics on postpartum PTSD: Rebecca Grekin and Michael W. O'Hara, "Prevalence and Risk Factors of Postpartum Posttraumatic Stress Disorder: A Meta-analysis," *Clinical Psychology Review* 34, no. 5 (2014): 389–401, https://doi.org/10.1016/j.cpr.2014.05.003.

169 is echoed in studies: K. Wijma, J. Soderquist, and B. Wijma, "Posttraumatic Stress Disorder After Childbirth: A Cross Sectional Study," *Journal of Anxiety Disorders* 11, no. 6 (1997): 587–97. Jo Czarnocka and Pauline Slade, "Prevalence and Predictors of Post-traumatic Stress Symptoms Following Childbirth," *British Journal of Clinical Psychology* 39, part 1 (March 2000): 35–51, https://doi.org/10.1348 /014466500163095. Susan Ayers, Rachel Harris, Alexandra Sawyer, et al., "Posttraumatic Stress Disorder After Childbirth: Analysis of Symptom Presentation and Sampling," *Journal of Affective Disorders* 119, nos. 1–3 (December 2009): 200–04, https://doi.org/10.1016/j .jad.2009.02.029.

Shame: The Cinderella Emotion

171 The difference between "I am bad" and "I did something bad." Brené Brown, "Listening to Shame," TED Talk, https://www.youtube.com/watch?time _continue=853&v=psN1DORYYV0.

176 our brains are hardwired: Terry F. Taylor, "The Influence of Shame on Posttrauma Disorders: Have We Failed to See the Obvious?," *European Journal of Psychotraumatology* 6 (September 22, 2015): 28847, https:// www.ncbi.nlm.nih.gov/pubmed/26399959.

176 In a University of London study: Bernice Andrews, Chris R. Brewin, Suzanna Rose, and Marilyn Kirk, "Predicting PTSD Symptoms in Victims of Violent Crime: The Role of Shame, Anger, and Childhood Abuse," *Journal of Abnormal Psychology* 109, no. 1 (February 2000): 69–73, https:// www.ncbi.nlm.nih.gov/pubmed/10740937.

177 modern researchers have found: Craig J. Bryan, Chad E. Morrow, Neysa Etienne, and Bobbie Ray-Sannerud, "Guilt, Shame, and Suicidal Ideation in a Military Outpatient Clinical Sample," *Depression and Anxiety* 30, no. 1 (January 2013): 55–60, doi: 10.1002/da.22002.

177 grief can be traumatic: Richard A. Bryant, "Prolonged Grief: Where to After Diagnostic and Statistical Manual of Mental Disorders, 5th Edition?," *Current Opinion in Psychiatry* 27, no. 1 (2014): 21–26, http://www.medscape .com/viewarticle/818619_6.

The Science of Suicide Prevention

181 The statistics are sobering: When discussing suicide statistics, it is important to note the distinction between *veterans*, i.e., retired military personnel, and *active-duty personnel*, i.e., persons who are still serving in the military. For the latter group suicide rates nearly doubled between 2005 and 2009. A recent and thoughtful analysis of this tragic situation can be found in Charles W. Hoge and Carl A. Castro, "Preventing Suicides in US Service Members and Veterans: Concerns After a Decade of War," *The Journal of the American Medical Association* 308, no. 7 (2012): 671–72, https://doi .org/10.1001/jama.2012.9955.

181 The "war is hell" camp: Michael Schoenbaum, Ronald C. Kessler, Stephen E. Gilman, et al., "Predictors of Suicide and Accident Death in the Army Study to Assess Risk and Resilience in Servicemembers (Army STARRS): Results from the Army Study to Assess Risk and Resilience in Servicemembers (Army STARRS)," *JAMA Psychiatry* 71, no. 5 (2014): 493–503, https://doi.org/10.1001/jamapsychiatry.2013.4417.

181 an exhaustive 2015 study: Mark A. Reger, Derek J. Smolenski, Nancy
     A. Skopp, et al., "Risk of Suicide Among US Military Service Members
     Following Operation Enduring Freedom or Operation Iraqi Freedom
     Deployment and Separation from the US Military," *JAMA Psychiatry* 72,
     no. 6 (2015): 561–69, https://doi.org/10.1001/jamapsychiatry.2014.3195.

182 death by suicide occurred: The rate of suicide attempts by soldiers in
     the US Army is elevated among those who have never been deployed. See
     Robert J. Ursano, Ronald C. Kessler, Murray B. Stein, et al., "Risk Factors,
     Methods, and Timing of Suicide Attempts Among US Army Soldiers,"
     JAMA Psychiatry 73, no. 7 (2016): 741–49, https://doi.org/10.1001/jama
     psychiatry.2016.0600

182 Having PTSD certainly puts veterans: T. A. Bullman and H. K. Kang,
     "Posttraumatic Stress Disorder and the Risk of Traumatic Deaths
     Among Vietnam Veterans," *The Journal of Nervous and Mental Disease*
     182, no. 11 (November 1994): 604–10, https://www.ncbi.nlm.nih.gov
     /pubmed/7964667. Jitender Sareen, Tanya Houlahan, Brian J. Cox, and
     Gordon J. G. Asmundson, "Anxiety Disorders Associated with Suicidal
     Ideation and Suicide Attempts in the National Comorbidity Survey," *The
     Journal of Nervous and Mental Disease* 193, no. 7 (July 2005): 450–54,
     https://pdfs.semanticscholar.org/b816/da72792851e86369a946c8b8
     afcea2b799e3.pdf.

182 anger: M. Kotler, I. Iancu, R. Efroni, and M. Amir, "Anger, Impulsivity,
     Social Support, and Suicide Risk in Patients with Posttraumatic Stress Dis-
     order," *The Journal of Nervous and Mental Disease* 189, no. 3 (March 2001):
     162–67, https://www.ncbi.nlm.nih.gov/pubmed/11277352.

182 impulsivity: M. Amir, Z. Kaplan, R. Efroni, and M. Kotler, "Suicide
     Risk and Coping Styles in Posttraumatic Stress Disorder Patients,"
     Psychotherapy and Psychosomatics 68, no. 2 (1999): 76–81, https://doi
     .org/10.1159/000012316.

182 Veterans with partial PTSD: Matthew Jakupcak, Katherine D. Hoerster,
     Alethea Varra, et al., "Hopelessness and Suicidal Ideation in Iraq and
     Afghanistan War Veterans Reporting Subthreshold and Threshold Post-
     traumatic Stress Disorder," *The Journal of Nervous and Mental Disease* 199,
     no. 4 (2011): 272–75, https://doi.org/10.1097/NMD.0b013e3182124604.

182 Combat veterans who feel guilt: H. Hendin and A. P. Haas, "Suicide
     and Guilt as Manifestations of PTSD in Vietnam Combat Veterans,"
     The American Journal of Psychiatry 148, no. 5 (1991): 586–91, https://doi
     .org/10.1176/ajp.148.5.586.

182 a scholarly construct: Brett T. Litz, Nathan Stein, Eileen Delaney, et al.,

"Moral Injury and Moral Repair in War Veterans: A Preliminary Model and Intervention Strategy," *Clinical Psychology Review* 29, no. 8 (2009): 695–706, https://doi.org/10.1016/j.cpr.2009.07.003.

182 In war, this might involve: K. D. Drescher, D. W. Foy, C. Kelly, et al., "An Exploration of the Viability and Usefulness of the Construct of Moral Injury in War Veterans," *Traumatology* 17, no. 1 (2011): 8–13, doi: 10.1177/1534765610395615.

182 In a 2013 study: Blair E. Wisco, Brian P. Marx, Casey L. May, et al., "Moral Injury in U.S. Combat Veterans: Results from the National Health and Resilience in Veterans Study," *Depression and Anxiety* 34, no. 4 (April 2017), https://doi.org/10.1002/da.22614.

183 Also at higher risk: T. A. Bullman and H. K. Kang, "A Study of Suicide Among Vietnam Veterans," *Federal Practitioner* 12, no. 3 (March 1995): 9–13. Craig J. Bryan and Tracy A. Clemans, "Repetitive Traumatic Brain Injury, Psychological Symptoms, and Suicide Risk in a Clinical Sample of Deployed Military Personnel," *JAMA Psychiatry* 70, no. 7 (2013): 686–91, https://doi.org/10.1001/jamapsychiatry.2013.1093. Lisa A. Brenner, Rosalinda V. Ignacio, and Frederic C. Blow, "Suicide and Traumatic Brain Injury Among Individuals Seeking Veterans Health Administration Services," *The Journal of Head Trauma Rehabilitation* 26, no. 4 (2011): 257–64, https://doi.org/10.1097/HTR.0b013e31821fdb6e.

183 traumatic brain injuries: Trine Madsen, Anette Erlangsen, Sonja Orlovska, et al., "Association Between Traumatic Brain Injury and Risk of Suicide," *JAMA* 320, no. 6 (2018): 580–88, doi:10.1001/jama.2018.10211, https://jamanetwork.com/journals/jama/article-abstract/2697009.

183 a team of researchers: Rachel Kimerling, Kerry Makin-Byrd, Samantha Louzon, et al., "Military Sexual Trauma and Suicide Mortality," *American Journal of Preventive Medicine* 50, no. 6 (2016): 684–91, https://doi.org/10.1016/j.amepre.2015.10.019.

183 the suicide rate of women veterans: Claire A. Hoffmire, Janet E. Kemp, and Robert M. Bossarte, "Changes in Suicide Mortality for Veterans and Nonveterans by Gender and History of VHA Service Use, 2000–2010," *Psychiatric Services* 66, no. 9 (2015): 959–65, https://doi.org/10.1176/appi.ps.201400031.

183 LGBT veterans who experience victimization: This echoes findings in the broader literature that it is not the sexual orientation of the individual per se but the negative life experiences he or she endures that take a negative toll on his or her mental health. See R. A. Burns, P. Butterworth, and A. F. Jorm, "The Long-Term Mental Health Risk Associated with Non-

heterosexual Orientation," *Epidemiology and Psychiatric Sciences* 27, no. 1 (February 2018): 71–83, https://doi.org/10.1017/S2045796016000962.

184 The key to suicide prevention: Keith S. Cox, Emily R. Mouilso, Margaret R. Venners, et al., "Reducing Suicidal Ideation Through Evidence-Based Treatment for Posttraumatic Stress Disorder," *Journal of Psychiatric Research* 80 (September 2016): 59–63, https://doi.org/10.1016/j.jpsychires .2016.05.011.

Talking Cures and Beyond

189 reach as many people as possible: in *Handbook of PTSD: Science and Practice,* 2nd ed., ed. Matthew J. Friedman, Terence Martin Keane, and Patricia A. Resick (New York: Guilford Press, 2014), 557–676.

189 a cognitive theory of PTSD: Anke Ehlers and David M. Clark, "A Cognitive Model of Posttraumatic Stress Disorder," *Behaviour Research and Therapy* 38, no. 4 (2000): 319–45.

190 Although CPT is most effective: Patricia A. Resick, Jennifer Schuster Wachen, Katherine A. Dondanville, et al., "Effect of Group vs Individual Cognitive Processing Therapy in Active-Duty Military Seeking Treatment for Posttraumatic Stress Disorder: A Randomized Clinical Trial," *JAMA Psychiatry* 74, no. 1 (2017): 28–36, https://doi.org/10.1001/jamapsychiatry .2016.2729.

190 CPT also focuses on: Darren L. Weber, "Information Processing Bias in Post-traumatic Stress Disorder," *The Open Neuroimaging Journal* 2 (June 2008): 29–51, https://doi.org/10.2174/1874440000802010029.

190 PE, which was developed: Edna B. Foa, Elizabeth Ann Hembree, and Barbara Olasov Rothbaum, *Prolonged Exposure Therapy for PTSD: Emotional Processing of Traumatic Experiences* (Oxford, UK: Oxford University Press, 2007).

191 "Trauma thoughts and memories": Personal communication with Dr. Craig Rosen, 12/15/2017.

192 PTSD symptoms improve: Bradley V. Watts, Paula P. Schnurr, Lorna Mayo, et al., "Meta-Analysis of the Efficacy of Treatments for Posttraumatic Stress Disorder," *The Journal of Clinical Psychiatry* 74, no. 6 (2013): e541–50, https://doi.org/10.4088/JCP.12r08225.

192 virtual reality exposure therapy: Barbara Olasov Rothbaum, Larry Hodges, and Rob Kooper, "Virtual Reality Exposure Therapy," *Journal of Psychotherapy Practice & Research* 6, no. 3 (Summer 1997): 219–26, https://www .ncbi.nlm.nih.gov/pubmed/9185067.

193 seven-day intensive treatment: Anke Ehlers, Ann Hackmann, Nick Grey, et al., "A Randomized Controlled Trial of 7-Day Intensive and Standard Weekly Cognitive Therapy for PTSD and Emotion-Focused Supportive Therapy," *American Journal of Psychiatry* 171, no. 3 (2014), https:///doi.org /10.1176/appi.ajp.2013.13040552.

193 In another British Study: Dominic Murphy, Georgina Hodgman, Carron Carson, et al., "Mental Health and Functional Impairment Outcomes Following a 6-Week Intensive Treatment Programme for UK Military Veterans with Post-Traumatic Stress Disorder (PTSD): A Naturalistic Study to Explore Dropout and Health Outcomes at Follow-up," *BMJ Open* 5 (2015): e007051, doi: 10.1136/bmjopen-2014-007051.

193 EMDR engages patients in a trauma memory: Francine Shapiro, "The Role of Eye Movement Desensitization and Reprocessing (EMDR) Therapy in Medicine: Adressing the Psychological and Physcial Symptoms Stemming from Adverse Life Experiences," *The Permanente Journal* 18.1 (2014): 17–77. *PMC*. Web. Sept. 12, 2018, https://www.ncbi.nlm.nih.gov /pmc/articles/PMC3951033/.

193 Brief eclectic psychotherapy: Berthold P. R. Gersons and Ulrich Schnyder, "Learning from Traumatic Experiences with Brief Eclectic Psychotherapy for PTSD," *European Journal of Psychotraumatology* 4, no. 1 (December 2013): 21369, https://www.tandfonline.com/doi/pdf/10.3402/ejpt.v4i0.21369.

193 On the global front: Shaili Jain, "The Role of Paraprofessionals in Providing Treatment for Posttraumatic Stress Disorder in Low-Resource Communities," *The Journal of the American Medical Association* 304, no. 5 (2010): 571–72, https://doi.org/10.1001/jama.2010.1096. Zachary Steel, Tien Chey, Derrick Silove, et al., "Association of Torture and Other Potentially Traumatic Events with Mental Health Outcomes Among Populations Exposed to Mass Conflict and Displacement: A Systematic Review and Meta-Analysis," *The Journal of the American Medical Association* 302, no. 5 (2009): 537–49, https://doi.org/10.1001/jama.2009.1132.

194 importance of acknowledging societal trauma: S. M. Weine, A. D. Kulenovic, I. Pavkovic, and R. Gibbons, "Testimony Psychotherapy in Bosnian Refugees: A Pilot Study," *The American Journal of Psychiatry* 155, no. 12 (1998): 1720–26, https://doi.org/10.1176/ajp.155.12.1720.

194 narrative exposure therapy: Maggie Schauer, Thomas Elbert, and Frank Neuner, *Narrative Exposure Therapy: A Short-Term Intervention for Traumatic Stress Disorders After War, Terror, or Torture* (Cambridge, MA: Hogrefe & Huber, 2005).

194 thus enabling survivors: I. Agger and S. Jensen, "Testimony as Ritual and Evidence in Psychotherapy for Political Refugees," *Journal of Traumatic Stress* 3, no. 1 (January 1990): 115–130, doi: 10.1002/jts.2490030109.

194 What impact: Josh M. Cisler, J. Scott Steele, Jennifer K. Lenow, et al., "Functional Reorganization of Neural Networks During Repeated Exposure to the Traumatic Memory in Posttraumatic Stress Disorder: An Exploratory fMRI Study," *Journal of Psychiatric Research* 48, no. 1 (2018): 47–55, https://doi.org/10.1016/j.jpsychires.2013.09.013.

194 On the molecular level: Julia Morath, Maria Moreno-Villanueva, Gilava Hamuni, et al., "Effects of Psychotherapy on DNA Strand Break Accumulation Originating from Traumatic Stress," *Psychotherapy and Psychosomatics* 83, no. 5 (2014): 289–97, https://doi.org/10.1159/000362739.

194 exposure therapy: Julia Morath, Hannah Gola, Annette Sommershof, et al., "The Effect of Trauma-Focused Therapy on the Altered T Cell Distribution in Individuals with PTSD: Evidence from a Randomized Controlled Trial," *Journal of Psychiatric Research* 54 (July 2014): 1–10, https://doi.org/10.1016/j.jpsychires.2014.03.016.

194 many sufferers are not seeking: Stephanie M. Keller and Peter W. Tuerk, "Evidence-Based Psychotherapy (EBP) Non-initiation Among Veterans Offered an EBP for Posttraumatic Stress Disorder," *Psychological Services* 13, no. 1 (2016): 42–48, https://doi.org/10.1037/ser0000064.

195 the dropout rate is high: Lisa M. Najavits, "The Problem of Dropout from 'Gold Standard' PTSD Therapies," *F1000 Prime Reports* 7 (April 2015): 43, https://doi.org/10.12703/P7-43.

195 Skills Training in Affective and Interpersonal Regulation: Marylene Cloitre, Christie Jackson, and Janet A. Schmidt, "Case Reports: STAIR for Strengthening Social Support and Relationships Among Veterans with Military Sexual Trauma and PTSD," *Military Medicine* 181, no. 2 (February 1, 2016): e183–87, https://doi.org/10.7205/MILMED-D-15-00209.

195 a powerful alternative: Marylene Cloitre, K. Chase Stovall-McClough, Kate Nooner, et al., "Treatment for PTSD Related to Childhood Abuse: A Randomized Controlled Trial," *The American Journal of Psychiatry* 167, no. 8 (2010): 915–24, https://doi.org/10.1176/appi.ajp.2010.09081247. STAIR may be especially well tolerated by individuals who dissociate; see Marylene Cloitre, Eva Petkova, Jing Wang, and Feihan Lu (Lassell), "An Examination of the Influence of a Sequential Treatment on the Course and Impact of Dissociation Among Women with PTSD Related to Childhood Abuse," *Depression and Anxiety* 29, no. 8 (2012): 709–17, https://doi

.org/10.1002/da.21920. STAIR may also lay an essential groundwork for the patient to be able to better tolerate a more traditional trauma-focused therapy in the future; see Marylene Cloitre, Karestan C. Koenen, Lisa R. Cohen, and Hyemee Han, "Skills Training in Affective and Interpersonal Regulation Followed by Exposure: A Phase-Based Treatment for PTSD Related to Childhood Abuse," *Journal of Consulting and Clinical Psychology* 70, no. 5 (2002): 1067–74, https://pdfs.semanticscholar.org/9f63/780cb 12262e8c599d69c32e3cc89524fd0eb.pdf.

195   Acceptance and commitment therapy: ACT is an effective treatment for depression and many other conditions, but a recent study showed limited evidence for how well it works as a PTSD treatment. See D. Ducasse and G. Fond, "Acceptance and commitment therapy," *L'Encephale* 41, no. 1 (2015): 1–9, https://doi.org/10.1016/j.encep.2013.04.017.

195   Integrating spiritual approaches: J. Irene Harris, Christopher R. Erbes, Brian E. Engdahl, et al., "The Effectiveness of a Trauma Focused Spiritually Integrated Intervention for Veterans Exposed to Trauma," *Journal of Clinical Psychology* 67, no. 4 (2011): 425–38, https://doi.org/10.1002/jclp.20777. Joseph M. Currier, Jason M. Holland, and Kent D. Drescher, "Spirituality Factors in the Prediction of Outcomes of PTSD Treatment for U.S. Military Veterans," *Journal of Traumatic Stress* 28, no. 1 (2015): 57–64, https://doi.org/10.1002/jts.21978.

196   Mind body treatments: Complementary therapies are widely used by patients with PTSD. Recent use estimates in PTSD populations range from 26 to 39 percent. See Gary N. Asher, Jonathan Gerkin, and Bradley N. Gaynes, "Complementary Therapies for Mental Health Disorders," *The Medical Clinics of North America* 101, no. 5 (2017): 847–64, https://doi .org/10.1016/j.mcna.2017.04.004. David Spiegel and Etzel Cardeña, "New Uses of Hypnosis in the Treatment of Posttraumatic Stress Disorder," *The Journal of Clinical Psychiatry* 51, suppl. (1990): 39–43.

196   massage, acupuncture, and hypnosis are widely used by patients with PTSD: Barbara Niles, DeAnna L. Mori, Craig Polizzi, et al., "A Systematic Review of Randomized Trials of Mind-Body Interventions for PTSD,"*Journal of Clinical Psychiatry* (2018):1–24, https://doi.org/10.1002/jclp.22634.

196   electroencephalographic (EEG) biofeedback: Kerstin Mayer and Martijn Arns, "Electroencephalogram Neurofeedback: Application in ADHD and Epilepsy," *Psychiatric Annals* 46, no. 10 (2016): 594–600, https://doi .org/10.3928/00485713-20160906-01.

196   A recent pilot study: Mark Gapen, Bessel A. van der Kolk, Ed Hamlin,

et al., "A Pilot Study of Neurofeedback for Chronic PTSD," *Applied Psychophysiology and Biofeedback* 41, no. 3 (2016): 251–61, https://doi .org/10.1007/s10484-015-9326-5.

196 A four-session mindfulness training program: Kyle Possemato, Dessa Bergen-Cico, Scott Treatman, et al., "A Randomized Clinical Trial of Primary Care Brief Mindfulness Training for Veterans with PTSD," *Journal of Clinical Psychology* 72, no. 3 (2016): 179–93, https://doi.org/10.1002 /jclp.22241.

197 Programs that harness the power of nature: Nick Caddick, Brett Smith, and Cassandra Phoenix, "The Effects of Surfing and the Natural Environment on the Well-Being of Combat Veterans," *Qualitative Health Research* 25, no. 1 (2014): 76–86, https://doi.org/10.1177/1049732314549477. Stephanie Westlund, "'Becoming Human Again': Exploring Connections Between Nature and Recovery from Stress and Post-traumatic Distress," *Work* 50, no. 1 (2015): 161–74, https://doi.org/10.3233/WOR-141934.

197 including horses: Michael D. Anestis, Joye C. Anestis, Laci L. Zawilinski, et al., "Equine-Related Treatments for Mental Disorders Lack Empirical Support: A Systematic Review of Empirical Investigations," *Journal of Clinical Psychology* 70, no. 12 (2014): 1115–32, https://doi.org/10.1002/ jclp.22113.

197 Dance programs: Sarah Wilbur, Hilary B. Meyer, Matthew R. Baker, et al., "Dance for Veterans: A Complementary Health Program for Veterans with Serious Mental Illness," *Arts & Health* 7, no. 2 (2015): 96–108, https:// doi.org/10.1080/17533015.2015.1019701.

197 the use of dogs: Cheryl A. Krause-Parello, Sarah Sarni, and Eleni Padden, "Military Veterans and Canine Assistance for Post-traumatic Stress Disorder: A Narrative Review of the Literature," *Nurse Education Today* 47, suppl. C (2016): 43–50, https://doi.org/https://doi.org/10.1016/j .nedt.2016.04.020.

197 they remain largely untested: Mark S. Bauer, Laura Damschroder, Hildi Hagedorn, et al., "An Introduction to Implementation Science for the Non-specialist," *BMC Psychology* 3, no. 1 (2015): 32, https://doi .org/10.1186/s40359-015-0089-9.

Psych Meds

202 Antidepressant medications are effective treatments: Mathew Hoskins, Jennifer Pearce, Andrew Bethell, et al., "Pharmacotherapy for Post-traumatic Stress Disorder: Systematic Review and Meta-analysis," *The British Journal of Psychiatry* 206, no. 2 (2015): 93–100, https://doi.org/10.1192/bjp.bp.114.148551.

202 it has been hypothesized: Hans-Peter Kapfhammer, "Patient-Reported Outcomes in Post-traumatic Stress Disorder. Part II: Focus on Pharmacological Treatment," *Dialogues in Clinical Neuroscience* 16, no. 2 (2014): 227–37, http://www.ncbi.nlm.nih.gov/pmc/articles/PMC4140515/.

203 which antidepressant to prescribe: Elisa F. Cascade, Amir H. Kalali, Ann M. Rasmusson, and Candice Monson, "What Treatments Are Prescribed for Posttraumatic Stress Disorder?," *Psychiatry* 4, no. 2 (2007): 25–26, http://www.ncbi.nlm.nih.gov/pmc/articles/PMC2922344/.

203 mirtazapine can be useful: Norio Watanabe, Ichiro M. Omori, Atsuo Nakagawa, et al., "Mirtazapine Versus Other Antidepressive Agents for Depression," *The Cochrane Database of Systematic Reviews*, no. 12 (December 2011): CD006528, https://doi.org/10.1002/14651858.CD006528.pub2.

203 The antidepressant venlafaxine: K. Taylor and M. C. Rowbotham, "Venlafaxine Hydrochloride and Chronic Pain," *Western Journal of Medicine* 165, no. 3 (1996): 147–48, http://www.ncbi.nlm.nih.gov/pmc/articles /PMC1303727/.

203 up to 60 percent of sufferers: K. Brady, T. Pearlstein, G. M. Asnis, et al., "Efficacy and Safety of Sertraline Treatment of Posttraumatic Stress Disorder: A Randomized Controlled Trial," *The Journal of the American Medical Association* 283, no. 14 (2000): 1837–44. J. R. Davidson, B. O. Rothbaum, B. A. van der Kolk, et al., "Multicenter, Double-Blind Comparison of Sertraline and Placebo in the Treatment of Posttraumatic Stress Disorder," *Archives of General Psychiatry* 58, no. 5 (2001): 485–92.

203 neuroimaging studies has shown: Kathleen Thomaes, Ethy Dorrepaal, Nel Draijer, et al., "Can Pharmacological and Psychological Treatment Change Brain Structure and Function in PTSD? A Systematic Review," *Journal of Psychiatric Research* 50, suppl. C (2014): 1–15, https://doi .org/10.1016/j.jpsychires.2013.11.002.

205 My own research has shown: One of the first research studies I was involved in as a fellow at the NCPTSD was a national study of almost 500 veterans with PTSD in which we gathered clinical data and pulled information about their prescription medications from a national pharmacy database. We found that mood stabilizers had been prescribed to almost 20 percent of the patients, SGA to 15 percent, and long-term benzodiazepines to 14 percent of the sample. These percentages are significant, especially considering the quality of evidence to support such prescribing for PTSD patients. See Shaili Jain, Mark A. Greenbaum, and Craig Rosen, "Concordance Between Psychotropic Prescribing for Veterans with PTSD and Clinical Practice Guidelines," *Psychiatric Services* 63, no. 2 (2012): 154–60, https://doi.org/10.1176/appi.ps.201100199.

205 Some studies suggest that topiramate: Steven L. Batki, David L. Pennington, Brooke Lasher, et al., "Topiramate Treatment of Alcohol Use Disorder in Veterans with Posttraumatic Stress Disorder: A Randomized Controlled Pilot Trial," *Alcoholism: Clinical & Experimental Research* 38, no. 8 (2014): 2169–77, https://doi.org/10.1111/acer.12496.

205 SGAs may be helpful: Erika J. Wolf, Karen S. Mitchell, Mark W. Logue, et al., "The Dopamine D(3) Receptor Gene and Posttraumatic Stress Disorder," *Journal of Traumatic Stress* 27, no. 4 (2014): 379–87, https://doi.org/10.1002/jts.21937.

206 Early studies found: Kapfhammer, "Patient-Reported Outcomes in Post-traumatic Stress Disorder. Part II: Focus on Pharmacological Treatment."

206 The study results: John H. Krystal, Robert A. Rosenheck, Joyce A. Cramer, et al., "Adjunctive Risperidone Treatment for Antidepressant-Resistant Symptoms of Chronic Military Service–Related PTSD: A Randomized Trial," *The Journal of the American Medical Association* 306, no. 5 (2011): 493–502, https://doi.org/10.1001/jama.2011.1080.

207 In a study of eighty veterans: Gerardo Villarreal, Mark B. Hamner, José M. Cañive, et al., "Efficacy of Quetiapine Monotherapy in Posttraumatic Stress Disorder: A Randomized, Placebo-Controlled Trial," *American Journal of Psychiatry* 173, no. 12 (2016): 1205–12, https://doi.org/10.1176/appi.ajp.2016.15070967.

207 Preliminary data suggest that: David Mataix-Cols, Lorena Fernandez de la Cruz, Benedetta Monzani, et al., "D-Cycloserine Augmentation of Exposure-Based Cognitive Behavior Therapy for Anxiety, Obsessive-Compulsive, and Posttraumatic Stress Disorders: A Systematic Review and Meta-analysis of Individual Participant Data," *JAMA Psychiatry* 74, no. 5 (2017): 501–10, https://doi.org/10.1001/jamapsychiatry.2016.3955. JoAnn Difede, Judith Cukor, Katarzyna Wyka, et al., "D-Cycloserine Augmentation of Exposure Therapy for Post-traumatic Stress Disorder: A Pilot Randomized Clinical Trial," *Neuropsychopharmacology* 39, no. 5 (2014): 1052–58, https://doi.org/10.1038/npp.2013.317.

207 Veterans who received hydrocortisone: Rachel Yehuda, Linda M. Bierer, Laura C. Pratchett, et al., "Cortisol Augmentation of a Psychological Treatment for Warfighters with Posttraumatic Stress Disorder: Randomized Trial Showing Improved Treatment Retention and Outcome," *Psychoneuroendocrinology* 51 (January 2015): 589–97, https://doi.org/10.1016/j.psyneuen.2014.08.004. Matthew A. Battista, Robert Hierholzer, Hani Raoul Khouzam, et al., "Pilot Trial of Memantine in the Treatment of Post-

traumatic Stress Disorder," *Psychiatry* 70, no. 2 (2007): 167–74, https://doi .org/10.1521/psyc.2007.70.2.167.

207 alpha 2 adrenergic receptor antagonist Yohimbine: Peter W. Tuerk, Bethany C. Wangelin, Mark B. Powers, et al., "Augmenting Treatment Efficiency in Exposure Therapy for PTSD: A Randomized Double-Blind Placebo-Controlled Trial of Yohimbine HCI," *Cognitive Behavior Therapy* 47, no. 5 (2018): 351–71, doi: 10.1080/16506073.2018.1432679.

207 Transcranial magnetic stimulation: F. Andrew Kozel, et al., "Repetitive TMS to augment cognitive processing therapy in combat veterans of recent conflicts with PTSD: A randomized clinical trial," *Journal of Affective Disorders* 229, 506–14, doi:https://doi.org/10.1016/j.jad.2017.12.046, https:// www.jad-journal.com/article/S0165-0327(17)31575-6/.

208 One class of medications: Jeffrey Guina, Sarah R. Rossetter, Bethany J. Derhodes, et al., "Benzodiazepines for PTSD: A Systematic Review and Meta-analysis," *Journal of Psychiatric Practice* 21, no. 4 (2015), http://journals .lww.com/practicalpsychiatry/Fulltext/2015/07000/Benzodiazepines_ for_PTSD__A_Systematic_Review_and.6.aspx.

208 increased odds of falling: Robert G. Cumming and David G. Le Conteur, "Benzodiazepines and Risk of Hip Fractures in Older People: A Review of the Evidence," *CNS Drugs* 17, no. 11 (September 2003): 825–37, https:// link.springer.com/article/10.2165%2F00023210-200317110-00004.

207 Benzodiazepines fell seriously out of favor: Daniel F. Kripke, Robert D. Langer, and Lawrence E. Kline, "Hypnotics' Association with Mortality or Cancer: A Matched Cohort Study," *BMJ Open* 2, no. 1 (2012), http://bm-jopen.bmj.com/content/2/1/e000850.abstract.

Medication Management

209 required to do more with less: Tait D. Shanafelt, Lotte N. Dyrbye, and Colin P. West, "Addressing Physician Burnout: The Way Forward," *The Journal of the American Medical Association* 317, no. 9 (2017): 901–02, https://doi.org/10.1001/jama.2017.0076.

209 the fundamentals of treatment: Lloyd Sederer, "Improving Public Mental Health: Four Secrets in Plain Sight," *Psychiatric Times*, December 13, 2016, http://psychnews.psychiatryonline.org/doi/full/10.1176/appi .pn.2016.12b2.

214 Eating a well-balanced, nutritious diet: Simon Rosenbaum, Anne Tiede-mann, Robert Stanton, et al., "Implementing Evidence-Based Physical Activity Interventions for People with Mental Illness: An Australian

Perspective," *Australasian Psychiatry* 24, no. 1 (2016): 49–54, https://doi
.org/10.1177/1039856215590252.

214 we seem to be forgetting: Shellene K. Dietrich, Coleen M. Francis-Jimenez,
Melida Delcina Knibbs, et al., "Effectiveness of Sleep Education Programs
to Improve Sleep Hygiene and/or Sleep Quality in College Students:
A Systematic Review," *JBI Database of Systematic Reviews and Imple-
mentation Reports* 14, no. 9 (2016): 108–34, https://doi.org/10.11124
/JBISRIR-2016-003088.

214 never filled the prescription: When I was a research fellow at the
NCPTSD, I was a coinvestigator on a national study of several hundred
veterans with PTSD that investigated whether they were getting first-line
medication treatment or not. First-line medication consisted of their not
only taking an antidepressant but also taking it for long enough (about six
to eight weeks) and at a strong enough dose for the medication to work;
in other words, did the veteran get a therapeutic trial of medication? Our
analysis found that veterans from the wars in Afghanistan and Iraq, though
they were just as likely to be provided with the medications, were less likely
to complete a therapeutic trial than were older veterans. Our findings echo
what I see on the ground in my clinic. See Shaili Jain, Mark A. Greenbaum,
and Craig S. Rosen, "Do Veterans with Posttraumatic Stress Disorder Receive First-Line Pharmacotherapy? Results from the Longitudinal Veterans Health Survey," *The Primary Care Companion for CNS Disorders* 14, no.
2 (2012), https://doi.org/10.4088/PCC.11m01162.

214 Why do people: Jessica A. Chen, Stephanie M. Keller, Lori A. Zoellner, and
Norah C. Feeny, "'How Will It Help Me?': Reasons Underlying Treatment Preferences Between Sertraline and Prolonged Exposure in PTSD,"
The Journal of Nervous and Mental Disease 201, no. 8 (2013): 691–97, https://
doi.org/10.1097/NMD.0b013e31829c50a9.

215 historical antecedents: Edward Shorter, *A History of Psychiatry: From
the Era of the Asylum to the Age of Prozac* (Hoboken, NJ: Wiley, 1998).

215 advocate for tried and tested treatments: Gregory E. Gray and Letitia A.
Pinson, "Evidence-Based Medicine and Psychiatric Practice," *Psychiatric
Quarterly* 74, no. 4 (December 2003): 387–99, https://link.springer.com
/article/10.1023/A:1026091611425.

215 As a group we are more diverse: Hermioni N. Lokko, Justin A. Chen,
Ranna I. Parekh, and Theodore A. Stern, "Racial and Ethnic Diversity in
the US Psychiatric Workforce: A Perspective and Recommendations,"
Academic Psychiatry 40, no. 6 (2016): 898–904, https://doi.org/10.1007

/s40596-016-0591-2. Nancy C. Andreasen, "Diversity in Psychiatry: Or, Why Did We Become Psychiatrists?," *American Journal of Psychiatry* 158, no. 5 (2001): 673–75, https://doi.org/10.1176/appi.ajp.158.5.673.

215 Regardless of their reasons: Lori A. Zoellner, Norah C. Feeny, and Joyce N. Bittinger, "What You Believe Is What You Want: Modeling PTSD-Related Treatment Preferences for Sertraline or Prolonged Exposure," *Journal of Behavior Therapy and Experimental Psychiatry* 40, no. 3 (2009): 455–67, https://doi.org/10.1016/j.jbtep.2009.06.001.

The Allure of Magic Bullets

216 In 2008, reports started to emerge: Eugene G. Lipov, Jay R. Joshi, Sergei Lipov, et al., "Cervical Sympathetic Blockade in a Patient with Post-traumatic Stress Disorder: A Case Report," *Annals of Clinical Psychiatry* 20, no. 4 (2008), https://doi.org/10.1080/10401230802435518.

216 led to immediate symptom relief: In 2013 a case series was reported in which treatment-resistant veterans with PTSD had been given the block. After the intervention, five of the nine veterans experienced a significant improvement in their PTSD symptoms, but those benefits diminished over time. See Eugene G. Lipov, Maryam Navaie, Peter R. Brown, et al., "Stellate Ganglion Block Improves Refractory Post-traumatic Stress Disorder and Associated Memory Dysfunction: A Case Report and Systematic Literature Review," *Military Medicine* 178 no. 2 (2013): e260–64, https://doi.org/10.7205/MILMED-D-12-00290.

217 first controlled study: Nancy A. Melville, "Stellate Ganglion Block No Better than Placebo for PTSD," Medscape, March 26, 2015, http://www.medscape.com/viewarticle/842095.

217 magic bullets: Ian A. Cook, Michelle Abrams, and Andrew F. Leuchter, "Trigeminal Nerve Stimulation for Comorbid Posttraumatic Stress Disorder and Major Depressive Disorder," *Neuromodulation* 19, no. 3 (2016): 299–305, https://doi.org/10.1111/ner.12399.

217 ketamine: Caroline Cassels, "Ketamine: New Potential as Rapid PTSD Treatment," Medscape, April 17, 2014, http://www.medscape.com/viewarticle/823760.

217 A 2014 paper: Adriana Feder, Michael K. Parides, James W. Murrough, et al., "Efficacy of Intravenous Ketamine for Treatment of Chronic Posttraumatic Stress Disorder: A Randomized Clinical Trial," *JAMA Psychiatry* 71, no. 6 (2014): 681–88, https://doi.org/10.1001/jamapsychiatry.2014.62.

218 The data remain thin: Andrea Cipriani, et al., "3,4 Methylenedioxy-

methamphetamine (MDMA)-Assisted Psychotherapy for Post-Traumatic Stress Disorder in Service Personnel," *The Lancet Pyschiatry* 5, no. 6, 453–55, doi:https://doi.org/10.1016/S2215-0366(18)30170-6.

218 only a couple of small randomized, controlled studies: Peter Oehen, Rafael Traber, Verena Widmer, and Ulrich Schnyder, "A Randomized, Controlled Pilot Study of MDMA (±3,4-Methylenedioxymethamphetamine)-Assisted Psychotherapy for Treatment of Resistant, Chronic Post-traumatic Stress Disorder (PTSD)," *Journal of Psychopharmacology* 27, no. 1 (2013): 40–52, https://doi.org/10.1177/0269881112464827.

218 Neuroscientists have put forth: Alexander Neumeister, Jordan Seidel, Benjamin J. Ragen, and Robert H. Pietrzak, "Translational Evidence for a Role of Endocannabinoids in the Etiology and Treatment of Posttraumatic Stress Disorder," *Psychoneuroendocrinology* 51 (January 2018): 577–84, https://doi.org/10.1016/j.psyneuen.2014.10.012.

218 In 2016, investigators: Samuel T. Wilkinson, Rajiv Radhakrishnan, and Deepak Cyril D'Souza, "A Systematic Review of the Evidence for Medical Marijuana in Psychiatric Indications," *The Journal of Clinical Psychiatry* 77, no. 8 (2016): 1050–64, https://doi.org/10.4088/JCP.15r10036.

220 downplay the downsides: Tista S. Ghosh, Michael Van Dyke, Ali Maffey, et al., "Medical Marijuana's Public Health Lessons—Implications for Retail Marijuana in Colorado," *The New England Journal of Medicine* 372, no. 11 (2015): 991–93, https://doi.org/10.1056/NEJMp1500043.

220 Marijuana also impairs: Alejandro Azofeifa, Margaret E. Mattson, and Althea Grant, "Monitoring Marijuana Use in the United States: Challenges in an Evolving Environment," *The Journal of the American Medical Association* 316, no. 17 (2016): 1765–66, https://doi.org/10.1001/jama.2016.13696.

220 one observational study: Samuel T. Wilkinson, Elina Stefanovics, and Robert A. Rosenheck, "Marijuana Use Is Associated with Worse Outcomes in Symptom Severity and Violent Behavior in Patients with Posttraumatic Stress Disorder," *The Journal of Clinical Psychiatry* 76, no. 9 (2015): 1174–80, https://doi.org/10.4088/JCP.14m09475.

219 Bonn-Miller reminded me: Personal communication with Dr. Marcel Bonn-Miller, January 21, 2017. See also Mallory J. E. Loflin, Kimberly A. Babson, and Marcel O. Bonn-Miller, "Cannabinoids as Therapeutic for PTSD," *Current Opinion in Psychology* 14, suppl. C (2017): 78–83, https://doi.org/https://doi.org/10.1016/j.copsyc.2016.12.001.

Trauma of the Masses: A Wicked Problem

225 "The term 'wicked'": Australian Public Service Commission, "Tackling Wicked

Problems: A Public Policy Perspective," May 31, 2012, http://www.apsc.gov.au/publications-and-media/archive/publications-archive/tackling-wicked-problems.

225 civilians reaching close to 200 million: Eric Hobsbawm, "War and Peace," *The Guardian, U.S. Edition,* February 22, 2002, accessed January 11, 2018, https://www.theguardian.com/education/2002/feb/23/artsandhumanities.highereducation.

225 Civilian rape has long been used: B. Allen, *Rape Warfare: The Hidden Genocide in Bosnia-Herzegovina and Croatia* (Minneapolis: University of Minnesota Press, 1996). K. Hirschfeld, J. Leaning, S. Crosby, et al., *Nowhere to Turn: Failure to Protect, Support and Assure Justice for Darfuri Women* (Cambridge, MA: Physicians for Human Rights and Harvard Humanitarian Initiative, 2009), http://hhi.harvard.edu/publications/nowhere-turn-failure-protect-support-and-assure-justice-darfuri-women.

225 Syria being a source of major concern: "Syria: The Story of the Conflict," BBC News, March 11, 2016, accessed January 1, 2018, http://www.bbc.com/news/world-middle-east-26116868.

225 children into refugees: Lydia DePillis, Kulwant Saluja, and Denise Lu, *The Washington Post,* December 21, 2015, accessed January 2, 2018. https://www.washingtonpost.com/graphics/world/historical-migrant-crisis/.

226 forced labor worldwide: ILO Special Action Programme to combat Forced Labour (SAP-FL), Programme for the Promotion of the Declaration on Fundamental Principles and Rights at Work, "ILO 2012 Global Estimate of Forced Labour: Executive Summary," 2012, accessed January 2, 2018, http://www.ilo.org/wcmsp5/groups/public/---ed_norm/---declaration/documents/publication/wcms_181953.pdf.

226 In a national survey of Americans: Ronald C. Kessler, Amanda Sonnega, Evelyn Bromet, et al., "Posttraumatic Stress Disorder in the National Comorbidity Survey," *Archives of General Psychiatry* 52, no. 12 (1995): 1048–60, https://www.ncbi.nlm.nih.gov/pubmed/7492257.

226 Comparable statistics: Craig L. Katz and Anand Pandya, "Disaster Psychiatry: A Closer Look," *Psychiatric Clinics of North America* 27, no. 3 (September 2004): 391–610, http://www.psych.theclinics.com/issue/S0193-953X(00)X0012-3.

224 tens of thousands of people were affected: Fatih Ozbay, Tanja Auf der Heyde, Dori Reissman, and Vansh Sharma, "The Enduring Mental Health Impact of the September 11th Terrorist Attacks: Challenges and Lessons Learned," *Psychiatric Clinics of North America* 36, no. 3 (2013): 417–29, https://doi.org/10.1016/j.psc.2013.05.011.

The 1947 Partition

231 During World War I: Cahal Milmo, "Forgotten Role of Indian Soldiers Who Served in First World War Marked at Last," *The Independent*, November 7, 2015, http://www.independent.co.uk/news/uk/home-news/forgotten -role-of-indian-soldiers-who-served-in-first-world-war-marked-at -last-a6725851.html.

231 tantamount to nothing: "Montagu-Chelmsford Report: United Kingdom-India [1918]," *Encyclopædia Britannica*, https://www.britannica.com/event /Montagu-Chelmsford-Report.

233 By 1947, the British had: For more on the reasons why Great Britain quit India, please see http://www.nationalarchives.gov.uk/education /empire/g3/cs3/background.htm.

236 "Up to two million people": C. Ryan Perkins, "1947 Partition of India & Pakistan," https://exhibits.stanford.edu/1947-partition/about/1947 -partition-of-india-pakistan.

237 As powerful as the desire is to deny: Judith Herman, *Trauma and Recovery: The Aftermath of Violence—From Domestic Abuse to Political Terror* (New York: Basic Books, 2015), 1.

237 "People were not well equipped": Yasmin Khan, *The Great Partition: The Making of India and Pakistan* (New Haven, CT: Yale University Press, 2017), 187.

237 More recently, the concerned voices: Urvashi Butalia, *The Other Side of Silence: Voices from the Partition of India* (Durham, NC: Duke University Press, 2003).

237 activists and scholars have been growing louder: Sanjeev Jain, Alok Sarin, *The Psychological Impact of the Partition of India* (Newbury Park, CA: SAGE Publishing, 2018).

War, Disaster, and Terror: Hard-Earned Knowledge and Lessons for the Future

239 Their results: J. T. de Jong, I. H. Komproe, M. van Ommeren, et al., "Lifetime Events and Posttraumatic Stress Disorder in 4 Postconflict Settings," *The Journal of the American Medical Association* 286, no. 5 (2001): 555–62. The percentages were close to 40 percent, 30 percent, 16 percent, and 18 percent in Algeria, Cambodia, Ethiopia, and Gaza, respectively.

239 A 2003 national survey: Barbara Lopes Cardozo, Oleg O. Bilukha, Carol A. Gotway Crawford, et al., "Mental Health, Social Functioning, and Disability in Postwar Afghanistan," *The Journal of the American Medical Association* 292, no. 5 (2004): 575–84, https://doi.org/10.1001/jama.292.5.575.

240 More recently, European scientists: Alison Abbott, "The Mental-Health

Crisis Among Migrants," *Nature* 538 (October 13, 2016): 158–160, http://www.nature.com/news/the-mental-health-crisis-among-migrants-1.20767.

240 it is safe to assume: Lisa R. Fortuna, Michelle V. Porche, and Margarita Alegria, "Political Violence, Psychosocial Trauma, and the Context of Mental Health Services Use Among Immigrant Latinos in the United States," *Ethnicity & Health* 13, no. 5 (2008): 435–63, https://doi.org/10.1080/13557850701837286.

240 Many have a history: N. M. Shrestha, B. Sharma, M. van Ommeren, et al., "Impact of Torture on Refugees Displaced Within the Developing World: Symptomatology Among Bhutanese Refugees in Nepal," *The Journal of the American Medical Association* 280, no. 5 (1998): 443–48. M. van Ommeren, J. T. de Jong, B. Sharma, et al., "Psychiatric Disorders Among Tortured Bhutanese Refugees in Nepal," *Archives of General Psychiatry* 58, no. 5 (2001): 475–82.

240 A 2017 study of over 300: H.E. Ainamani, T. Elbert, D.K. Olema, et al., "PTSD Symptom Severity Relates to Cognitive and Psycho-social Dysfunction —A Study with Congoloese Refugees in Uganda," *European Journal of Psychotraumatology* 14, no. 8 (2017), doi: 10.1080/20008198.2017.1283086.

240 Stable settlement and social support: Mina Fazel, Ruth V. Reed, Catherine Panter-Brick, and Alan Stein, "Mental Health of Displaced and Refugee Children Resettled in High-Income Countries: Risk and Protective Factors," *The Lancet* 379, no. 9812 (2018): 266–82, https://doi.org/10.1016/S0140-6736(11)60051-2.

240 Holocaust survivors, as a group, proved resilient: Ora Nakash, Irena Liphshitz, Lital Keinan-Boker, and Itzhak Levav, "The Effect of Cancer on Suicide Among Elderly Holocaust Survivors," *Suicide & Life-Threatening Behavior* 43, no. 3 (2013): 290–95, https://doi.org/10.1111/sltb.12015. Efrat Barel, Marinus H. van IJzendoorn, Abraham Sagi-Schwartz, and Marian J. Bakermans-Kranenburg, "Surviving the Holocaust: A Meta-Analysis of the Long-Term Sequelae of a Genocide," *Psychological Bulletin* 136, no. 5 (2010): 677–98, https://doi.org/10.1037/a0020339.

241 PTSD was rampant: R. Yehuda, B. Kahana, J. Schmeidler, et al., "Impact of Cumulative Lifetime Trauma and Recent Stress on Current Posttraumatic Stress Disorder Symptoms in Holocaust Survivors," *The American Journal of Psychiatry* 152, no. 12 (1995): 1815–18, https://doi.org/10.1176/ajp.152.12.1815. K. Kuch and B. J. Cox, "Symptoms of PTSD in 124 Survivors of the Holocaust," *The American Journal of Psychiatry* 149, no. 3 (1992): 337–40, https://doi.org/10.1176/ajp.149.3.337. Survivors who had

been exposed to atrocities (e.g., in concentration camps) were more likely to have PTSD, and, as would be expected for that period of history, when PTSD was not formally recognized as a medical condition, many had not received adequate psychiatric care for their condition.

241 This guilt-ridden melancholia: R. Yehuda, B. Kahana, S. M. Southwick, and E. L. Giller Jr., "Depressive Features in Holocaust Survivors with Post-traumatic Stress Disorder," *Journal of Traumatic Stress* 7, no. 4 (1994): 699–704.

241 In a thoughtful analysis: Cendrine Bursztein Lipsicas, Itzhak Levav, and Stephen Z. Levine, "Holocaust Exposure and Subsequent Suicide Risk: A Population-Based Study," *Social Psychiatry and Psychiatric Epidemiology* 52, no. 3 (2017): 311–17, https://doi.org/10.1007/s00127-016-1323-3.

241 Feelings of guilt: A. L. Beal, "Post-traumatic Stress Disorder in Prisoners of War and Combat Veterans of the Dieppe Raid: A 50-Year Follow-up," *Canadian Journal of Psychiatry* 40, no. 4 (May 1995): 177–84, https://www.ncbi.nlm.nih.gov/pubmed/7621386. F. A. Allodi, "Post-traumatic Stress Disorder in Hostages and Victims of Torture," *Psychiatric Clinics of North America* 17, no. 2 (1994): 279–88.

241 As might be expected: Ligia Kiss, Nicola S. Pocock, Varaporn Naisanguansri, et al., "Health of Men, Women, and Children in Post-trafficking Services in Cambodia, Thailand, and Vietnam: An Observational Cross-sectional Study," *The Lancet Global Health* 3, no. 3 (2015): e154–61, https://doi.org/10.1016/S2214-109X(15)70016-1.

241 In a small study: Retina Rimal and Chris Papadopoulos, "The Mental Health of Sexually Trafficked Female Survivors in Nepal," *The International Journal of Social Psychiatry* 62, no. 5 (2016): 487–95, https://doi.org 10.1177/0020764016651457.

241 Similar results were found: Melanie Abas, Nicolae V. Ostrovschi, Martin Prince, et al., "Risk Factors for Mental Disorders in Women Survivors of Human Trafficking: A Historical Cohort Study," *BMC Psychiatry* 13 (August 2013): 204, https://doi.org/10.1186/1471-244X-13-204.

242 Such downstream consequences: Dorothy Neriah Muraya and Deborah Fry, "Aftercare Services for Child Victims of Sex Trafficking: A Systematic Review of Policy and Practice," *Trauma, Violence & Abuse* 17, no. 2 (2016): 204–20, https://doi.org/10.1177/1524838015584356.

242 rates of PTSD after natural disasters: Thomas M. Stein, "Mass Shootings," in *Disaster Medicine*, ed. David E. Hogan and Jonathan L. Burstein (Philadelphia: Lippincott Williams & Wilkins, 2011), 444–52, at 451.

242 PTSD remains sufficiently frequent: C. S. North, S. J. Nixon, S. Shariat, et

al., "Psychiatric Disorders Among Survivors of the Oklahoma City Bombing," *The Journal of the American Medical Association* 282, no. 8 (1999): 755–62.

242 their home being destroyed: Sandro Galea, Arijit Nandi, and David Vlahov, "The Epidemiology of Post-traumatic Stress Disorder After Disasters," *Epidemiologic Reviews* 27 (2005): 78–91, https://doi.org/10.1093/epirev /mxi003. Craig L. Katz and Anand Pandya, "Disaster Psychiatry: A Closer Look," *Psychiatric Clinics of North America* 27, no. 3 (September 2004): 391–610, http://www.psych.theclinics.com/issue/S0193-953X(00)X0012-3.

242 This variability explains: Most statistics reported are in the lower half of this range, however. See Galea et al., "The Epidemiology of Post-traumatic Stress Disorder After Disasters."

242 One study found: Alexander C. McFarlane, "The Longitudinal Course of Posttraumatic Morbidity: The Range of Outcomes and Their Predictors," *The Journal of Nervous and Mental Disease* 176, no. 1 (1988), http://journals .lww.com/jonmd/Fulltext/1988/01000/The_Longitudinal_Course_of _Posttraumatic_Morbidity.4.aspx.

242 Other research: Chia-Ming Chang, Li-Ching Lee, Kathryn M. Connor, et al., "Posttraumatic Distress and Coping Strategies Among Rescue Workers After an Earthquake," *The Journal of Nervous and Mental Disease* 191, no. 6 (2003): 391–98, https://doi.org/10.1097/01.NMD .0000071588.73571.3D.

243 Four years after the hurricane: Howard J. Osofsky, Joy D. Osofsky, Mindy Kronenberg, et al., "Posttraumatic Stress Symptoms in Children After Hurricane Katrina: Predicting the Need for Mental Health Services," *American Journal of Orthopsychiatry* 79, no. 2 (2009): 212–20, https://doi .org/10.1037/a0016179. Mindy E. Kronenberg, Tonya Cross Hansel, Adrianne M. Brennan, et al., "Children of Katrina: Lessons Learned About Postdisaster Symptoms and Recovery Patterns," *Child Development* 81, no. 4 (2010): 1241–59, https://doi.org/10.1111/j.1467-8624.2010.01465.x.

243 Not surprisingly, vulnerable older adults: Joan M. Cook, Avron Spiro III, and Danny G. Kaloupek, "Trauma in Older Adults," in *Handbook of PTSD: Science and Practice*, 2nd ed., ed. Matthew J. Friedman, Terence Martin Keane, and Patricia A. Resick (New York: Guilford Press, 2014), 351–69, at 354.

243 Mental health professionals reported: Jun Yamashita and Jun Shigemura, "The Great East Japan Earthquake, Tsunami, and Fukushima Daiichi Nuclear Power Plant Accident," *Psychiatric Clinics of North America* 36, no. 3 (2018): 351–70, https://doi.org/10.1016/j.psc.2013.05.004.

243 One year after the disaster: Takuya Tsujiuchi, Maya Yamaguchi, Kazutaka
     Masuda, et al., "High Prevalence of Post-traumatic Stress Symptoms in
     Relation to Social Factors in Affected Population One Year After the
     Fukushima Nuclear Disaster," *PLOS One* 11, no. 3 (2016): e0151807,
     https://doi.org/10.1371/journal.pone.0151807.

243 The reality of pre-Katrina poverty: Howard J. Osofsky and Joy D.
     Osofsky, "Hurricane Katrina and the Gulf Oil Spill: Lessons Learned,"
     Psychiatric Clinics of North America 36, no. 3 (2013): 371–83, https://doi.
     org/10.1016/j.psc.2013.05.009.

244 In Sri Lanka: Daya Somasundaram, "Recent Disasters in Sri Lanka,"
     Psychiatric Clinics of North America 36, no. 3 (2018): 321–38, https://doi
     .org/10.1016/j.psc.2013.05.001.

244 most survivors did *not* develop PTSD: Edna B. Foa and Shawn P. Ca-
     hill, "Psychological Treatments for PTSD: An Overview," in *9/11: Mental
     Health in the Wake of Terrorist Attacks*, ed. Yuval Neria, Raz Gross, Randall
     D. Marshall, and Ezra S. Susser (Cambridge, UK: Cambridge University
     Press, 2006), 457–74, at 470.

244 their distress diminished: Shaili Jain, "Complex PTSD, STAIR,
     Social Ecology and Lessons Learned from 9/11—A Conversation with
     Dr. Marylene Cloitre," *PLOS Blogs*, March 29, 2017, http://blogs.plos
     .org/mindthebrain/2017/03/29/complex-ptsd-stair-social-ecology-and
     -lessons-learned-from-911-a-conversation-with-dr-marylene-cloitre/.

244 These findings have been replicated: Maria Paz Garcia-Vera, Jesus Sanz,
     and Sara Gutierrez, "A Systematic Review of the Literature on Posttraumatic
     Stress Disorder in Victims of Terrorist Attacks," *Psychological Reports* 119,
     no. 1 (2016): 328–59, https://doi.org/10.1177/0033294116658243.

244 low percentages can still translate: Robert Henley, Randall Marshall,
     and Stefan Vetter, "Integrating Mental Health Services into Humanitarian
     Relief Responses to Social Emergencies, Disasters, and Conflicts: A Case
     Study," *The Journal of Behavioral Health Services & Research* 38, no. 1 (2011):
     132–41, https://doi.org/10.1007/s11414-010-9214-y.

244 Terror also seeps beyond: Paz Garcia-Vera et al., "A Systematic Review
     of the Literature on Posttraumatic Stress Disorder in Victims of Terrorist
     Attacks."

245 In one study: E. J. Bromet, M. J. Hobbs, S. A. P. Clouston, et al.,
     "DSM-IV Post-traumatic Stress Disorder Among World Trade Center
     Responders 11–13 Years After the Disaster of 11 September 2001 (9/11),"
     Psychological Medicine 46, no. 4 (2016): 771–83, https://doi.org/10.1017
     /S0033291715002184.

245 Psychological First Aid: The National Child Traumatic Stress Center, "Psychological First Aid," http://www.nctsn.org/content/psychological -first-aid.

245 A version of Psychological First Aid: Lisa Schlein, "Psychological First Aid Helps People Affected by Crisis," VOA [Voice of America], October 10, 2016, http://www.voanews.com/a/psychological-first-aid-helps-people -affected-by-crisis/3543841.html.

245 Haiti: Alison Schafer, Leslie M. Snider, and Mark van Ommeren, "Psychological First Aid Pilot: Haiti Emergency Response," *Intervention* 8, no. 3 (2010): 245–54, http://www.interventionjournal.com/sites/default/files /Schafer_2010_Int_PFA_Haiti.pdf.

245 Psychological First Aid is a first step: Fran H. Norris, Susan P. Stevens, Betty Pfefferbaum, et al., "Community Resilience as a Metaphor, Theory, Set of Capacities, and Strategy for Disaster Readiness," *American Journal of Community Psychology* 41, nos. 1–2 (2008): 127–50, https://doi.org /10.1007/s10464-007-9156-6.

245 It holds the promise of curbing: Richard A. Bryant, H. Colin Gallagher, Lisa Gibbs, et al., "Mental Health and Social Networks After Disaster," *American Journal of Psychiatry* 174, no. 3 (2016): 277–85, https://doi .org/10.1176/appi.ajp.2016.15111403.

246 Another outreach program: D. Whybrow, N. Jones, and N. Greenberg, "Promoting Organizational Well-being: A Comprehensive Review of Trauma Risk Management," *Occupational Medicine* 65, no. 4 (2015): 331–36, https://doi.org/10.1093/occmed/kqv024.

246 July 7, 2005, suicide bombs: G. James Rubin and Simon Wessely, "The Psychological and Psychiatric Effects of Terrorism," *Psychiatric Clinics of North America* 36, no. 3 (2013): 339–50, https://doi.org/10.1016/j.psc .2013.05.008.

246 Trauma Response Programme: C. R. Brewin, N. Fuchkan, Z. Huntley, et al., "Outreach and Screening Following the 2005 London Bombings: Usage and Outcomes," *Psychological Medicine* 40, no. 12 (2010): 2049–57, https://doi.org/10.1017/S0033291710000206.

247 Other programs deployed: Lise Eilin Stene and Grete Dyb, "Health Service Utilization After Terrorism: A Longitudinal Study of Survivors of the 2011 Utøya Attack in Norway," *BMC Health Services Research* 15 (April 2015): 158, https://doi.org/10.1186/s12913-015-0811-6.

248 The scientific findings are clear: Michael Duffy, Kate Gillespie, and David M. Clark, "Post-traumatic Stress Disorder in the Context of Terrorism and Other Civil Conflict in Northern Ireland: Randomised Controlled

Trial," *The British Medical Journal* 334, no. 7604 (2007): 1147, http://www.bmj.com/content/334/7604/1147.abstract.

248 Unfortunately, the PTSD epidemic: Abbott, "The Mental-Health Crisis Among Migrants," *Nature* 538 (2016): 158–60.

248 the mental health community has developed: More information about narrative exposure therapy can be found in the Treating Traumatic Stress section. A recent small study suggests that NET may also be a feasible treatment for PTSD in survivors of human trafficking. See Katy Robjant, Jackie Roberts, and Cornelius Katona, "Treating Posttraumatic Stress Disorder in Female Victims of Trafficking Using Narrative Exposure Therapy: A Retrospective Audit," *Frontiers in Psychiatry* 8 (June 1, 2017): 63, https://doi.org/10.3389/fpsyt.2017.00063.

248 all civilian survivors of war: Christopher T. Thompson, Andrew Vidgen, Neil Roberts, Psychological Interventions for Post-Traumatic Stress Disorder in Refugees and Asylum Seekers: A Systematic Review and Meta-analysis, *Clinical Psychology Review* 63 (July 2018): 66–79.

248 specifically tailored to meet: Michela Nose, Francesca Ballette, Irene Bighelli, et al., "Psychosocial Interventions for Post-traumatic Stress Disorder in Refugees and Asylum Seekers Resettled in High-Income Countries: Systematic Review and Meta-analysis," *PLOS One* 12, no. 2 (2017): e0171030, https://doi.org/10.1371/journal.pone.0171030.

249 In a 2002 study: Phuong N. Pham, Harvey M. Weinstein, and Timothy Longman, "Trauma and PTSD Symptoms in Rwanda: Implications for Attitudes Toward Justice and Reconciliation," *The Journal of the American Medical Association* 292, no. 5 (2004): 602–12, https://doi.org/10.1001/jama.292.5.602.

249 In a 2005 study: Patrick Vinck, Phuong N. Pham, Eric Stover, and Harvey M. Weinstein, "Exposure to War Crimes and Implications for Peace Building in Northern Uganda," *The Journal of the American Medical Association* 298, no. 5 (2007): 543–54, https://doi.org/10.1001/jama.298.5.543.

An Americanization of Human Suffering?

250 India's vulnerability to natural disasters: Nilamadhab Kar, "Indian Research on Disaster and Mental Health," *Indian Journal of Psychiatry* 52, suppl. 1 (2010): S286–90, https://doi.org/10.4103/0019-5545.69254.

250 rape and domestic violence were up: B. L. Himabindu, Radhika Arora, and N. S. Prashanth, "Whose Problem Is It Anyway? Crimes Against Women in India," *Global Health Action* 7 (July 21, 2014), https://doi.org/10.3402/gha.v7.23718.

250 India accounts for nearly: Chaitanya Undavalli, Piyush Das, Taru Dutt, et al., "PTSD in Post–Road Traffic Accident Patients Requiring Hospitalization in Indian Subcontinent: A Review on Magnitude of the Problem and Management Guidelines," *Journal of Emergencies, Trauma, and Shock* 7, no. 4 (2014): 327–31, https://doi.org/10.4103/0974-2700.142775.

252 All rates significantly lower: Fran H. Norris and Laurie B. Slone, "Epidemiology of Trauma and PTSD," in *Handbook of PTSD: Science and Practice,* 2nd ed, ed. Matthew J. Friedman, Terence Martin Keane, and Patrica A. Resick (New York: Guilford Press, 2014), 100–20.

252 The controversy surrounding: Michel L. A. Duckers, Eva Alisic, and Chris R. Brewin, "A Vulnerability Paradox in the Cross-National Prevalence of Post-traumatic Stress Disorder," *The British Journal of Psychiatry* 209, no. 4 (2016): 300–05, https://doi.org/10.1192/bjp.bp.115.176628.

253 Examples of how various cultures: Roberto Lewis-Fernández, Devon E. Hinton, and Luana Marques, "Culture and PTSD," in *Handbook of PTSD: Science and Practice,* 2nd ed., ed. Matthew J. Friedman, Terence Martin Keane, and Patricia A. Resick (New York: Guilford Press, 2014), 522–540, at 531.

253 "The meaningfulness of diagnosing": Rupinder K. Legha, "Culture and PTSD: Trauma in Global and Historical Perspective," *American Journal of Psychiatry* 173, no. 9 (2016): 943–44, https://doi.org/10.1176/appi.ajp.2016.16040475.

Prevention with Precision

257 for centuries, prevention was actually deemed: Matthew Smith, "An Ounce of Prevention," *The Lancet* 386, no. 9992 (2018): 424–25, https://doi.org/10.1016/S0140-6736(15)61437-4.

257 By the mid-1950s: David Henderson, cited in Joshua Bierer, "Introduction to the Second Volume," *International Journal of Social Psychiatry* 2, no. 1 (1956): 5–11.

257 But in the ensuing decades: Glen P. Mays and Sharla A. Smith, "Evidence Links Increases in Public Health Spending to Declines in Preventable Deaths," *Health Affairs* 30, no. 8 (2011): 1585–93, https://doi.org/10.1377/hlthaff.2011.0196.

257 But in recent years: Dilip V. Jeste and Carl C. Bell, "Preface to Prevention in Mental Health: Lifespan Perspective," *Psychiatric Clinics of North America* 34, no. 1 (2018): xiii–xvi, https://doi.org/10.1016/j.psc.2011.01.001.

258 biological adversity: Arvin Garg, Renee Boynton-Jarrett, and Paul H. Dworkin, "Avoiding the Unintended Consequences of Screening for Social

Determinants of Health," *The Journal of the American Medical Association* 316, no. 8 (2016): 813–14, https://doi.org/10.1001/jama.2016.9282.

258   how factors such as: Sandro Galea and George J. Annas, "Aspirations and Strategies for Public Health," *The Journal of the American Medical Association* 315, no. 7 (2016): 655–56, https://doi.org/10.1001/jama.2016.0198. Kristine A. Campbell, Tonya Myrup, and Lina Svedin, "Parsing Language and Measures Around Child Maltreatment," *Pediatrics* 139, no. 1 (January 2017), https://doi.org/10.1542/peds.2016-3475.

258   Through this strategy: Muin J. Khoury and Sandro Galea, "Will Precision Medicine Improve Population Health?," *The Journal of the American Medical Association* 316, no. 13 (2016): 1357–58, https://doi.org/10.1001 /jama.2016.12260.

258   Mass shootings traumatize: Jacob Bor, et al., Police Killings and Their Spillover Effects on the Mental Health of Black Americans: A Population-Based, Quasi-experimental Study, *The Lancet* 392, no. 10144, 302–10, doi:https://doi.org.10.1016/S0140-6736(18)31130-9.

         Fran H. Norris, "Impact of Mass Shootings on Survivors, Families, and Communities," *PTSD Research Quarterly* 18, no. 3 (2007): 1–4, http:// www.ptsd.va.gov/professional/newsletters/research-quarterly/V18N3 .pdf.

259   gun violence to be a public health crisis: David E. Stark and Nigam H. Shah, "Funding and Publication of Research on Gun Violence and Other Leading Causes of Death," *The Journal of the American Medical Association* 317, no. 1 (2017): 84–85, https://doi.org/10.1001/jama.2016.16215.

259   Effective solutions: James M. Shultz, Siri Thoresen, and Sandro Galea, "The Las Vegas Shootings—Underscoring Key Features of the Firearm Epidemic," *The Journal of the American Medical Association* 318, no. 18 (2017): 1753–54, https://doi.org/10.1001/jama.2017.16420.

259   need to incorporate: Edward W. Campion, Stephen Morrissey, Debra Malina, et al., "After the Mass Shooting in Las Vegas—Finding Common Ground on Gun Control," *The New England Journal of Medicine* 377, no. 17 (2017): 1679–80, https://doi.org/10.1056/NEJMe1713203.

259   "The whole issue of guns": Personal communication with Dr. Renee Binder, 2/23/2017.

260   The Nurse-Family Partnership: Coalition for Evidence-Based Policy, "Social Programs That Work: Nurse-Family Partnership—Top Tier," http://evidencebasedprograms.org/1366-2/nurse-family-partnership.

260   child abuse and neglect cost: Centers for Disease Control and Prevention, "Child Abuse and Neglect: Consequences," April 5, 2016, https://

www.cdc.gov/violenceprevention/childmaltreatment/consequences
.html.

260 Globally, a variety: Wendy Knerr, Frances Gardner, and Lucie Cluver, "Improving Positive Parenting Skills and Reducing Harsh and Abusive Parenting in Low- and Middle-Income Countries: A Systematic Review," *Prevention Science* 14, no. 4 (2013): 352–63, https://doi.org/10.1007/s11121-012-0314-1.

260 Strength at Home: Casey T. Taft, Suzannah K. Creech, Matthew W. Gallagher, et al., "Strength at Home Couples Program to Prevent Military Partner Violence: A Randomized Controlled Trial," *Journal of Consulting and Clinical Psychology* 84, no. 11 (2016): 935–45, https://doi.org/10.1037/ccp0000129. Furthermore, as the researchers pointed out, their intervention could also have utility in other populations exposed to stress and trauma, such as refugees, inner-city residents, and war-exposed civilians.

261 the Stanford researchers involved: Clea Sarnquist, Benjamin Omondi, Jake Sinclair, et al., "Rape Prevention Through Empowerment of Adolescent Girls," *Pediatrics* 133, no. 5 (2014): e1226–32, https://doi.org/10.1542/peds.2013-3414. Also, personal communication with Mike Baiocchi, February 10, 2017. See also Charlene Y. Senn, Misha Eliasziw, Paula C. Barata, et al., "Efficacy of a Sexual Assault Resistance Program for University Women," *The New England Journal of Medicine* 372, no. 24 (2015): 2326–35, https://doi.org/10.1056/NEJMsa1411131.

261 For every dollar we spend: Kleinman touches on this in this essay; see Arthur Kleinman, "Rebalancing Academic Psychiatry: Why It Needs to Happen—and Soon," *The British Journal of Psychiatry* 201, no. 6 (December 2012): 421–22, at http://bjp.rcpsych.org/content/201/6/421.abstract.

The Golden Hours

262 The Golden Hours: Nils C. Westfall and Charles B. Nemeroff, "State-of-the-Art Prevention and Treatment of PTSD: Pharmacotherapy, Psychotherapy, and Nonpharmacological Somatic Therapies," *Psychiatric Annals* 46, no. 9 (2016): 533–49, https://doi.org/10.3928/00485713-20160808-01. Heather M. Sones, Steven R. Thorp, and Murray Raskind, "Prevention of Posttraumatic Stress Disorder," *Psychiatric Clinics of North America* 34, no. 1 (2011): 79–94, https://doi.org/https://doi.org/10.1016/j.psc.2010.11.001.

262 Secondary prevention intervenes: Roger K. Pitman, Kathy M. Sanders, Randall M. Zusman, et al., "Pilot Study of Secondary Prevention of Posttraumatic Stress Disorder with Propranolol," *Biological Psychiatry* 51, no. 2

(2002): 189–92. There was low-quality evidence for preventing the onset of PTSD in three trials with 118 participants treated with propranolol (RR 0.62; 95% CI 0.24 to 1.59; P value = 0.32). See Taryn Amos, Dan J. Stein, and Jonathan C. Ipser, "Pharmacological Interventions for Preventing Post-traumatic Stress Disorder (PTSD)," *The Cochrane Database of Systematic Reviews*, no. 7 (July 2014), https://doi.org/10.1002/14651858 .CD006239.pub2.

262 This window of time: Shaili Jain, "Cortisol, the Intergenerational Transmission of Stress, and PTSD: An Interview with Dr. Rachel Yehuda," *PLOS Blogs*, June 8, 2016, http://blogs.plos.org/blog/2016/06/08 /cortisol-the-intergenerational-transmission-of-stress-and-ptsd-an -interview-with-dr-rachel-yehuda/.

262 Dr. Gustav Schelling: Gustav Schelling, Benno Roozendaal, and Dominique J.-F. de Quervain, "Can Posttraumatic Stress Disorder Be Prevented with Glucocorticoids?," *Annals of the New York Academy of Sciences* 1032 (December 2004): 158–66, https://doi.org/10.1196/annals.1314.013.

262 He observed that patients: John Griffiths, Gillian Fortune, Vicki Barber, and J. Duncan Young, "The Prevalence of Post Traumatic Stress Disorder in Survivors of ICU Treatment: A Systematic Review," *Intensive Care Medicine* 33, no. 9 (2007): 1506–18, https://doi.org/10.1007/s00134-007 -0730-z.

262 scientists have hypothesized: D. J. de Quervain, B. Roozendaal, and J. L. McGaugh, "Stress and Glucocorticoids Impair Retrieval of Long-Term Spatial Memory," *Nature* 394, no. 6695 (1998): 787–90, https://doi. org/10.1038/29542.

262 Schelling tested his observation: Gustav Schelling, Benno Roozendaal, Till Krauseneck, et al., "Efficacy of Hydrocortisone in Preventing Post-traumatic Stress Disorder Following Critical Illness and Major Surgery," *Annals of the New York Academy of Sciences* 1071, no. 1 (July 2006): 46–53, https://doi.org/10.1196/annals.1364.005.

263 Another cutting edge approach: Shaili Jain, "Cortisol, the Intergenerational Transmission of Stress, and PTSD: An Interview with Dr. Rachel Yehuda," *POLS Blogs Network*, June 8, 2016, http://blogs .plos.org/blog/2016/06/08/cortisol-the-intergenerational-transmission -of-stress-and-ptsd-an-interview-with-dr-rachel-yehuda/.

263 Scientists have known: S. B. Norman, M. B. Stein, J. E. Dimsdale, and D. B. Hoyt, "Pain in the Aftermath of Trauma Is a Risk Factor for Post-traumatic Stress Disorder," *Psychological Medicine* 38, no. 4 (2008): 533–42, https://doi.org/10.1017/S0033291707001389. Marit Sijbrandij,

Annet Kleiboer, Jonathan I. Bisson, et al., "Pharmacological Prevention of Post-traumatic Stress Disorder and Acute Stress Disorder: A Systematic Review and Meta-analysis," *The Lancet Psychiatry* 2, no. 5 (2015): 413–21, https://doi.org/10.1016/S2215-0366(14)00121-7.

263 Opioids also act to reduce: R. Shiekhattar and G. Aston-Jones, "Modulation of Opiate Responses in Brain Noradrenergic Neurons by the Cyclic AMP Cascade: Changes with Chronic Morphine," *Neuroscience* 57, no. 4 (1993): 879–85.

263 recent molecular studies hint: Raül Andero, Shaun P. Brothers, Tanja Jovanovic, et al., "Amygdala-Dependent Fear Is Regulated by Oprl1 in Mice and Humans with PTSD," *Science Translational Medicine* 5, no. 188 (2013): 188ra73, http://stm.sciencemag.org/content/5/188/188ra73. abstract.

263 Early work suggests: Troy Lisa Holbrook, Michael R. Galarneau, Judy L. Dye, et al., "Morphine Use After Combat Injury in Iraq and Post-traumatic Stress Disorder," *The New England Journal of Medicine* 362, no. 2 (2010): 110–17, https://doi.org/10.1056/NEJMoa0903326.

263 Less progress has been made: J. T. Mitchell, "When Disaster Strikes . . . the Critical Incident Stress Debriefing Process," *JEMS* 8, no. 1 (January 1983): 36–39.

264 subsequent studies found: Bryan E. Bledsoe, "Critical Incident Stress Management (CISM): Benefit or Risk for Emergency Services?," *Prehospital Emergency Care* 7, no. 2 (2003): 272–79.

264 some explanations point: Heather M. Sones, Steven R. Thorp, and Murray Raskind, "Prevention of Posttraumatic Stress Disorder," *Psychiatric Clinics of North America* 34, no. 1 (2011): 79–94, https://doi.org/10.1016/j.psc.2010.11.001.

264 "watchful waiting" approach: National Institute for Health and Care Excellence, "Post-traumatic Stress Disorder: Management: Clinical Guideline [CG26]," March 2005, https://www.nice.org.uk/guidance/cg26/chapter/1-guidance?unlid=425484881201641163558.

264 that is, until a team: Barbara Olasov Rothbaum, Megan C. Kearns, Matthew Price, et al., "Early Intervention May Prevent the Development of Posttraumatic Stress Disorder: A Randomized Pilot Civilian Study with Modified Prolonged Exposure," *Biological Psychiatry* 72, no. 11 (2012): 957–63, https://doi.org/10.1016/j.biopsych.2012.06.002.

265 These results: L. Iyadurai, S. E. Blackwell, R. Meiser-Stedman, et al., "Preventing Intrusive Memories After Trauma Via a Brief Intervention Involving Tetris Computer Game Play in the Emergency Department: A

Proof-of-Concept Randomized Controlled Trial," *Molecular Pyschiatry* 23, (2018): 674–82, https://www.nature.com/articles/mp201723/.

Reaching the Hard to Reach: Making PTSD Treatment More Accessible: Location, Location, Location

266 The effect of not getting: Fran H. Norris and Laurie B. Slone, "Epidemiology of Trauma and PTSD," in *Handbook of PTSD: Science and Practice*, 2nd ed., ed. Matthew J. Friedman, Terence Martin Keane, and Patricia A. Resick (New York: Guilford Press, 2014), 100–121, at 108.

266 From an economic standpoint: R. C. Kessler, "Posttraumatic Stress Disorder: The Burden to the Individual and to Society," *The Journal of Clinical Psychiatry* 61, suppl. 5 (2000): 4–12, https://www.ncbi.nlm.nih.gov /pubmed/10761674.

266 only a minority of PTSD sufferers get treatment: Rene Soria-Saucedo, Janice Haechung Chung, Heather Walter, et al., "Factors That Predict the Use of Psychotropics Among Children and Adolescents with PTSD: Evidence From Private Insurance Claims," *Psychiatric Services* 69, no. 9 (2018): 1007–14, https://doi.org/10.1176/appi.ps.201700167.

266 Since the 1990s: R. J. Gatchel and M. S. Oordt, *Clinical Health Psychology and Primary Care: Practical Advice and Clinical Guidance for Successful Collaboration* (Washington, DC: American Psychological Association, 2003). This states that "up to 70%" of primary care medical appointments are for psychosocial-related problems.

267 There has also been a push: Thomas L. Schwenk, "Integrated Behavioral and Primary Care: What Is the Real Cost?," *The Journal of the American Medical Association* 316, no. 8 (2016): 822–23, https://doi.org/10.1001 /jama.2016.11031.

267 Though such initiatives remain: Andrew S. Pomerantz, Lisa K. Kearney, Laura O. Wray, et al., "Mental Health Services in the Medical Home in the Department of Veterans Affairs: Factors for Successful Integration," *Psychological Services* 11, no. 3 (2014): 243–53, https://doi.org/10.1037 /a0036638. Peter A. Coventry, Joanna L. Hudson, Evangelos Kontopantelis, et al., "Characteristics of Effective Collaborative Care for Treatment of Depression: A Systematic Review and Meta-regression of 74 Randomised Controlled Trials," *PLOS One* 9, no. 9 (2014): e108114, https:// doi.org/10.1371/journal.pone.0108114. Ranak B. Trivedi, Edward P. Post, Haili Sun, et al., "Prevalence, Comorbidity, and Prognosis of Mental Health Among US Veterans," *American Journal of Public Health* 105, no. 12 (2015): 2564–69, https://doi.org/10.2105/AJPH.2015.302836.

Brenda Reiss-Brennan, Kimberly D. Brunisholz, Carter Dredge, et al., "Association of Integrated Team-Based Care with Health Care Quality, Utilization, and Cost," *The Journal of the American Medical Association* 316, no. 8 (2016): 826–34, https://doi.org/10.1001/jama.2016.11232. Jarrad Aguirre and Victor G. Carrion, "Integrated Behavioral Health Services: A Collaborative Care Model for Pediatric Patients in a Low-Income Setting," *Clinical Pediatrics* 52, no. 12 (2013): 1178–80, https://doi .org/10.1177/0009922812470744.

268 Such programs are yielding: Doyanne Darnell, Stephen O'Connor, Amy Wagner, et al., "Enhancing the Reach of Cognitive-Behavioral Therapy Targeting Posttraumatic Stress in Acute Care Medical Settings," *Psychiatric Services* 68, no. 3 (2016): 258–63, https://doi.org/10.1176/appi .ps.201500458. Kelly C. Young-Wolff, Krista Kotz, and Brigid McCaw, "Transforming the Health Care Response to Intimate Partner Violence: Addressing 'Wicked Problems,'" *The Journal of the American Medical Association* 315, no. 23 (2016): 2517–18, https://doi.org/10.1001 /jama.2016.4837. Douglas Zatzick, Peter Roy-Byrne, Joan Russo, et al., "A Randomized Effectiveness Trial of Stepped Collaborative Care for Acutely Injured Trauma Survivors," *Archives of General Psychiatry* 61, no. 5 (2004): 498–506, https://doi.org/10.1001/archpsyc.61.5.498.

268 Similar success has been seen: Richard J. Shaw, Nick St John, Emily Lilo, et al., "Prevention of Traumatic Stress in Mothers of Preterms: 6-Month Outcomes," *Pediatrics* 134, no. 2 (2014): e481–88, https://doi.org/10.1542 /peds.2014-0529.

268 Students are now being taught: Stephanie B. Gold, Larry A. Green, and C. J. Peek, "From Our Practices to Yours: Key Messages for the Journey to Integrated Behavioral Health," *Journal of the American Board of Family Medicine* 30, no. 1 (2017): 25–34, https://doi.org/10.3122 /jabfm.2017.01.160100.

269 Veterans who have gone through: Shaili Jain, Kaela Joseph, Hannah Holt, et al., "Implementing a Peer Support Program for Veterans: Seeking New Models for the Provision of Community-Based Outpatient Services for Posttraumatic Stress Disorder and Substance Use Disorders," in *Partnerships for Mental Health*, ed. Laura Weiss Roberts, Daryn Reicherter, Steven Adelsheim, and Shashank V. Joshi (Cham, Switzerland: Springer International Publishing, 2015), 125–35, https://doi.org/10.1007/978 -3-319-18884-3_10. S. Jain, C. McLean, E. P. Adler, et al., "Does the Integration of Peers into the Treatment of Adults with Posttraumatic Stress Disorder Improve Access to Mental Health Care? A Literature Review

and Conceptual Model," *Journal of Traumatic Stress Disorders & Treatment* 2 (2013): 3, https://www.scitechnol.com/2324-8947/2324-8947-2-109. pdf. Shaili Jain, "The Role of Paraprofessionals in Providing Treatment for Posttraumatic Stress Disorder in Low-Resource Communities," *The Journal of the American Medical Association* 304, no. 5 (2010): 571–72, https:// doi.org/10.1001/jama.2010.1096. Shaili Jain, Julia M. Hernandez, Steven E. Lindley, et al., "Peer Support Program for Veterans in Rural Areas," *Psychiatric Services* 65, no. 9 (2014): 1177, https://doi.org/10.1176/appi .ps.650704. Shaili Jain, Caitlin McLean, Emerald P. Adler, and Craig S. Rosen, "Peer Support and Outcome for Veterans with Posttraumatic Stress Disorder (PTSD) in a Residential Rehabilitation Program," *Community Mental Health Journal* 52, no. 8 (2016): 1089–92, https://doi.org/10.1007 /s10597-015-9982-1.

Rebeccah Sokol and Edwin Fisher, "Peer Support for the Hardly Reached: A Systematic Review," *American Journal of Public Health* 106, no. 7 (2016): 1308, https://doi.org/10.2105/AJPH.2016.303180a. Subsequent research done by others also showed that peers were valuable resources for military personnel with mental health issues. See Paul Y. Kim, Robin L. Toblin, Lyndon A. Riviere, et al., "Provider and Nonprovider Sources of Mental Health Help in the Military and the Effects of Stigma, Negative Attitudes, and Organizational Barriers to Care," *Psychiatric Services* 67, no. 2 (2016): 221– 26, https://doi.org/10.1176/appi.ps.201400519. Melba A.Hernandez-Tejada, Stephanie Hamski, and David Sanchez-Carracedo, "Incorporating Peer Support During In Vivo Exposure to Reverse Dropout from Prolonged Exposure Therapy for Posttraumatic Stress Disorder: Clinical Outcomes," *International Journal of Psychiatry in Medicine* 52, no.4–6(2017):366–380.

269 Many studies have shown: Autumn Backhaus, Zia Agha, Melissa L. Maglione, et al., "Videoconferencing Psychotherapy: A Systematic Review," *Psychological Services* 9, no. 2 (2012): 111–31, https://doi.org/10.1037 /a0027924. Leslie A. Morland, Margaret-Anne Mackintosh, Carolyn J. Greene, et al., "Cognitive Processing Therapy for Posttraumatic Stress Disorder Delivered to Rural Veterans via Telemental Health: A Randomized Noninferiority Clinical Trial," *The Journal of Clinical Psychiatry* 75, no. 5 (2014): 470–76, https://doi.org/10.4088/JCP.13m08842. Ron Acierno, Rebecca Knapp, Peter Tuerk, et al., "A Non-inferiority Trial of Prolonged Exposure for Posttraumatic Stress Disorder: In Person versus Home-Based Telehealth," *Behaviour Research and Therapy* 89, suppl. C (2017): 57–65, https://doi.org/https://doi.org/10.1016/j.brat.2016.11.009. Kathryn J. Azevedo, Brandon J. Weiss, Katie Webb, et al., "Piloting Specialized

Mental Health Care for Rural Women Veterans Using STAIR Delivered via Telehealth: Implications for Reducing Health Disparities," *Journal of Health Care for the Poor and Underserved* 27, no. 4A (2016): 1–7, https://doi .org/10.1353/hpu.2016.0189.

270 In attempts to save therapists time: Jennifer Wild, Emma Warnock-Parkes, Nick Grey, et al., "Internet-Delivered Cognitive Therapy for PTSD: A Development Pilot Series," *European Journal of Psychotraumatology* 7 (2016): 31019, https://www.ncbi.nlm.nih.gov/pmc/articles/PMC5106866/. Christine Knaevelsrud, Janine Brand, Alfred Lange, et al., "Web-Based Psychotherapy for Posttraumatic Stress Disorder in War-Traumatized Arab Patients: Randomized Controlled Trial," *Journal of Medical Internet Research* 17, no. 3 (March 2015): e71, https://doi.org/10.2196/jmir.3582. Shaili Jain, "Treating Posttraumatic Stress Disorder via the Internet: Does Therapeutic Alliance Matter?," *The Journal of the American Medical Association* 306, no. 5 (2011): 543–44, https://doi.org/10.1001/jama.2011.1097.

270 Preliminary studies have found: Eric Kuhn, Carolyn Greene, Julia Hoffman, et al., "Preliminary Evaluation of PTSD Coach, a Smartphone App for Post-traumatic Stress Symptoms," *Military Medicine* 179, no. 1 (2014): 12–18, https://doi.org/10.7205/MILMED-D-13-00271.

271 "I'm excited about": Personal communication with Dr. Eric Kuhn, 1/23/2017.

269 "In ten years": Personal communication with Dr. Josef Ruzek, 6/23/2017.

The Power of Social Networks

272 receiving social support after traumatic events: Joseph A. Boscarino, "Post-traumatic Stress and Associated Disorders Among Vietnam Veterans: The Significance of Combat Exposure and Social Support," *Journal of Traumatic Stress* 8, no. 2 (April 1995): 317–36, https://link.springer.com /article/10.1007/BF02109567.

272 a positive social network can help: Krzysztof Kaniasty, "Social Support and Traumatic Stress," *PTSD Research Quarterly* 16, no. 2 (2005): 1–3, http://www.ptsd.va.gov/professional/newsletters/research-quarterly/ V16N2.pdf.

272 optimizing social support: Nils C. Westfall and Charles B. Nemeroff, "State-of-the-Art Prevention and Treatment of PTSD: Pharmacotherapy, Psychotherapy, and Nonpharmacological Somatic Therapies," *Psychiatric Annals* 46, no. 9 (2016): 533–49, https://doi.org/10.3928/00485713 -20160808-01.

272 The power of positive social networks: Another topic in the research on

social support is the influence of negative social interactions. For example, veterans who return home from war to unsympathetic, judgmental, and possibly hostile social environments show greater vulnerability to developing psychopathology. See A. J. E. Dirkzwager, I. Bramsen, and H. M. van der Ploeg, "Social Support, Coping, Life Events, and Posttraumatic Stress Symptoms Among Former Peacekeepers: A Prospective Study," *Personality and Individual Differences* 34 (2003): 1545–59. Y. Neria, Z. Solomon, and R. Dekel, "An Eighteen-Year Follow-up Study of Israeli Prisoners of War and Combat Veterans," *The Journal of Nervous and Mental Disease* 186, no. 3 (1998): 174–82. R. H. Stretch, "Incidence and Etiology of Post-traumatic Stress Disorder Among Active Duty Army Personnel," *Journal of Applied Social Psychology* 16 (1986): 464–81.

272 National Vietnam Veterans' Readjustment Study: D. W. King, L. A. King, J. A. Fairbank, et al., "Resilience-Recovery Factors in Posttraumatic Stress Disorder Among Female and Male Vietnam Veterans: Hardiness, Postwar Social Support, and Additional Stressful Life Events," *Journal of Personality and Social Psychology* 74 (1998): 420–34.

273 "The community around survivors": Shaili Jain, "Complex PTSD, STAIR, Social Ecology and Lessons Learned from 9/11—A Conversation with Dr. Marylene Cloitre," *PLOS Blogs*, March 29, 2017, http://blogs.plos.org /mindthebrain/2017/03/29/complex-ptsd-stair-social-ecology-and -lessons-learned-from-911-a-conversation-with-dr-marylene-cloitre/.

273 Indeed, social media: Tamer A. Hadi and Keren Fleshler, "Integrating Social Media Monitoring into Public Health Emergency Response Operations," *Disaster Medicine and Public Health Preparedness* 10, no. 5 (2016): 775–80, https://doi.org/10.1017/dmp.2016.39.

273 Social media have been used: Courtney Stokes and Jason C. Senkbeil, "Facebook and Twitter, Communication and Shelter, and the 2011 Tuscaloosa Tornado," *Disasters* 41, no. 1 (2017): 194–208, https://doi .org/10.1111/disa.12192.

274 These virtual instantiations: Irina Shklovski, Moira Burke, Sara Kiesler, and Robert Kraut, "Technology Adoption and Use in the Aftermath of Hurricane Katrina in New Orleans," *American Behavioral Scientist* 53, no. 8 (2010): 1228–46, https://doi.org/10.1177/0002764209356252.

274 After the shootings: Amanda M. Vicary and R. Chris Fraley, "Student Reactions to the Shootings at Virginia Tech and Northern Illinois University: Does Sharing Grief and Support over the Internet Affect Recovery?," *Personality & Social Psychology Bulletin* 36, no. 11 (2010): 1555–63, https://doi.org/10.1177/0146167210384880.

274 Social media rely: Mark E. Keim and Eric Noji, "Emergent Use of Social Media: A New Age of Opportunity for Disaster Resilience," *American Journal of Disaster Medicine* 6, no. 1 (2011): 47–54.

The Science of Resilience

276 In recent decades: Steven M. Southwick and Dennis S. Charney, *Resilience: The Science of Mastering Life's Greatest Challenges* (Cambridge, UK: Cambridge University Press, 2012).

277 Childhoods filled with repeated exposure: Parents who endured "toxic stress" during childhood may be more likely to have kids with developmental delays and have a harder time coping with their children's health issues. Nicole Racine, Andre Plamondon, Sheri Madigan, et al., "Maternal Adverse Childhood Experiences and Infant Development," *Pediatrics* (2018): 2017–495.

277 Researchers have also identified: Margaret Haglund, Nicole Cooper, Steven Southwick, and Dennis Charney, "6 Keys to Resilience for PTSD and Everyday Stress," *Current Psychiatry* 6, no. 4 (2007): 23–30.

279 A recent study examined data: Sungrok Kang, Carolyn M. Aldwin, Soyoung Choun, and Avron Spiro III, "A Life-Span Perspective on Combat Exposure and PTSD Symptoms in Later Life: Findings from the VA Normative Aging Study," *The Gerontologist* 56, no. 1 (2016): 22–32, https://doi .org/10.1093/geront/gnv120.

282 Big-data studies have identified: Emily J. Ozer, Suzanne R. Best, Tami L. Lipsey, and Daniel S. Weiss, "Predictors of Posttraumatic Stress Disorder and Symptoms in Adults: A Meta-analysis," *Psychological Bulletin* 129, no. 1 (2003): 52–73. C. R. Brewin, B. Andrews, and J. D. Valentine, "Meta-Analysis of Risk Factors for Posttraumatic Stress Disorder in Trauma-Exposed Adults," *Journal of Consulting and Clinical Psychology* 68, no. 5 (2000): 748–66. Arieh Shalev, Israel Liberzon, and Charles Marmar, "Post-traumatic Stress Disorder," *The New England Journal of Medicine* 376, no. 25 (2017): 2459–69, https://doi.org/10.1056/NEJMra1612499.

283 Hardiness training: Salvatore R. Maddi, "The Courage and Strategies of Hardiness as Helpful in Growing Despite Major, Disruptive Stresses," *American Psychologist* 63, no. 6 (2008): 563–64, https://doi .org/10.1037/0003-066X.63.6.563.

283 Stress inoculation training: M. Deahl, M. Srinivasan, N. Jones, et al., "Preventing Psychological Trauma in Soldiers: The Role of Operational Stress Training and Psychological Debriefing," *British Journal of Medical Psychology* 73, part 1 (March 2000): 77–85.

283 The Aban Aya Youth Project: Kobie Douglas and Carl C. Bell, "Youth Homicide Prevention," *Psychiatric Clinics of North America* 34, no. 1 (2018): 205–16, https://doi.org/10.1016/j.psc.2010.11.013. C. C. Bell, S. Gamm, P. Vallas, and P. Jackson, "Strategies for the Prevention of Youth Violence in Chicago Public Schools," in *School Violence: Contributing Factors, Management, and Prevention*, ed. M. Shafii and S. Shafii (Washington, DC: American Psychiatric Press, 2001), 251–272.

How This Book Was Written

291 Rita Charon: R. Charon, "Narrative Medicine: Form, Function, and Ethics," *Annals of Internal Medicine* 134, no. 1 (2001): 83–87, http://annals.org /aim/article-abstract/714105.

291 Jack Coulehan: Jack Coulehan and Anne Hunsaker Hawkins, "Keeping Faith: Ethics and the Physician-Writer," *Annals of Internal Medicine* 139, no. 4 (2003): 307–11, http://annals.org/aim/article-abstract/716679 /keeping-faith-ethics-physician-writer.

291 Danielle Ofri: Danielle Ofri, "Danielle Ofri," *The Lancet* 361, no. 9368 (2018): 1572, https://doi.org/10.1016/S0140-6736(03)13181-9.

GLOSSARY

ACE: Adverse childhood experience. The landmark ACE study renewed public awareness about the devastating impact of childhood adversity on human well-being.

Amygdala: An almond-shaped set of neurons located in the temporal lobe of the brain that plays a key role in the processing of emotions such as fear and pleasure.

Benzodiazepines: A class of psychotropic medications shown to be harmful to PTSD sufferers.

Biomarkers/biological markers: Biochemical, genetic, or molecular characteristics or substances that indicate a particular biological condition or process.

CBT: Cognitive behavior therapy, the gold standard in PTSD treatment. It typically involves meeting with a mental health professional weekly for up to four months, with each session lasting anywhere from sixty to ninety minutes. Note that CBT for PTSD is an overarching banner term that encompasses many therapies, including cognitive processing therapy (CPT) and prolonged exposure (PE).

CDC: Centers for Disease Control and Prevention, the health protection agency of the United States.

Chromosomes: Chromosomes carry genes in a linear order. Chromosomal studies have shown that PTSD patients have shorter telomeres—the segments on the ends of chromosomes that are a measure of cellular age—than their healthy counterparts, which suggests a link between PTSD and accelerated aging, a biological process that leads to many physical illnesses.

Cognition: The mental process of acquiring knowledge through thought, experience, and the senses.

Cortisol: A stress hormone.

CPT: Cognitive processing therapy, a treatment for PTSD.

DSM: The Diagnostic and Statistical Manual of Mental Disorders, the standard classification of mental disorders used by US mental health professionals.

EMDR: Eye movement desensitization and reprocessing, a form of therapy that involves engaging patients in a trauma memory in brief sequential doses while they simultaneously focus on an external stimulus. The external stimulus may be the therapist directing the patient in lateral eye movements, hand tapping, or audio stimulation.

Epigenetics: A manner in which PTSD can possibly alter the way genes express themselves in a trauma survivor. Such alterations can then be passed on from parents to children on a cellular level, in the form of changes in neurons, brain chemistry, neuroanatomy, and genes.

Explicit memory: Memory of autobiographical facts, such as a birth date or phone number, that is deliberately retrieved.

False positive: Screening positive for a condition but not having the diagnosis.

fMRI: Functional magnetic resonance imaging, a noninvasive brain scan that measures and maps brain activity. fMRI scans measure changes in blood flow in the brain to detect areas of activity. The computer images that result help decipher what is going on in the PTSD brain.

Frontal lobe: The part of the brain that helps in decision making, thinking problems through, and planning daily activities.

Glucocorticoid: A type of hormone that is synthesized by the adrenal cortex with anti-inflammatory action.

Hippocampus: A part of the brain that is crucial to memory formation.

HPA: Hypothalamic-pituitary-adrenal axis, the brain's central coordinator of the response to stress.

Implicit memory: Memory activated through environmental or internal cues, such as driving a car, which does not require deliberate recall.

Insula: An area of the brain that detects cues from the body and processes emotions and empathy. It helps to integrate one's feelings and actions and typically becomes smaller as the brain matures with age.

IPV: Intimate partner violence (formerly known as domestic violence).

IRT: Imagery rehearsal therapy, a talk treatment that specifically targets nightmares by having patients recall the nightmare, write it down, and change the theme into a more positive story line. Patients rehearse the rewritten dream scenario ten to twenty minutes a day so that they can displace the traumatic content when the dream recurs.

MEG: Magnetoencephalography, a brain scan that measures the magnetic fields generated by brain cell activity. It is a direct measure of brain function.

Munchausen syndrome: A disorder in which a person simulates illness or psychological trauma for attention, sympathy, or reassurance.

NCPTSD: National Center for PTSD.

NMDA: N-methyl-D-aspartate, a brain receptor that plays an essential role in learning and memory.

Noradrenaline/norepinephrine: The main neurotransmitter of the body's sympathetic nervous system, vital to mounting the body's response to a threat (i.e., the "fight-or-flight" reaction).

Partial PTSD: A condition in which a patient does not meet the full criteria for a diagnosis of PTSD but is still suffering.

PE: Prolonged exposure, a type of therapy used to treat PTSD.

PET: Positron emission tomography, a scan that examines the brain by detecting gamma rays emitted from a tracer, which is introduced into the body on a biologically active molecule. Using a special camera and computer, researchers can generate images of the way the brain functions by monitoring the brain's metabolism.

Prefrontal cortex: A region of the brain that is involved in the planning and the execution of human actions.

Prevalence: How many people in any given population have a condition at a given time.

Psychological first aid: An approach for assisting people after incidents of disaster and terrorism.

Secondary injuries: Injuries that may occur after a trauma, for example if the survivor experiences blame for the event or faces questions regarding the survivor's character.

Serotonin: A neurotransmitter made from the amino acid tryptophan that can be found all over the brain, including regions of the brain implicated in the neurobiology of PTSD, such as the hippocampus, prefrontal cortex, and amygdala.

SSRI: Selective serotonin reuptake inhibitor, a psychotropic medication such as fluoxetine, paroxetine, or sertraline, that has the strongest scientific evidence for effectiveness in treating PTSD.

STAIR: Skills Training in Affective and Interpersonal Regulation, a therapy that focuses on the practical consequences of living with PTSD day to day by teaching simple skills to manage negative emotions and improve personal relationships.

Sympathetic nervous system: A body system that stimulates the fight-or-flight response.

TBI: Traumatic brain injury, a potential result of head injuries that may occur simultaneously with PTSD.

Telomeres: The segments on the ends of chromosomes that are a measure of cellular age.

Temporal lobe: A portion of the brain that receives sensory information such as sounds and speech from the ears and is a key component of comprehension.

WHO: World Health Organization, an agency of the United Nations whose mission is to improve the health of the world's people and prevent or control communicable diseases worldwide.

RESOURCES

These resources are not an alternative to getting personal medical advice or having a medical consultation about any condition. Always make decisions about diagnosis and treatment in consultation with a trusted health care practitioner.

General Information About PTSD

National Center for PTSD (https://www.ptsd.va.gov/): The website of the Department of Veterans Affairs' National Center for PTSD shares information with veterans, their families and friends, and the general public. Resources include videos by veterans who have experienced PTSD, a guide to helpful mobile applications, and an online PTSD coach. The site also includes information for researchers and health care providers, such as an index of the professional research literature, a directory of manuals and videos, and assessment tools.

American Psychiatric Association (https://www.psychiatry.org/patients -families/ptsd/what-is-ptsd): The American Psychiatric Association (APA), an organization that works with psychiatrists to ensure that patients are well cared for and effectively treated, details symptoms and diagnostic information, as well as treatment modalities, on its PTSD site.

Coping After Disaster, Trauma (https://www.psychiatry.org/patients -families/coping-after-disaster-trauma): A section of the APA website that outlines steps to cope with stress after a tragic experience.

American Psychological Association (http://www.apa.org/topics /ptsd/): The American Psychological Association, an organization with a scientific and professional focus for psychologists in the United States, provides the latest news about PTSD on its website, along with information on ways for people with PTSD and their friends and family members to get help, such as how to find a therapist and how to choose between many treatment options.

International Society for Traumatic Stress Studies (https://www .istss.org/public-resources.aspx): The International Society for Traumatic Stress Studies (ISTSS) provides educational materials that help people and communities facing traumatic events.

PC-PTSD-5 (https://goo.gl/m1CzQe): Paula Schnurr and Teri Brister's site assists visitors to gain a deeper understanding of PTSD on Google through PC-PTSD-5, a screening questionnaire that is clinically validated to assess one's likelihood of having PTSD.

National Institute for Health and Care Excellence (https://www.nice .org.uk/guidance/cg26/informationforpublic): The United Kingdom's National Institute for Health and Care Excellence (NICE) provides information for the general public about treating PTSD in adults and children.

National Institute of Mental Health (https://www.nimh.nih.gov /health/topics/post-traumatic-stress-disorder-ptsd/index.shtml): The National Institute of Mental Health (NIMH) is the foremost US agency funding research on mental illness. Its PTSD site overviews the condition, details the signs and symptoms of PTSD, outlines the risk factors for PTSD, and describes treatment options. It also provides information about joining research studies about PTSD.

Resources for Addressing Trauma in Children

Child Trauma Research Program, University of California, San Francisco (http://childtrauma.ucsf.edu/resources-0): This site offers interventions for families with children up to age five who have witnessed or directly experienced traumatic events.

Cue-Centered Treatment, California Evidence-Based Clearinghouse for Child Welfare (http://www.cebc4cw.org/program/cue-centered -treatment-cct/detailed): This site describes a trauma treatment program for children and adolescents that promotes resiliency.

National Center for PTSD: In Children and Teens (https://www.ptsd .va.gov/public/family/ptsd-children-adolescents.asp): This site presents facts regarding the effect of trauma on children and teenagers and describes treatment options.

Help in Times of Crisis

National Suicide Prevention Lifeline (https://suicidepreventionlife line.org/): The National Suicide Prevention Lifeline provides free, confidential support around the clock for anyone in distress, with prevention and crisis resources also for family and friends and best practices for mental health professionals through online chat and a call center (1-800-273-8255).

Veterans Crisis Line (https://www.veteranscrisisline.net/): A tool that confidentially connects veterans who are experiencing a crisis, such as suicidal thoughts, as well as their families and friends, with VA responders through online chat, text (838255), and a toll-free hotline (1-800-273-8255; press 1).

Information About PTSD Treatment Options

Cognitive processing therapy (http://cptforptsd.com/): Cognitive processing therapy (CPT) helps people with PTSD understand the relationship between traumatic experiences and thoughts and consider the ways their thought patterns might affect their symptoms and recovery. This website provides CPT resources for patients and training information for health care providers.

Eye movement desensitization and reprocessing (http://www.emdr .com/): Eye movement desensitization and reprocessing (EMDR) is a psychotherapy treatment that helps people with PTSD process their traumatic memories in a way that lessens the distress the memories cause. This site describes the treatment in session-by-session details for patients, for example, and provides clinicians with resources and training opportunities.

Prolonged exposure (http://www.med.upenn.edu/ctsa/workshops _pet.html): Prolonged exposure (PE) is a method of therapy developed by Edna Foa, PhD, to help people with PTSD process traumatic events and reduce the symptoms of PTSD. This site describes the therapy in detail and provides information on outpatient and inpatient options for therapy. It also has links for professional training for health care providers.

Trauma-Focused Cognitive Behavioral Therapy National Therapist Certification Program (https://tfcbt.org/about-tfcbt/): This site describes an evidence-based treatment to help children who have experienced trauma and provides information, for health care professionals, on earning certification as a therapist.

Mayo Clinic (http://www.mayoclinic.org/diseases-conditions/post
-traumatic-stress-disorder/diagnosis-treatment/treatment/ptc
-20308558): This site provides resources for patients in its section on
PTSD therapies and medications. It also has helpful information on
preparing for appointments with health care providers.

WebMD (http://www.webmd.com/drugs/condition-1020-Post+
Traumatic+Stress+Disorder): This site lists common medications
prescribed for treating PTSD and includes user reviews for patients
to consider.

INDEX

ABOUT THE AUTHOR

SHAILI JAIN, M.D., is a British-born American physician of Indian ancestry. She is a psychiatrist and PTSD specialist currently serving as Medical Director for Integrated Care at the VA Palo Alto Healthcare System. She is a trauma scientist affiliated with the National Center for Posttraumatic Stress Disorder, a consortium widely regarded as the world's leading center of excellence on PTSD; and a clinical associate professor affiliated with the Department of Psychiatry and Behavioral Sciences at the Stanford University School of Medicine.

Dr. Jain's work is widely accredited for elucidating the role of paraprofessionals and peers in the treatment of American veterans with PTSD. Her work has been published in some of the most prestigious medical journals, such as the *Journal of the American Medical Association, Psychiatric Services,* and the *Journal of Traumatic Stress,* in addition to being featured in national publications such as the *New York Times.* Her medical essays and commentary have appeared in the *New England Journal of Medicine, Psychology Today, Kevin MD, STAT,* public radio, and elsewhere.